BIRTH COUNTS

Statistics of pregnancy and childbirth

Tables

Alison Macfarlane
Miranda Mugford

National Perinatal Epidemiology Unit
(in collaboration with Office of Population Censuses and
Surveys)

London: Her Majesty's Stationery Office

© Crown copyright 1984
First published 1984

ISBN 0 11 691084 4

Birth Counts: Statistics of pregnancy and childbirth
First volume. ISBN 0 11 690965 X. £9.95 net

Foreword to tables

This book brings together statistics collected by government departments and the National Health Service about pregnancy, childbirth and newborn babies, the health services provided for them and the social, economic and environmental factors which can affect the outcome of pregnancy. As our brief at the National Perinatal Epidemiology Unit covers England and Wales, we have presented the data for these two countries more comprehensively than for Scotland and Northern Ireland.

It is intended that this book should be used alongside the first volume of *Birth counts*. This offers a critical appraisal of the data, showing how their strengths and limitations arise from the context in which they are collected, and also contains an index to both volumes.

Alison Macfarlane
Miranda Mugford

Contents

Notes on Tables

Symbols and conventions used:

Numbers		*Rates*	
0	zero	0.0 or 0.00	< 0.5 or < 0.05
—	empty cell	—	empty cell
..	not available	..	not available

Table A3.1 Live births 1838-1981 and infant and childhood mortality 1846-1981, by year and age, England and Wales

Year	Live births		Infant and childhood deaths					
	Number	Rate per 1,000 women aged 15-44	Numbers			Rates		
			Under 1 year	1-4 years	5-9 years	Under 1 year*	1-4 years†	5-9 years†
1838	463,787	126.9	..	..	..	..	..	..
1839	492,574	132.8	..	..	..	..	..	..
1840	502,303	133.1	..	..	..	..	..	..
1841	512,158	134.4	..	..	..	..	..	..
1842	517,739	134.4	..	..	..	..	..	..
1843	527,325	135.4	..	..	..	..	..	..
1844	540,763	137.0	..	..	..	..	..	..
1845	543,521	136.6	..	..	..	..	..	..
1846	572,625	142.3	93,644	66,976	16,190	164	40.4	8.1
1847	539,965	132.8	88,508	69,863	19,120	164	40.7	9.5
1848	563,059	136.6	86,407	70,098	20,586	153	40.6	10.1
1849	578,159	139.1	92,171	68,929	22,794	159	39.9	11.1
1850	593,422	141.2	86,302	58,359	16,832	145	33.6	8.1
1851	615,865	145.0	94,753	65,192	18,122	154	37.4	8.6
1852	624,012	145.0	98,660	67,454	18,932	158	38.0	8.9
1853	612,391	141.1	97,931	67,147	17,807	160	37.0	8.3
1854	634,405	144.6	99,299	78,886	20,202	157	43.2	9.3
1855	635,043	143.2	97,503	68,240	17,832	154	36.7	8.1
1856	657,453	146.2	94,407	64,660	16,165	144	34.4	7.2
1857	663,071	146.3	103,227	70,777	17,441	156	37.2	7.8
1858	655,481	143.1	103,837	83,092	23,813	158	42.7	10.5
1859	689,881	149.0	105,629	78,635	21,417	153	40.4	9.3
1860	684,048	145.7	100,984	65,800	15,967	148	33.0	6.8
1861	696,406	147.2	106,428	74,701	15,890	153	37.1	6.8
1862	712,684	149.0	101,373	77,140	17,992	142	38.0	7.5
1863	727,417	150.5	108,089	93,921	24,380	149	45.8	10.1
1864	740,275	151.2	112,935	86,868	23,635	153	41.7	9.6
1865	748,069	151.6	119,810	80,033	19,733	160	38.0	7.9
1866	753,870	151.2	120,299	82,720	19,029	160	38.7	7.5
1867	768,349	152.5	117,261	71,337	16,177	153	33.1	6.3
1868	786,858	154.1	122,075	81,054	19,750	155	37.1	7.6
1869	773,381	150.3	120,274	83,288	21,183	156	37.4	8.0
1870	792,787	152.4	126,638	85,056	23,051	160	37.8	8.6
1871	797,428	151.6	125,868	80,745	21,445	158	35.3	7.9
1872	825,907	154.6	123,596	73,843	18,658	150	32.0	6.7
1873	829,778	153.8	123,768	70,611	16,195	149	30.2	5.8
1874	854,956	156.2	128,858	84,941	20,636	151	36.1	7.3
1875	850,607	153.4	134,614	81,936	19,119	158	34.1	6.6

Table A3.1 **Live births 1838-1981 and infant and childhood mortality 1846-1981, by year and age, England and Wales** *continued*

Year	Live births		Infant and childhood deaths					
	Number	Rate per 1,000 women aged 15-44	Numbers			Rates		
			Under 1 year	1-4 years	5-9 years	Under 1 year*	1-4 years†	5-9 years†
1876	887,968	157.5	129,940	76,613	17,917	146	31.6	6.1
1877	888,200	155.9	120,817	75,757	17,310	136	30.8	5.8
1878	891,906	154.5	135,927	88,408	19,177	152	35.4	6.4
1879	880,389	150.5	119,252	80,423	18,527	135	31.4	6.0
1880	881,643	148.3	134,686	89,755	19,352	153	34.5	6.2
1881	883,642	147.0	114,976	69,206	18,084	130	26.2	5.7
1882	889,014	145.8	125,020	82,729	19,540	141	31.4	6.1
1883	890,722	144.1	122,226	75,654	19,225	137	28.7	6.0
1884	906,750	144.2	133,128	79,167	18,888	147	30.0	5.8
1885	894,270	140.7	123,130	74,219	16,609	138	28.1	5.1
1886	903,760	140.2	134,870	75,193	15,707	149	28.5	4.8
1887	886,331	135.5	128,277	75,930	16,845	145	28.6	5.1
1888	879,868	132.3	120,079	67,985	15,665	136	25.4	4.7
1889	885,944	131.7	127,198	74,604	15,802	144	28.0	4.7
1890	869,937	127.6	130,955	75,437	16,773	151	28.1	5.0
1891	914,157	132.1	135,801	74,477	16,000	149	28.2	4.7
1892	897,957	127.3	132,463	73,401	15,865	148	27.3	4.6
1893	914,572	127.9	145,061	71,772	17,330	159	26.8	5.1
1894	890,289	122.4	121,799	64,777	14,607	137	23.8	4.3
1895	922,291	124.8	148,093	71,546	14,144	161	26.5	4.1
1896	915,331	121.5	135,013	72,140	15,423	148	26.4	4.5
1897	921,683	120.7	143,589	66,483	13,716	156	24.3	4.0
1898	923,165	118.9	148,013	66,752	13,202	160	24.3	3.8
1899	928,646	117.7	150,975	64,797	14,400	163	23.5	4.1
1900	927,062	115.6	142,912	67,048	14,644	154	24.1	4.2
1901	929,807	114.2	140,648	61,099	14,162	151	21.9	4.1
1902	940,509	114.4	124,996	60,028	14,225	133	21.5	4.1
1903	948,271	114.1	124,718	55,622	12,424	132	19.9	3.5
1904	945,389	112.3	137,392	62,286	12,780	145	22.0	3.6
1905	929,293	109.6	119,091	55,167	12,431	128	19.4	3.5
1906	935,081	109.2	123,895	54,786	12,904	132	19.2	3.6
1907	918,042	106.1	107,978	55,275	12,609	118	19.2	3.5
1908	940,383	107.3	113,254	51,065	12,255	120	17.7	3.4
1909	914,472	103.6	99,430	50,834	12,555	109	17.4	3.4
1910	896,962	100.6	94,579	45,267	11,216	105	15.4	3.0
1911	881,138	97.8	114,600	54,470	12,668	130	18.3	3.4
1912	872,737	95.8	82,779	44,295	11,486	95	14.6	3.1
1913	881,890	95.9	95,608	45,349	11,822	108	14.8	3.2
1914	879,096	95.4	91,971	46,006	12,763	105	15.0	3.4
1915	814,614	87.1	89,380	55,607	14,388	110	17.4	3.8

Table A3.1 **Live births 1838-1981 and infant and childhood mortality 1846-1981, by year and age, England and Wales** – *continued*

Year	Live births		Infant and childhood deaths					
	Number	Rate per 1,000 women aged 15-44	Numbers			Rates		
			Under 1 year	1-4 years	5-9 years	Under 1 year*	1-4 years†	5-9 years†
1916	785,520	83.2	71,646	38,320	12,101	91	12.3	3.2
1917	668,346	70.0	64,483	40,511	12,009	96	13.7	3.2
1918	662,661	68.9	64,386	59,767	20,866	97	21.6	5.7
1919	692,438	72.0	61,715	31,924	12,876	89	12.7	3.5
1920	957,782	99.8	76,552	29,186	11,799	80	12.1	3.3
1921	848,814	89.7	70,250	26,391	9,707	83	10.3	2.8
1922φ	780,124	82.0	60,121	33,641	8,730	77	12.4	2.6
1923	758,131	79.3	52,582	25,992	7,228	69	9.1	2.3
1924	729,933	75.8	54,813	28,919	6,971	75	9.7	2.3
1925	710,582	73.6	53,316	27,764	7,687	75	9.8	2.5
1926	694,563	71.9	48,757	23,001	7,755	70	8.4	2.4
1927	654,172	67.5	45,610	24,306	7,846	70	9.2	2.3
1928	660,267	67.9	42,960	19,822	8,174	65	7.7	2.3
1929	643,673	65.9	47,868	26,629	8,923	74	10.7	2.5
1930	648,811	66.2	38,908	16,756	7,871	60	6.9	2.3
1931	632,081	64.4	41,939	18,038	7,073	65.7	7.6	2.1
1932	613,972	62.6	39,933	16,542	6,601	64.5	7.0	2.1
1933	580,413	59.4	36,960	15,507	6,827	62.7	6.6	2.2
1934	597,642	61.4	35,017	15,278	7,402	59.3	6.7	2.4
1935	598,756	60.9	34,092	11,509	6,105	57.0	5.2	2.0
1936	605,292	61.0	35,425	12,254	5,877	58.7	5.6	2.0
1937	610,557	61.2	35,175	11,311	5,459	57.7	5.2	1.9
1938	621,204	62.2	32,724	10,215	5,379	52.8	4.7	1.9
1939	614,479	61.3	31,190	7,924	4,197	50.6	3.5	1.5
1940	590,120	58.7	33,892	11,104	5,491	56.8	4.8	2.0
1941	579,091	57.9	34,550	12,149	5,677	60.0	5.3	2.1
1942	651,503	65.2	32,258	7,772	4,129	50.6	3.5	1.5
1943	684,334	68.6	33,431	7,583	3,904	49.1	3.4	1.4
1944	751,478	75.7	33,455	6,612	3,895	45.4	2.8	1.4
1945	679,937	68.8	31,959	6,441	3,360	46.0	2.6	1.2
1946	820,719	83.3	33,451	5,334	2,427	42.9	2.2	0.9
1947	881,026	90.6	36,849	5,765	2,549	41.4	2.2	0.9
1948	775,306	80.2	26,766	5,019	2,174	33.9	1.7	0.8
1949	730,518	76.0	23,882	4,641	2,045	32.4	1.6	0.7
1950	697,097	73.0	20,817	4,087	1,971	29.6	1.3	0.6
1951	677,529	71.6	20,223	4,133	1,771	29.7	1.4	0.6
1952	673,735	71.8	18,555	3,356	1,715	27.6	1.2	0.5
1953	684,372	73.5	18,324	3,204	1,763	26.8	1.2	0.5
1954	673,651	72.9	17,160	2,501	1,503	25.4	0.9	0.4
1955	667,811	72.8	16,613	2,638	1,579	24.9	1.0	0.4

3

Table A3.1 Live births 1838-1981 and infant and childhood mortality 1846-1981, by year and age, England and Wales – *continued*

Year	Live births		Infant and childhood deaths					
	Number	Rate per 1,000 women aged 15-44	Numbers			Rates		
			Under 1 year	1-4 years	5-9 years	Under 1 year*	1-4 years†	5-9 years†
1956	700,335	77.0	16,554	2,376	1,456	23.7	0.9	0.4
1957	723,381	80.0	16,720	2,554	1,426	23.1	1.0	0.4
1958	740,715	82.2	16,685	2,348	1,351	22.5	0.9	0.4
1959	748,501	83.0	16,629	2,461	1,351	22.2	0.9	0.4
1960	785,005	86.8	17,118	2,431	1,426	21.8	0.9	0.4
1961	811,281	89.2	17,393	2,662	1,320	21.4	0.9	0.4
1962	838,736	90.8	18,187	2,550	1,271	21.7	0.9	0.4
1963	854,055	91.3	18,042	2,780	1,365	21.1	0.9	0.4
1964	875,972	93.0	17,445	2,552	1,345	19.9	0.8	0.4
1965	862,725	91.2	16,395	2,665	1,396	19.0	0.8	0.4
1966	849,823	90.2	16,147	2,783	1,341	19.0	0.8	0.4
1967	832,164	88.5	15,266	2,574	1,386	18.3	0.8	0.4
1968	819,272	87.9	14,982	2,687	1,441	18.3	0.8	0.4
1969	797,538	85.7	14,391	2,559	1,337	18.0	0.8	0.3
1970	784,486	84.3	14,267	2,326	1,354	18.2	0.7	0.3
1971	783,155	84.0	13,720	2,204	1,484	17.5	0.7	0.4
1972	725,440	77.5	12,498	2,308	1,426	17.2	0.7	0.4
1973	675,953	71.7	11,407	2,099	1,327	16.9	0.7	0.3
1974	639,885	67.6	10,459	1,922	1,225	16.3	0.7	0.3
1975	603,445	63.4	9,488	1,699	1,140	15.7	0.6	0.3
1976	584,270	60.8	8,334	1,469	1,127	14.3	0.6	0.3
1977	569,259	58.7	7,841	1,383	1,008	13.8	0.6	0.3
1978	596,418	60.7	7,881	1,346	1,045	13.2	0.6	0.3
1979	638,028	64.1	8,178	1,168	970	12.8	0.5	0.3
1980	656,234	65.0	7,899	1,186	866	12.0	0.5	0.3
1981	634,456	61.8	7,030	1,186	751	11.1	0.5	0.2

* *Rates per 1,000 live births*

† *Rates per 1,000 population*

ϕ *Population derived from an estimate published in 1921*

Rates are based on the female home population aged 15-44 years except for the years 1939-1947 when they are based on the female total population aged 15-44 years.

Source: *Registrar General's Annual Reports*
Registrar General's Statistical Reviews
OPCS *Birth Statistics, Series FM1* and *Mortality Statistics, Series DH1 and DH3*

Table A3.2 Fertility and infant and childhood mortality, by year and age, Scotland, 1855-1981

| Year | Live births | | Infant and childhood deaths | | | | | |
| | Number | Rate per 1,000 women aged 15-44φ | Numbers | | | Rates | | |
			Under 1 year	1-4 years	5-9 years	Under 1 year*	1-4 years†	5-9 years†
1855	93,349	. .	11,691	10,980	2,838	125.2	37.4+	8.0
1856	101,821	. .	12,058	11,314	2,995	118.4	40.3+	8.6
1857	103,415	. .	12,191	11,652	2,954	117.9	41.4+	8.4
1858	104,018	. .	12,622	12,223	3,217	121.3	38.0	9.0
1859	106,543	. .	11,523	11,972	3,493	108.2	37.0	9.7
1860	105,629	. .	13,413	12,780	3,405	127.0	39.3	9.4
1861	107,009	. .	11,869	11,232	3,059	110.9	34.3	8.4
1862	107,069	. .	12,556	12,641	3,293	117.3	38.4	9.0
1863	109,341	. .	13,125	15,926	4,185	120.0	48.1	11.4
1864	112,333	. .	14,180	14,195	4,118	126.2	42.7	11.1
1865	113,070	. .	14,099	12,238	3,345	124.7	36.6	8.8
1866	113,667	. .	13,915	12,027	3,437	122.4	35.8	9.2
1867	114,044	. .	13,521	11,598	3,209	118.6	34.3	8.5
1868	115,514	. .	13,600	12,755	3,431	117.7	37.5	9.1
1869	113,354	. .	14,654	14,387	4,105	129.3	. .	. .
1870	115,390	. .	14,166	12,497	4,076	122.8	. .	. .
1871	116,128	. .	15,134	12,801	3,779	130.3	. .	. .
1872	118,765	. .	14,720	12,242	3,772	123.9	. .	. .
1873	119,700	. .	14,950	12,391	3,618	124.9	. .	. .
1874	123,711	. .	15,447	14,376	4,911	124.9	. .	. .
1875	123,578	. .	16,320	14,007	4,202	132.1	. .	. .
1876	126,534	. .	15,340	12,125	3,382	121.2	. .	. .
1877	126,822	. .	14,571	11,233	3,042	114.9	. .	. .
1878	126,773	. .	15,599	13,342	3,446	123.0	. .	. .
1879	125,730	. .	13,571	11,299	3,191	107.9	. .	. .
1880	124,570	. .	15,523	13,011	3,667	124.6	. .	. .
1881	126,171	. .	14,198	10,382	3,142	112.5	. .	. .
1882	126,158	. .	14,883	11,665	3,339	118.0	. .	. .
1883	124,458	. .	14,812	11,813	3,296	119.0	. .	. .
1884	129,157	. .	15,228	11,490	3,335	117.9	. .	. .
1885	126,100	. .	15,200	10,891	2,968	120.5	. .	. .
1886	127,890	. .	14,797	10,185	2,901	115.7	. .	. .
1887	124,418	. .	15,202	11,537	3,111	122.2	. .	. .
1888	123,269	. .	13,945	9,649	2,734	113.1	. .	. .
1889	122,783	. .	14,895	10,807	2,693	121.3	. .	. .
1890	121,526	. .	15,877	11,847	2,886	130.6	. .	. .
1891	125,986	. .	16,110	10,409	2,862	127.9	. .	. .
1892	125,043	. .	14,693	10,095	2,651	117.5	. .	. .
1893	127,110	. .	17,286	11,922	2,836	136.0	. .	. .
1894	124,367	. .	14,516	9,041	2,401	116.7	. .	. .

5

Table A3.2 Fertility and infant and childhood mortality, by year and age, Scotland, 1855-1981 – *continued*

Year	Live births		Infant and childhood deaths					
	Number	Rate per 1,000 women aged 15-44φ	Numbers			Rates		
			Under 1 year	1-4 years	5-9 years	Under 1 year*	1-4 years†	5-9 years†
1895	126,494	. .	16,874	10,868	2,515	133.4	. .	. .
1896	129,172	. .	14,924	8,965	2,270	115.5	. .	. .
1897	128,877	. .	17,773	10,354	2,331	137.9	. .	. .
1898	130,861	. .	17,566	10,412	2,296	134.2	. .	. .
1899	130,733	. .	17,132	9,354	2,202	131.0	. .	. .
1900	131,401	. .	16,888	9,509	2,252	128.5	. .	. .
1901	132,192	. .	17,104	9,880	2,334	129.4	. .	. .
1902	132,267	120.6	15,004	8,433	2,148	113.4	. .	. .
1903	133,525	120.6	15,693	8,139	2,058	117.5	. .	. .
1904	132,603	118.6	16,329	9,199	2,086	123.1	. .	. .
1905	131,410	116.4	15,275	8,677	1,968	116.2	. .	. .
1906	132,005	115.8	15,174	8,075	2,113	115.0	. .	. .
1907	128,840	111.9	14,140	9,002	2,225	109.7	. .	. .
1908	131,362	113.0	15,900	9,543	2,073	121.0	. .	. .
1909	128,669	112.7	13,856	7,992	2,146	107.7	. .	. .
1910	124,059	108.0	13,436	8,124	2,066	108.3	. .	. .
1911	121,850	106.6	13,707	7,333	1,934	112.5	17.3	3.8
1912	122,790	107.6	12,949	7,368	1,828	105.5	17.4	3.6
1913	120,516	105.9	13,214	7,133	1,833	109.6	16.9	3.6
1914	123,934	108.5	13,710	7,148	1,887	110.6	16.9	3.7
1915	114,181	99.1	14,441	9,120	2,060	126.5	21.4	4.0
1916	109,942	94.7	10,674	6,650	1,846	97.1	15.5	3.5
1917	97,441	83.4	10,473	7,245	1,704	107.5	16.7	3.3
1918	98,554	83.8	9,836	8,015	2,407	99.8	18.4	4.6
1919	106,268	90.2	10,795	6,506	1,928	101.6	14.9	3.7
1920	136,546	116.6	12,565	4,361	1,530	92.0	10.1	2.9
1921	123,201	105.0	11,130	4,461	1,377	90.3	10.3	2.6
1922	115,085	96.4	11,664	7,524	1,282	101.4	19.9	2.8
1923	111,902	93.8	8,825	4,926	1,178	78.9	12.3	2.7
1924	106,900	90.0	10,446	6,570	1,190	97.7	15.6	2.9
1925	104,137	87.4	9,430	4,819	1,182	90.6	12.0	2.8
1926	102,449	86.0	8,514	4,228	1,143	83.1	10.8	2.6
1927	96,672	81.2.	8,576	4,103	1,212	88.7	10.9	2.7
1928	96,822	82.2	8,299	4,247	1,240	85.7	11.6	2.6
1929	92,880	78.7	8,061	4,140	1,160	86.8	11.9	2.4
1930	94,549	80.2	7,852	3,426	1,195	83.0	10.1	2.6
1931	92,220	79.8	7,544	3,306	1,107	81.8	9.8	2.4
1932	91,000	78.4	7,840	3,386	1,108	86.2	10.2	2.5
1933	86,546	74.5	7,019	2,638	995	81.1	8.0	2.3
1934	88,836	76.5	6,901	2,961	1,137	77.7	9.0	2.7

Table A3.2   Fertility and infant and childhood mortality, by year and age, Scotland, 1855-1981 – *continued*

Year	Live births		Infant and childhood deaths					
	Number	Rate per 1,000 women aged 15-44φ	Numbers			Rates		
			Under 1 year	1-4 years	5-9 years	Under 1 year*	1-4 years†	5-9 years†
1935	87,928	74.9	6,754	2,202	918	76.8	6.8	2.2
1936	88,928	75.1	7,315	2,437	877	82.3	7.6	2.1
1937	87,810	73.7	7,050	2,195	851	80.3	6.9	2.1
1938	88,627	74.0	6,163	2,098	769	69.5	6.6	1.9
1939	86,913	72.1	5,955	1,422	699	68.5	4.5	1.8
1940	86,392	71.4	6,766	2,182	897	78.3	6.7	2.2
1941	89,748	73.5	7,426	2,186	929	82.7	6.5	2.3
1942	90,703	74.2	6,283	1,429	639	69.3	4.3	1.6
1943	94,669	78.7	6,174	1,360	718	65.2	4.1	1.7
1944	95,920	79.9	6,237	1,191	652	65.0	3.6	1.6
1945	86,924	73.1	4,889	1,092	534	56.2	3.3	1.3
1946	104,413	89.5	5,621	1,052	499	53.8	3.2	1.2
1947	113,147	97.1	6,309	995	480	55.8	3.0	1.2
1948	100,344	86.6	4,486	805	388	44.7	2.2	1.0
1949	95,674	83.4	3,961	751	357	41.4	2.0	0.9
1950	92,530	81.0	3,569	694	279	38.6	1.8	0.7
1951	90,639	79.8	3,391	664	309	37.4	1.7	0.8
1952	90,422	80.1	3,181	539	282	35.2	1.5	0.7
1953	90,913	81.3	2,800	499	286	30.8	1.4	0.6
1954	92,315	83.2	2,861	435	229	31.0	1.3	0.5
1955	92,539	84.1	2,811	411	252	30.4	1.2	0.6
1956	95,313	·87.5	2,727	371	189	28.6	1.1	0.4
1957	97,977	90.8	2,802	364	236	28.6	1.0	0.5
1958	99,481	92.8	2,758	338	190	27.7	1.0	0.4
1959	99,251	93.2	2,816	432	161	28.4	1.2	0.4
1960	101,292	96.4	2,673	379	218	26.4	1.0	0.5
1961	101,169	96.9	2,615	406	189	25.8	1.1	0.4
1962	104,334	99.0	2,768	391	196	26.5	1.0	0.5
1963	102,691	97.1	2,624	408	199	25.6	1.1	0.5
1964	104,355	98.6	2,508	347	173	24.0	0.9	0.4
1965	100,660	96.3	2,327	350	205	23.1	0.9	0.5
1966	96,536	93.5	2,239	354	199	23.2	0.9	0.4
1967	96,221	94.3	2,024	323	192	21.0	0.8	0.4
1968	94,786	93.5	1,970	356	202	20.8	0.9	0.4
1969	90,290	89.5	1,902	330	177	21.1	0.9	0.4
1970	87,335	86.6	1,714	315	207	19.6	0.9	0.4
1971	86,728	85.6	1,722	262	164	19.9	0.7	0.4
1972	78,550	77.7	1,477	279	195	18.8	0.8	0.4
1973	74,392	73.4	1,412	276	194	19.0	0.8	0.4
1974	70,093	68.3	1,326	257	156	18.9	0.8	0.3

Table A3.2 Fertility and infant and childhood mortality, by year and age, Scotland, 1855-1981 – *continued*

Year	Live births		Infant and childhood deaths					
	Number	Rate per 1,000 women aged 15-44φ	Numbers			Rates		
			Under 1 year	1-4 years	5-9 years	Under 1 year*	1-4 years†	5-9 years†
1975	67,943	66.1	1,168	217	168	17.2	0.7	0.4
1976	64,895	62.4	959	196	132	14.8	0.7	0.3
1977	62,342	59.4	1,004	176	126	16.1	0.6	0.3
1978	64,295	60.7	830	160	100	12.9	0.6	0.2
1979	68,366	63.9	878	148	116	12.8	0.6	0.3
1980	68,892	63.7	831	144	106	12.1	0.6	0.3
1981	69,054	63.8	780	117	85	11.3	0.5	0.2

* ·Rates per 1,000 live births

† Rates per 1,000 population

φ The rates for 1902-1930 are based on the numbers of women aged 15-45 years.

+ Denominators derived by subtracting numbers of live births from population aged 0-4 years.

Source: Registrar General, Scotland *Annual Reports*

Table A3.3 Age-specific fertility, England and Wales, 1939-80

Year	Total births per 1,000 women in each age group						
	15-44	15-19	20-24	25-29	30-34	35-39	40-44
1939	63.7	16.3	95.8	117.3	85.1	49.3	16.5
1940	61.0	16.2	94.9	114.6	80.1	46.4	16.1
1941	60.0	15.3	93.2	107.7	74.4	45.0	16.4
1942	67.4	15.5	101.0	122.9	87.5	50.5	17.7
1943	70.8	16.0	103.4	125.9	95.9	55.8	18.7
1944	77.8	16.7	109.9	137.3	109.4	65.4	20.4
1945	70.8	17.4	104.7	119.9	96.0	59.8	19.5
1946	85.6	17.1	121.7	156.3	121.0	68.5	20.1
1947	92.8	19.6	148.2	172.6	120.3	67.7	20.3
1948	82.1	21.7	139.1	147.8	101.5	57.9	18.1
1949	77.8	23.0	134.4	140.6	94.4	52.3	16.0
1950	74.7	22.5	128.2	138.5	91.3	49.8	14.8
1951	73.3	21.6	128.1	136.0	90.7	47.4	14.0
1952	73.4	21.7	131.2	137.5	90.9	45.9	13.7
1953	75.2	22.4	137.2	142.3	91.2	45.8	13.6
1954	74.7	23.1	138.9	142.1	87.2	45.9	13.6
1955	74.6	24.0	139.7	144.6	86.5	45.7	13.0
1956	78.8	27.8	149.5	153.7	90.4	47.1	13.0
1957	81.9	30.2	155.6	160.5	93.6	48.1	12.8
1958	84.0	31.6	161.1	164.6	95.9	47.3	12.5
1959	84.7	32.1	163.0	166.9	96.9	45.5	12.9
1960	88.5	34.6	168.3	174.9	103.1	47.8	14.4
1961	90.9	37.9	175.3	179.9	105.2	49.6	14.7
1962	92.4	39.7	181.5	184.5	106.6	50.0	14.6
1963	92.9	40.7	183.0	187.6	107.7	49.7	13.9
1964	94.1	42.9	182.0	187.9	109.1	51.3	13.6
1965	92.7	45.4	178.5	180.7	103.4	49.7	13.0
1966	91.6	48.1	176.6	174.7	98.0	46.7	12.2
1967	89.8	49.1	167.6	167.1	93.5	44.4	11.7
1968	89.1	49.8	165.3	165.4	90.7	41.2	10.8
1969	86.8	50.4	159.3	160.3	86.2	38.1	9.8
1970	85.4	50.4	158.0	156.5	81.3	35.4	8.9
1971	85.1	51.5	156.2	156.2	78.8	33.5	8.4
1972	78.4	48.6	143.3	144.2	70.8	29.6	7.4
1973	72.5	44.3	132.4	136.7	64.4	25.1	6.3
1974	68.3	40.9	125.1	131.0	61.0	22.1	5.5
1975	64.1	36.8	116.3	124.3	59.1	20.3	5.0
1976	61.5	32.7	111.6	120.9	58.4	19.0	4.5
1977	59.3	30.0	105.7	120.0	59.6	18.6	4.2
1978	61.2	30.1	108.8	124.8	64.4	19.9	4.3
1979	64.6	31.0	101.3	133.8	70.5	21.7	4.4
1980	65.5	31.1	115.0	136.7	71.8	22.8	4.4
1981	61.7	28.2	106.0	129.9	69.0	21.9	4.5

Source: OPCS *Birth statistics, Series FM1* and *Registrar General's Statistical Reviews*

Table A3.4 Live births, stillbirths and infant mortality, England and Wales, 1928-81

Year	Numbers		Sex ratio	Rates							
	Live births	Stillbirths	Males Females (total births)	Still-births*	Perinatal deaths*	Neonatal deaths†			Post neonatal deaths†	Infant deaths†
						Early	Late	Total		
1928	660,267	27,580	1.050	40.1	60.8	21.6	9.5	31.1	34.0	65.1
1929	643,673	26,847	1.051	40.0	61.4	22.3	10.6	3.28	41.5	74.4
1930	648,811	27,577	1.051	40.8	61.9	22.0	8.9	30.9	29.1	60.0
1931	632,081	26,933	1.056	40.9	62.1	22.1	9.5	31.6	34.8	66.4
1932	613,972	26,471	1.056	41.3	62.8	22.4	9.1	31.6	33.5	65.0
1933	580,413	25,084	1.051	41.4	63.4	22.9	9.3	32.2	31.5	63.7
1934	597,642	25,128	1.060	40.5	62.2	22.6	8.7	31.3	27.3	58.6
1935	598,756	25,435	1.061	40.7	61.9	22.0	8.4	30.4	26.6	56.9
1936	605,292	25,045	1.059	39.7	60.8	21.9	8.3	30.2	28.4	58.5
1937	610,557	24,806	1.061	39.0	60.2	22.0	7.7	29.8	27.9	57.6
1938	621,204	24,729	1.056	38.3	58.6	21.1	7.2	28.3	24.4	52.7
1939	614,479	24,320	1.060	38.1	58.5	21.3	7.0	28.3	22.4	50.8
1940	590,120	22,779	1.057	37.2	57.7	21.4	8.3	29.7	27.8	57.4
1941	579,091	20,876	1.057	34.8	54.7	20.6	8.3	28.9	30.7	59.7
1942	651,503	22,383	1.066	33.2	52.1	19.5	7.6	27.1	22.4	49.5
1943	684,334	21,262	1.067	30.1	47.9	18.3	6.9	25.2	23.6	48.9
1944	751,478	21,306	1.068	27.6	44.5	17.4	6.8	24.2	20.3	44.5
1945	679,937	19,333	1.064	27.6	45.2	18.1	6.8	24.9	22.1	47.0
1946	820,719	22,915	1.063	27.2	44.3	17.6	6.6	24.2	16.7	40.9
1947	881,026	21,795	1.064	24.1	40.3	16.6	6.2	22.8	19.0	41.8
1948	775,306	18,399	1.063	23.2	38.5	15.7	4.1	19.8	14.8	34.5
1949	730,518	16,947	1.063	22.7	38.0	15.6	3.7	19.3	13.4	32.7
1950	697,097	16,084	1.063	22.6	37.4	15.2	3.3	18.5	11.3	29.9
1951	677,529	15,985	1.063	23.0	38.2	15.5	3.4	18.9	11.0	29.8
1952	673,735	15,636	1.057	22.7	37.5	15.1	3.2	18.3	9.2	27.5
1953	684,372	15,681	1.061	22.4	36.9	14.8	2.9	17.7	9.1	26.8
1954	673,651	16,200	1.060	23.5	38.0	14.9	2.8	17.7	7.7	25.5
1955	667,811	15,829	1.061	23.2	37.4	14.6	2.6	17.2	7.6	24.9
1956	700,335	16,405	1.058	22.9	36.7	14.2	2.6	16.8	6.8	23.6
1957	723,381	16,615	1.061	22.5	36.2	14.1	2.4	16.5	6.7	23.1
1958	740,715	16,288	1.059	21.5	35.0	13.8	2.4	16.2	6.4	22.5
1959	748,501	15,901	1.063	20.8	34.1	13.6	2.3	15.9	6.3	22.2
1960	785,005	15,819	1.061	19.8	32.8	13.3	2.2	15.5	6.3	21.8
1961	811,281	15,727	1.062	19.0	32.0	13.3	2.1	15.3	6.1	21.4
1962	838,736	15,464	1.060	18.1	30.8	13.0	2.1	15.1	6.6	21.7
1963	854,055	14,989	1.056	17.2	29.3	12.3	2.0	14.3	6.9	21.1
1964	875,972	14,546	1.062	16.3	28.2	12.0	1.8	13.8	6.1	19.9
1965	862,725	13,841	1.057	15.8	26.9	11.3	1.7	13.0	6.0	19.0
1966	849,823	13,243	1.060	15.3	26.3	11.1	1.7	12.9	6.1	19.0
1967	832,164	12,528	1.059	14.8	25.4	10.7	1.8	12.5	5.8	18.3
1968	819,272	11,848	1.058	14.3	24.7	10.6	1.8	12.4	5.9	18.3
1969	797,538	10,654	1.059	13.2	23.4	10.3	1.7	12.0	6.0	18.0
1970	784,486	10,345	1.058	13.0	23.5	10.6	1.7	12.3	5.9	18.2

Table A3.4 Live births, stillbirths and infant mortality, England and Wales, 1928-81 - *continued*

Year	Numbers		Sex ratio Males Females (total births)	Rates							
	Live births	Stillbirths		Still-births*	Perinatal deaths*	Neonatal deaths†			Post neonatal deaths†	Infant deaths†
						Early	Late	Total		
1971	783,155	9,899	1.061	12.5	22.3	9.9	1.7	11.6	5.9	17.5
1972	725,440	8,799	1.063	12.0	21.7	9.8	1.7	11.5	5.7	17.2
1973	675,953	7,936	1.065	11.6	21.0	9.5	1.6	11.1	5.7	16.9
1974	639,885	7,175	1.061	11.1	20.4	9.4	1.7	11.0	5.3	16.3
1975	603,445	6,295	1.061	10.3	19.3	9.1	1.7	10.7	5.0	15.7
1976	584,270	5,709	1.058	9.7	17.7	8.2	1.5	9.7	4.6	14.3
1977	569,259	5,405	1.061	9.4	17.0	7.6	1.6	9.3	4.5	13.8
1978	596,418	5,108	1.061	8.5	15.5	7.1	1.6	8.7	4.5	13.2
1979	638,028	5,125	1.060	8.0	14.7	6.8	1.5	8.2	4.6	12.8
1980	656,234	4,773	1.049	7.2	13.3	6.2	1.5	7.7	4.4	12.0
1981	634,492	4,207	1.055	6.6	11.8	5.3	1.4	6.7	4.4	11.1

* Per 1,000 total births
† Per 1,000 live births
Source: OPCS *Birth statistics, Series FM1* and *Mortality statistics: childhood, Series DH3*

Table A3.5 Live births, stillbirths and infant mortality, Scotland, 1928-81

Year	Numbers		Sex ratio Males Females (total births)	Rates							
	Live births	Stillbirths		Still-births*	Perinatal deaths*	Neonatal deaths†			Post neonatal deaths†	Infant deaths†
						Early	Late	Total		
1928	96,822	-	1.05	-	-	23.5	13.2	36.7	49.0	85.7
1929	92,880	-	1.06	-	-	24.6	12.7	37.3	49.5	86.8
1930	94,549	-	1.03	-	-	23.6	11.6	35.2	47.8	83.0
1931	92,220	-	1.04	-	-	24.7	11.1	35.8	46.0	81.8
1932	91,000	-	1.05	-	-	23.8	12.3	36.1	50.1	86.2
1933	86,546	-	1.07	-	-	26.1	11.5	37.6	43.5	81.1
1934	88,836	-	1.05	-	-	24.7	11.5	36.2	41.5	77.7
1935	87,928	-	1.05	-	-	24.8	13.7	38.5	38.3	76.8
1936	88,928	-	1.04	-	-	24.9	12.7	37.6	44.7	82.3
1937	87,810	-	1.05	-	-	25.2	13.1	38.3	42.0	80.3
1938	88,627	-	1.05	-	-	24.3	10.7	35.0	34.5	69.5
1939	86,913	3,832	1.06	42.2	67.5	26.3	10.2	36.6	31.9	68.5
1940	86,392	3,799	1.05	42.1	66.5	25.5	11.8	37.3	41.1	78.3

Table A3.5 Live births, stillbirths and infant mortality, Scotland, 1928-81 - *continued*

Year	Numbers		Sex ratio	Rates							
	Live births	Stillbirths	Males Females (total births)	Still-births*	Perinatal deaths*	Neonatal deaths†			Post neonatal deaths†	Infant deaths†
						Early	Late	Total		
1941	89,748	3,698	1.06	39.6	64.4	25.8	14.1	39.9	42.8	82.7
1942	90,703	3,602	1.05	38.2	60.7	23.5	11.6	35.0	34.2	69.3
1943	94,669	3,494	1.05	35.6	56.9	22.1	10.8	32.9	32.3	65.2
1944	95,920	3,221	1.07	32.5	53.2	21.4	11.4	32.8	32.2	65.0
1945	86,924	2,949	1.06	32.8	52.8	20.7	7.8	28.5	27.7	56.2
1946	104,413	3,483	1.07	32.3	53.9	22.3	7.5	29.9	24.0	53.8
1947	113,147	3,563	1.05	30.5	49.9	20.0	8.5	28.5	27.2	55.8
1948	100,344	2,966	1.07	28.7	46.8	18.7	6.4	25.1	19.6	44.7
1949	95,674	2,666	1.06	27.1	44.9	18.3	4.9	23.2	18.2	41.4
1950	92,530	2,557	1.07	26.9	45.1	18.7	4.3	23.0	15.5	38.6
1951	90,639	2,479	1.06	26.6	44.2	18.0	4.2	22.3	15.1	37.4
1952	90,422	2,430	1.05	26.2	43.7	18.0	3.7	21.7	13.5	35.2
1953	90,913	2,308	1.06	24.8	40.6	16.3	3.0	19.3	11.5	30.8
1954	92,315	2,401	1.06	25.3	42.7	17.8	2.8	20.6	10.4	31.0
1955	92,539	2,330	1.06	24.6	41.1	16.9	2.8	19.7	10.6	30.4
1956	95,313	2,329	1.06	23.9	39.8	16.3	2.8	19.1	9.5	28.6
1957	97,977	2,378	1.06	23.7	40.0	16.7	2.9	19.6	9.0	28.6
1958	99,481	2,324	1.05	22.8	38.6	16.2	2.5	18.7	9.0	27.7
1959	99,251	2,252	1.06	22.2	38.4	16.6	2.8	19.4	9.0	28.4
1960	101,292	2,252	1.05	21.7	37.2	15.8	2.4	18.2	8.1	26.4
1961	101,169	2,147	1.06	20.8	35.9	15.6	2.4	17.9	7.9	25.8
1962	104,334	2,122	1.07	19.9	34.8	15.2	2.7	17.9	8.6	26.5
1963	102,691	1,997	1.05	19.1	33.4	14.6	2.3	16.8	8.7	25.6
1964	104,355	1,900	1.06	17.9	32.1	14.5	1.9	16.4	7.6	24.0
1965	100,660	1,835	1.07	17.9	31.5	13.8	2.1	15.9	7.2	23.1
1966	96,536	1,589	1.06	16.2	29.3	13.3	1.9	15.2	8.0	23.2
1967	96,221	1,544	1.07	15.8	27.5	11.9	2.0	13.8	7.2	21.0
1968	94,786	1,425	1.06	14.8	25.9	11.2	2.1	13.3	7.5	20.8
1969	90,290	1,283	1.07	14.0	25.2	11.4	2.1	13.5	7.6	21.1
1970	87,335	1,234	1.06	13.9	24.8	11.1	1.7	12.8	6.9	19.6
1971	86,728	1,155	1.05	13.1	24.5	11.5	2.0	13.5	6.4	19.9
1972	78,550	1,053	1.05	13.2	23.7	10.6	1.8	12.4	6.4	18.8
1973	74,392	873	1.08	11.6	22.5	11.0	1.7	12.7	6.3	19.0
1974	70,093	850	1.05	12.0	22.8	10.9	1.9	12.8	6.1	18.9
1975	67,943	765	1.06	11.1	21.1	10.1	1.7	11.8	5.4	17.2
1976	64,895	629	1.07	9.6	18.3	8.8	1.5	10.3	4.5	14.8
1977	62,342	553	1.05	8.8	18.3	9.6	1.7	11.3	4.8	16.1
1978	64,295	524	1.06	8.1	15.4	7.4	1.4	8.8	4.1	12.9
1979	68,366	475	1.07	6.9	14.1	7.3	1.4	8.7	4.2	12.8
1980	68,892	463	1.06	6.7	13.1	6.5	1.3	7.8	4.3	12.1
1981	69,054	436	1.05	6.3	11.6	5.4	1.5	6.9	4.4	11.3

Per 1,000 total births
†*Per 1,000 live births*
Source: Registrar General, Scotland *Annual Reports*

Table A3.6 Incidence of low birthweight, England and Wales

(a) Total births, 1955-81

| Year | Percentage of total births with birthweight g | | | | | | | Numbers | |
	1,000 and under	1,001-1,500	1,500 and under	1,501-2,000	2,001-2,250	2,251-2,500	2,500 and under	2,500 g and under	All weights (=100%)
1955			1.31	1.57	1.49	3.59	7.96	54,193	680,841
1956			1.28	1.54	1.50	3.51	7.83	55,817	713,274
1957			1.32	1.56	1.49	3.61	7.98	58,891	737,704
1958			1.27	1.53	1.48	3.57	7.84	59,407	757,390
1959			1.25	1.45	1.46	3.52	7.68	58,648	763,294
1960			1.23	1.47	1.45	3.49	7.64	61,060	799,710
1961			1.25	1.47	1.45	3.48	7.65	63,211	825,873
1962			1.20	1.42	1.47	3.48	7.57	64,535	853,014
1963	0.45	0.74	1.18	1.44	1.48	3.35	7.45	64,658	867,362
1964	0.45	0.71	1.16	1.36	1.40	3.27	7.20	64,054	890,234
1965	0.42	0.68	1.10	1.35	1.39	3.31	7.15	62,511	874,360
1966	0.43	0.66	1.09	1.38	1.47	3.36	7.30	62,899	861,496
1967	0.41	0.68	1.09	1.36	1.45	3.38	7.28	61,172	840,057
1968	0.43	0.69	1.12	1.39	1.49	3.38	7.38	60,989	826,367
1969	0.41	0.66	1.07	1.37	1.55	3.40	7.39	59,599	806,341
1970	0.41	0.70	1.11	1.39	1.58	3.45	7.53	59,685	792,451
1971	0.40	0.64	1.03	1.30	1.48	3.21	7.03	55,667	792,191
1972	0.38	0.64	1.02	1.33	1.55	3.32	7.22	53,102	735,597
1973	0.37	0.64	1.01	1.31	1.54	3.23	7.09	48,491	683,623
1974	0.39	0.63	1.02	1.30	1.52	3.21	7.06	45,579	646,004
1975	0.36	0.64	1.00	1.28	1.52	3.13	6.94	42,304	609,922
1976	0.35	0.65	1.00	1.31	1.52	3.11	6.94	40,958	590,152
1977	0.36	0.63	0.99	1.35	1.53	3.15	7.03	40,374	574,692
1978	0.34	0.67	1.01	1.34	1.50	3.18	7.03	42,301	602,042
1979	0.36	0.65	1.00	1.36	1.56	3.26	7.18	46,183	643,188
1980	0.34	0.66	1.01	1.39	1.56	3.27	7.22	47,750	661,549
1981	0.34	0.65	0.99	1.38	1.55	3.21	7.16	45,830	640,103

13

Table A3.6 Incidence of low birthweight, England and Wales - *continued*

(b) Live births, 1953-81

Year	Percentage of all live births with birthweight g							Numbers	
	1,000 and under	1,001-1,500	1,500 and under	1,501-2,000	2,001-2,250	2,251-2,500	2,500 and under	2,500 g and under	All weights
1953			0.78	1.25	1.30	3.28	6.60	45,472	688,999
1954			0.77	1.26	1.35	3.47	6.86	46,042	671,063
1955			0.81	1.27	1.38	3.47	6.93	46,132	665,414
1956			0.78	1.25	1.39	3.39	6.82	47,512	697,141
1957			0.80	1.26	1.39	3.50	6.95	50,168	721,511
1958			0.76	1.24	1.37	3.47	6.84	50,742	741,364
1959			0.77	1.17	1.36	3.42	6.73	50,310	747,891
1960			0.76	1.21	1.35	3.39	6.71	52,633	784,268
1961			0.79	1.21	1.36	3.38	6.74	54,632	810,595
1962			0.75	1.17	1.38	3.39	6.68	55,999	837,852
1963	0.27	0.47	0.74	1.19	1.40	3.25	6.59	56,172	852,708
1964	0.27	0.46	0.73	1.14	1.32	3.19	6.38	55,852	875,800
1965	0.26	0.44	0.70	1.13	1.30	3.23	6.36	54,743	860,716
1966	0.26	0.43	0.69	1.15	1.38	3.28	6.51	55,205	848,408
1967	0.24	0.45	0.69	1.15	1.37	3.29	6.50	53,804	827,762
1968	0.27	0.46	0.73	1.19	1.41	3.31	6.65	54,180	814,609
1969	0.26	0.45	0.71	1.19	1.47	3.34	6.71	53,406	795,842
1970	0.26	0.49	0.75	1.21	1.50	3.38	6.84	53,514	782,357
1971	0.24	0.44	0.68	1.13	1.42	3.15	6.38	49,886	782,396
1972	0.23	0.45	0.68	1.16	1.48	3.27	6.59	47,941	726,959
1973	0.22	0.44	0.67	1.14	1.47	3.18	6.45	43,599	675,927
1974	0.25	0.45	0.70	1.14	1.45	3.17	6.47	41,330	639,113
1975	0.23	0.47	0.71	1.14	1.46	3.08	6.40	38,612	603,726
1976	0.23	0.47	0.70	1.17	1.47	3.07	6.40	37,435	584,512
1977	0.23	0.46	0.69	1.21	1.48	3.11	6.48	36,915	569,368
1978	0.23	0.51	0.74	1.21	1.45	3.14	6.54	39,020	597,003
1979	0.25	0.50	0.75	1.24	1.52	3.22	6.72	42,888	638,124
1980	0.24	0.53	0.77	1.27	1.51	3.23	6.79	44,629	656,812
1981	0.25	0.54	0.78	1.28	1.51	3.18	6.77	43,079	635,942

Source: DHSS, annual summaries of LHS 27/1 returns

Table A3.7 Birthweight-specific mortality, England and Wales, 1953-81

Birthweight g		1953	1954	1955	1956	1957	1958	1959	1960	1961	1962
1,000 and under	Stillbirths*	..	..	..	..	..	..	..	..	..	..
	Under 24 hrs*	..	..	..	..	..	..	..	..	..	..
	1-6 days†	..	..	..	..	..	..	..	..	..	..
	7-27 days†	..	..	..	..	..	..	..	..	..	..
	Neonatal†	..	..	..	..	..	..	..	..	..	..
1,001-1,500	Stillbirths*	..	..	..	..	..	..	..	..	..	..
	Under 24 hrs*	..	..	..	..	..	..	..	..	..	..
	1-6 days†	..	..	..	..	..	..	..	..	..	..
	7-27 days†	..	..	..	..	..	..	..	..	..	..
	Neonatal†	..	..	..	..	..	..	..	..	..	..
1,500 and under	Stillbirths*	..	..	398.1	404.0	406.2	409.6	393.5	390.7	379.9	389.4
	Under 24 hrs*	441.4	449.1	445.2	442.0	447.9	449.2	461.6	468.7	447.5	475.1
	1-6 days†	..	..	..	..	..	..	..	..	..	..
	7-27 days†	..	..	..	..	..	..	..	..	..	..
	Neonatal†	686.8	684.8	681.8	666.2	665.3	668.6	662.6	665.2	651.3	655.6
1,501-2,000	Stillbirths*	..	..	208.1	206.9	207.0	201.3	208.5	192.1	194.0	188.7
	Under 24 hrs*	96.9	91.0	90.2	93.4	93.2	93.4	99.9	95.3	96.0	92.4
	1-6 days†	..	..	..	..	..	..	..	..	..	..
	7-27 days†	..	..	..	..	..	..	..	..	..	..
	Neonatal†	201.1	198.6	188.5	184.1	177.3	182.7	183.7	173.3	169.9	163.4
2,001-2,250	Stillbirths*	..	..	93.2	90.1	90.8	92.8	87.4	83.3	81.8	81.2
	Under 24 hrs*	31.6	33.9	30.5	32.3	31.1	31.4	31.4	36.0	34.2	30.2
	1-6 days†	..	..	..	..	..	..	..	..	..	..
	7-27 days†	..	..	..	..	..	..	..	..	..	..
	Neonatal†	78.8	81.1	77.8	80.3	71.4	69.3	71.4	72.6	69.9	64.2
2,251-2,500	Stillbirths*	..	..	54.8	54.9	52.2	50.7	48.1	49.3	46.0	42.2
	Under 24 hrs*	15.1	15.6	14.9	14.5	15.1	15.6	15.7	15.6	15.8	14.6
	1-6 days†	..	..	..	..	..	..	..	..	..	..
	7-27 days†	..	..	..	..	..	..	..	..	..	..
	Neonatal†	40.4	44.0	39.3	38.8	41.1	40.8	38.0	33.8	35.9	36.1
2,500 and under	Stillbirths*	140.1	150.4	148.7	148.8	148.1	145.9	142.2	138.0	135.7	132.3
	Under 24 hrs*	84.0	82.0	81.9	81.7	82.3	81.3	84.9	85.5	84.4	82.8
	1-6 days†	..	..	..	..	..	..	..	..	..	..
	7-27 days†	..	..	..	..	..	..	..	..	..	..
	Neonatal†	154.4	152.0	149.2	145.9	143.8	142.4	142.1	138.4	138.8	133.3
Over 2,500	Stillbirths*	..	..	12.3	12.3	11.6	10.9	10.7	10.0	9.4	8.8
	Under 24 hrs*	1.9	2.1	2.1	2.0	2.0	2.1	2.0	1.9	2.1	2.0
	1-6 days†	..	..	..	..	..	..	..	..	..	..
	7-27 days†	..	..	..	..	..	..	..	..	..	..
	Neonatal†	8.0	7.9	7.5	7.4	7.0	6.9	6.8	6.7	6.4	6.6

Birthweight g		1963	1964	1965	1966	1967	1968	1969	1970	1971	1972
1,000 and under	Stillbirths*	400.5	406.6	399.2	404.0	414.2	376.0	382.9	383.1	397.8	396.9
	Under 24 hrs*	666.7	653.1	628.5	674.4	677.6	595.7	627.8	603.1	592.4	609.5
	1-6 days†	163.4	162.4	193.5	161.9	196.6	189.5	173.5	167.9	181.0	139.2
	7-27 days†	21.1	24.2	23.2	19.4	29.4	24.0	29.2	37.8	26.5	25.2
	Neonatal†	851.2	839.7	845.1	855.7	903.7	809.1	830.4	808.7	799.9	773.8
1,001-1,500	Stillbirths*	369.1	361.8	364.8	356.1	347.5	335.2	328.2	311.9	319.3	304.0
	Under 24 hrs*	314.3	310.4	296.2	317.5	297.9	285.0	274.5	282.6	290.7	272.8
	1-6 days†	155.0	148.4	145.3	149.4	142.9	142.2	147.3	133.6	118.1	130.3
	7-27 days†	26.5	28.0	26.2	25.5	22.2	23.3	25.2	22.5	26.2	34.1
	Neonatal†	495.9	486.8	467.7	492.4	463.0	450.5	447.1	438.7	435.0	435.6
1,500 and under	Stillbirths*	380.9	379.1	377.9	374.9	372.5	350.9	349.3	338.3	349.4	338.3
	Under 24 hrs*	443.0	436.7	418.4	451.4	430.3	399.7	403.7	393.2	397.7	386.1
	1-6 days†	158.1	153.6	159.7	154.1	152.9	159.7	156.9	145.4	140.4	133.3
	7-27 days†	24.6	26.6	25.1	23.2	24.7	23.6	26.7	27.8	26.3	31.1
	Neonatal†	625.7	616.9	606.5	628.7	608.0	582.9	587.2	566.5	564.4	550.5
1,501-2,000	Stillbirths*	187.4	179.9	176.4	177.8	170.9	156.8	144.2	143.1	145.3	137.9
	Under 24 hrs*	89.8	88.3	88.3	82.6	79.9	81.8	72.8	78.8	84.9	75.1
	1-6 days†	62.9	60.8	56.5	51.6	51.5	47.4	58.7	47.7	44.6	50.4
	7-27 days†	9.6	10.4	12.9	10.1	12.1	10.8	11.8	9.4	9.9	12.5
	Neonatal†	162.3	159.5	157.6	144.4	143.5	140.0	143.3	135.8	139.4	138.0
2,001-2,250	Stillbirths*	73.8	75.4	75.1	74.1	73.8	65.3	60.4	61.2	57.7	51.1
	Under 24 hrs*	30.1	31.2	26.9	28.6	28.1	24.5	24.7	26.9	25.7	26.0
	1-6 days†	23.8	25.0	22.2	19.7	18.1	22.3	16.7	18.5	16.8	16.2
	7-27 days†	6.4	6.9	9.5	7.2	6.0	6.5	7.5	6.2	5.9	5.1
	Neonatal†	60.3	63.1	58.6	55.5	52.3	53.3	48.9	51.5	48.3	47.3
2,251-2,500	Stillbirths*	44.3	40.2	39.1	38.4	38.8	34.6	30.0	30.9	29.2	26.9
	Under 24 hrs*	14.0	15.0	11.9	12.6	11.7	10.7	10.0	11.6	11.5	10.2
	1-6 days†	11.8	11.8	11.2	9.1	9.9	9.4	8.4	8.5	8.8	8.2
	7-27 days†	5.0	3.9	7.9	4.3	4.7	4.6	4.1	4.2	3.8	5.8
	Neonatal†	30.8	30.7	31.0	26.0	26.2	24.7	22.6	24.4	24.0	24.2
2,500 and under	Stillbirths*	131.2	128.0	124.3	122.3	120.4	111.6	103.9	103.4	103.8	97.2
	Under 24 hrs*	79.8	79.7	73.2	75.4	72.0	69.5	66.0	73.4	68.9	64.0
	1-6 days†	40.2	39.5	38.2	34.4	34.3	35.6	34.9	34.9	31.0	30.4
	7-27 days†	8.4	8.3	11.0	8.0	8.4	8.2	8.6	8.7	7.7	9.4
	Neonatal†	128.3	127.5	122.4	117.7	114.7	113.3	109.5	117.1	107.6	103.8
Over 2,500	Stillbirths*	7.7	7.5	7.2	6.7	6.3	6.5	5.8	5.4	5.4	5.1
	Under 24 hrs*	2.1	2.2	2.1	1.7	1.7	1.8	1.7	1.7	1.7	1.7
	1-6 days†	2.6	2.5	2.4	2.5	2.3	2.1	2.1	2.2	2.1	2.2
	7-27 days†	1.6	1.4	1.1	1.3	1.3	1.3	1.2	1.2	1.3	1.2
	Neonatal†	6.3	6.1	5.6	5.6	5.4	5.2	5.0	5.2	5.1	5.0

Table A3.7   Birthweight-specific mortality, England and Wales, 1953-81-_continued_

Birthweight g		1973	1974	1975	1976	1977	1978	1979	1980	1981
1,000 and under	Stillbirths*	403.8	356.3	368.7	356.3	351.2	335.6	309.2	227.0	288.2
	Under 24 hrs*	614.2	572.1	591.1	545.2	540.5	495.6	517.7	462.6	393.5
	1-6 days†	173.1	155.4	157.8	175.7	172.7	197.7	163.1	173.9	165.8
	7-27 days†	21.1	21.7	37.3	36.2	47.3	60.7	58.2	63.6	65.1
	Neonatal†	808.4	749.2	786.2	757.2	760.5	754.0	738.9	700.1	624.4
1,001-1,500	Stillbirths*	313.1	301.4	267.9	277.5	278.9	246.7	237.0	172.6	179.8
	Under 24 hrs*	255.7	238.4	223.3	193.3	197.9	165.7	138.3	115.9	90.5
	1-6 days†	128.8	131.9	124.6	108.2	107.2	88.8	97.7	77.9	58.8
	7-27 days†	23.8	25.8	25.8	26.3	31.3	36.8	38.4	31.9	28.2
	Neonatal†	408.3	396.2	373.7	327.8	336.4	291.3	274.4	225.7	177.5
1,500 and under	Stillbirths*	346.6	322.2	304.3	305.0	305.0	276.7	262.6	237.6	217.4
	Under 24 hrs*	376.5	358.7	343.7	307.1	313.4	267.9	264.5	225.3	186.1
	1-6 days†	143.8	140.4	135.4	130.0	129.2	122.5	119.4	108.2	92.5
	7-27 days†	22.9	24.3	29.6	29.5	36.7	44.2	45.0	41.9	39.8
	Neonatal†	543.2	523.4	508.7	466.7	479.3	434.7	428.9	375.4	318.4
1,501-2,000	Stillbirths*	139.9	131.7	118.2	116.7	117.7	104.6	92.8	80.6	80.0
	Under 24 hrs*	74.6	69.6	63.8	51.9	46.3	46.4	36.9	36.6	27.4
	1-6 days†	45.9	39.6	40.1	37.9	34.8	29.9	27.9	25.6	17.6
	7-27 days†	11.4	10.5	8.8	11.1	9.9	9.6	9.2	7.9	8.0
	Neonatal†	131.8	119.7	112.7	100.9	91.0	85.8	74.0	70.1	53.0
2,001-2,250	Stillbirths*	59.5	52.0	48.3	43.7	43.1	40.2	38.5	33.1	30.0
	Under 24 hrs*	26.9	22.4	23.8	16.9	15.8	14.6	10.5	11.6	10.6
	1-6 days†	16.7	15.1	15.7	13.1	13.8	9.8	8.8	6.7	6.8
	7-27 days†	6.2	5.5	4.5	5.6	5.8	5.3	4.1	3.8	3.9
	Neonatal†	49.9	42.9	44.0	35.6	35.4	29.7	23.5	22.1	21.2
2,251-2,500	Stillbirths*	28.1	24.1	23.9	23.4	23.7	20.5	19.2	17.3	16.2
	Under 24 hrs*	10.2	11.2	12.1	7.4	8.1	6.0	6.3	5.6	4.5
	1-6 days†	7.5	8.1	8.1	6.4	5.9	5.5	5.1	4.3	4.1
	7-27 days†	4.0	4.1	3.1	4.2	3.3	3.6	2.5	2.7	1.8
	Neonatal†	21.7	23.3	23.3	18.0	17.3	15.2	13.9	12.6	10.3
2,500 and under	Stillbirths*	100.9	93.2	87.3	86.0	85.7	77.6	71.3	65.4	60.0
	Under 24 hrs*	62.9	61.4	60.4	50.6	49.7	45.8	42.6	38.3	32.0
	1-6 days†	30.2	29.0	29.9	27.3	26.3	24.5	23.2	21.3	17.9
	7-27 days†	7.7	7.7	7.4	8.6	8.7	9.8	8.9	8.6	8.0
	Neonatal†	100.9	98.1	97.8	86.5	84.6	80.2	74.6	68.3	57.9
Over 2,500	Stillbirths*	4.4	4.4	4.4	3.9	3.5	3.1	2.5	2.6	2.5
	Under 24 hrs*	1.5	1.2	1.2	1.6	1.0	0.8	1.0	0.9	0.9
	1-6 days†	2.2	2.5	2.3	1.9	1.9	1.9	1.6	1.5	1.2
	7-27 days†	1.2	1.3	1.3	1.0	1.1	1.0	1.0	1.0	0.9
	Neonatal†	4.9	4.9	4.8	4.5	4.1	3.8	3.5	3.4	3.0

* _Rates per 1,000 total births in each weight group_

† _Rates per 1,000 live births in each weight group_

Source: Derived from DHSS annual summaries of LHS 27/1 returns.
    OPCS birth and death registration data were used to impute rates for live-born babies weighing over 2,500 gms.

17

Table A3.8 Mortality in the first year of life by year of birth, England and Wales, 1970-79

Year of birth	Number of live births	Deaths per 1,000 live births							
		Early neonatal	Late neonatal	1-2 months	3-5 months	1-5 months	6-11 months	Post neonatal	Infant
(a) All causes									
1970	785,163	10.6	1.7	2.7	2.0	4.7	1.4	6.1	18.3
1971	782,602	9.9	1.7	2.4	1.8	4.2	1.3	5.5	17.1
1972	725,114	9.9	1.7	2.5	1.9	4.4	1.3	5.6	17.2
1973	673,766	9.5	1.6	2.4	1.9	4.3	1.1	5.4	16.5
1974	639,699	9.4	1.7	2.2	1.7	4.0	1.0	5.0	16.0
1975	603,493	9.1	1.6	2.1	1.8	3.9	1.1	4.9	15.6
1976	584,390	8.1	1.5	1.8	1.5	3.3	1.1	4.4	14.1
1977	569,068	7.7	1.6	1.8	1.7	3.5	1.0	4.6	13.9
1978	596,650	7.1	1.6	2.0	1.6	3.7	1.0	4.7	13.4
1979	637,797	6.7	1.5	1.9	1.6	3.5	1.1	4.6	12.8
(b) Congenital malformations (ICD 740-759)									
1970	785,163	1.7	0.7	0.6	0.4	1.0	0.3	1.3	3.7
1971	782,602	1.8	0.8	0.6	0.3	0.9	0.3	1.2	3.7
1972	725,114	1.8	0.9	0.6	0.4	0.9	0.3	1.2	3.8
1973	673,766	1.7	0.8	0.5	0.3	0.9	0.3	1.2	3.7
1974	639,699	1.9	0.9	0.5	0.4	0.8	0.3	1.1	3.9
1975	603,493	1.8	0.9	0.5	0.3	0.8	0.2	1.0	3.7
1976	584,390	1.7	0.8	0.4	0.3	0.7	0.3	0.9	3.4
1977	569,068	1.7	0.8	0.5	0.3	0.7	0.2	1.0	3.5
1978	596,650	1.8	0.7	0.5	0.3	0.7	0.2	0.9	3.4
1979	637,797	1.7	0.7	0.4	0.3	0.6	0.2	0.9	3.3
(c) Causes other than congenital malformations									
1970	785,163	8.8	1.0	2.1	1.6	3.7	1.1	4.8	14.6
1971	782,602	8.1	1.0	1.8	1.5	3.3	1.0	4.3	13.4
1972	725,114	8.1	0.8	1.9	1.5	3.5	1.0	4.4	13.4
1973	673,766	7.8	0.8	1.9	1.5	3.4	0.9	4.2	12.8
1974	639,699	7.5	0.8	1.7	1.4	3.1	0.8	3.9	12.2
1975	603,493	7.2	0.8	1.6	1.5	3.1	0.8	3.9	11.9
1976	584,390	6.4	0.8	1.4	1.3	2.6	0.8	3.5	10.6
1977	569,068	5.9	0.8	1.4	1.4	2.8	0.8	3.6	10.4
1978	596,650	5.4	0.9	1.6	1.4	3.0	0.8	3.8	10.0
1979	637,797	5.0	0.8	1.5	1.4	2.9	0.8	3.7	9.5

Source: Authors' analysis of OPCS data

Table A3.9 Age distribution of infant deaths, England and Wales, 1888-1980

Year	Percentage of infant deaths by age at death			Total infant deaths	
	0-2 months	3-5 months	6-11 months	Number	Rate†
1888-1890*	48.1	20.4	31.5	378,232	143.5
1891-1895*	48.9	20.7	30.5	683,217	150.5
1896-1900*	47.7	21.5	30.8	720,502	156.1
1901-1905	50.5	20.2	29.3	646,845	137.8
1906-1910	53.8	18.8	27.4	539,136	117.1

Year	Early neonatal (Under 1 week)	Late neonatal (1 week to under 4 weeks)	Neonatal (Under 4 weeks)	Post-neonatal (4 weeks to under 1 year	Number	Rate†
1906-1910	20.9	13.4	34.3	65.7	539,136	117.1
1911-1915	22.0	13.6	35.6	64.4	474,338	108.7
1916-1920	26.0	15.2	41.2	58.8	338,782	90.0
1921-1925	28.6	15.3	43.9	56.1	291,082	74.9
1926-1930	32.2	14.7	46.8	53.2	224,103	67.6
1931-1935	36.1	14.5	50.5	49.5	187,941	61.9
1936-1940	38.9	13.9	52.8	47.2	168,406	55.3
1941-1945	37.8	14.6	52.4	47.6	165,653	49.8
1946-1950	44.6	13.4	58.0	42.0	141,855	36.3
1951-1955	55.7	11.1	66.8	33.2	90,875	26.9
1956-1960	60.9	10.5	71.4	28.6	83,706	22.6
1961 1965	59.9	9.3	69.3	30.7	87,462	20.6
1966-1970	58.1	9.5	67.6	32.4	75,053	18.4
1971-1975	57.0	10.0	67.0	33.0	57,572	16.8
1976-1980*	54.1	11.7	65.8	34.2	40,133	13.2

* Data for 1888-97 are for England only.
† Per 1,000 live births
Source: Derived from data in *Mortality statistics: childhood, Series DH3* and the *Registrar General's Annual Reports* for 1888-1905

Table A3.10 Stillbirths by cause, England and Wales, 1968-78

(a) Numbers

ICD No.	Cause	1968	1969	1970	1971	1972	1973	1974	1975	1976	1977	1978
000-999	All causes	11,848	10,654	10,345	9,899	8,799	7,936	7,175	6,295	5,709	5,405	5,108
740-759	Congenital anomalies	2,153	2,058	2,010	2,123	1,976	1,735	1,605	1,422	1,246	1,143	1,050
740	Anencephalus	1,225	1,208	1,201	1,259	1,118	973	927	835	691	624	553
741	Spina bifida	270	240	207	252	209	200	166	161	129	146	130
742	Congenital hydrocephalus	319	270	259	268	251	241	185	164	160	129	137
743-744	Other congenital anomalies of central nervous system and eye	46	33	34	45	27	35	37	34	41	36	27
46-747	Congenital anomalies of circulatory system	38	41	33	40	34	23	39	27	29	25	22
760-779	Certain causes of perinatal morbidity and mortality	9,695	8,596	8,335	7,776	6,823	6,201	5,570	4,873	4,463	4,262	4,058
760-761	Maternal conditions	428	424	420	435	378	362	283	267	228	250	272
762	Toxaemias of pregnancy	1,290	1,110	955	946	793	668	651	562	501	491	438
763	Maternal ante and post partum infection	30	24	21	16	16	11	14	15	18	26	16
764-768	Difficult labour	537	516	485	415	380	298	272	212	186	151	139
769	Other complications of pregnancy and childbirth	711	545	606	593	541	455	417	408	370	354	341
769.4	Multiple pregnancy	126	110	108	130	102	98	96	97	124	139	136
770	Conditions of the placenta	3,012	2,700	2,668	2,428	2,173	2,114	1,816	1,675	1,490	1,447	1,405
771	Conditions of the cord	1,014	883	867	850	755	706	624	505	492	445	400
772	Birth injury without mention of cause	121	117	87	86	76	49	45	31	36	40	33
774-775	Haemolytic disease of newborn	496	439	418	338	272	207	171	124	108	92	85
776	Anoxic and hypoxic conditions not elsewhere classified	619	530	581	569	460	451	410	373	373	343	337
777	Immaturity	134	111	122	112	81	70	74	55	58	43	31
778-779	Other conditions of fetus and newborn	1,303	1,197	1,105	988	898	810	793	645	602	580	561

Table A3.10 Stillbirths by cause, England and Wales, 1968-78-continued

(b) Rates per 1,000 total births

ICD No.	Cause	1968	1969	1970	1971	1972	1973	1974	1975	1976	1977	1978
000-999	All causes	14.26	13.18	13.02	12.48	11.98	11.60	11.09	10.32	9.68	9.41	8.49
740-759	Congenital anomalies	2.59	2.55	2.53	2.68	2.69	2.54	2.48	2.33	2.11	1.99	1.75
740	Anencephalus	1.47	1.49	1.51	1.59	1.62	1.42	1.43	1.37	1.17	1.09	0.92
741	Spina bifida	0.32	0.30	0.26	0.32	0.28	0.29	0.26	0.26	0.22	0.25	0.22
742	Congenital hydrocephalus	0.38	0.33	0.33	0.34	0.34	0.35	0.29	0.27	0.27	0.22	0.23
743-744	Other congenital anomalies of central nervous system and eye	0.06	0.04	0.04	0.06	0.04	0.05	0.06	0.06	0.07	0.06	0.04
746-747	Congenital anomalies of circulatory system	0.05	0.05	0.04	0.05	0.05	0.03	0.06	0.04	0.05	0.04	0.04
760-779	Certain causes of perinatal morbidity and mortality	11.66	10.64	10.49	9.81	9.29	9.07	8.61	7.99	7.56	7.42	6.75
760-761	Maternal conditions	0.51	0.52	0.53	0.55	0.51	0.53	0.44	0.44	0.39	0.44	0.45
762	Toxaemias of pregnancy	1.55	1.37	1.20	1.19	1.08	0.98	1.01	0.92	0.85	0.85	0.73
763	Maternal ante and post partum infection	0.04	0.03	0.03	0.02	0.02	0.02	0.02	0.02	0.03	0.05	0.03
764-768	Difficult labour	*.65	0.64	0.61	0.52	0.52	0.44	0.42	0.35	0.32	0.26	0.23
769	Other complications of pregnancy and childbirth	0.86	0.67	0.76	0.75	0.74	0.67	0.64	0.67	0.63	0.62	0.57
769.4	Multiple pregnancy	0.15	0.14	0.14	0.16	0.14	0.14	0.15	0.16	0.21	0.24	0.23
770	Conditions of the placenta	3.62	3.34	3.36	3.06	2.96	3.09	2.81	2.75	2.53	2.52	2.34
771	Conditions of the cord	1.22	1.09	1.09	1.07	1.03	1.03	0.96	0.83	0.83	0.77	0.66
772	Birth injury without mention of causes	0.15	0.14	0.11	0.11	0.10	0.07	0.07	0.05	0.06	0.07	0.05
774-775	Haemolytic disease of newborn	0.60	0.54	0.53	0.43	0.37	0.30	0.26	0.20	0.18	0.16	0.14
776	Anoxic and hypoxic conditions not elsewhere classified	0.74	0.66	0.73	0.72	0.63	0.66	0.63	0.61	0.63	0.60	0.56
777	Immaturity	0.16	0.14	0.15	0.14	0.11	0.11	0.11	0.09	0.10	0.07	0.05
778-779	Other conditions of fetus and newborn	1.57	1.48	1.39	1.25	1.22	1.18	1.23	1.06	1.02	1.01	0.93

Source: OPCS unpublished data

Table A3.11 Perinatal deaths by cause, England and Wales, 1968-78

ICD No.	Cause	1968	1969	1970	1971	1972	1973	1974	1975	1976	1977	1978
		(a) Numbers										
000-999	All causes	20,530	18,886	18,633	17,631	15,980	14,374	13,157	11,716	10,416	9,717	9,313
000-136	Infective and parasitic diseases	32	32	32	45	41	46	45	45	48	52	62
460-519	Diseases of the respiratory system	235	201	213	163	170	127	130	109	103	74	74
480-486	Pneumonia	220	188	195	150	159	117	121	107	99	71	71
740-759	Congenital anomalies	3,612	3,431	3,372	3,524	3,263	2,893	2,800	2,529	2,236	2,115	2,078
740	Anencephalus	1,408	1,366	1,372	1,419	1,335	1,084	1,041	914	781	696	620
741	Spina bifida	441	389	377	455	412	384	389	373	292	329	278
742	Congenital hydrocephalus	378	320	299	313	288	291	229	203	191	160	165
743-744	Other congenital anomalies of central nervous system and eye	107	97	97	108	79	77	91	85	97	93	77
746-747	Congenital anomalies of circulatory system	504	492	465	477	432	391	353	361	309	281	323
760-779	Certain causes of perinatal morbidity and mortality	16,336	14,957	14,704	13,623	12,234	11,060	9,950	8,818	7,870	7,345	6,923
760-761	Maternal conditions	472	457	468	473	418	393	306	290	243	269	289
762	Toxaemias of pregnancy	1,380	1,226	1,030	1,024	870	734	711	602	540	517	467
763	Maternal ante and post partum infection*	37	30	28	20	20	19	17	25	21	31	26
764-768	Difficult labour	724	677	606	532	505	403	350	296	252	211	194
769	Other complications of pregnancy and childbirth	1,418	1,255	1,260	1,204	1,119	957	907	868	739	668	652
769.4	Multiple pregnancy	660	664	644	626	550	489	516	479	426	390	389
770	Conditions of the placenta	3,140	2,819	2,787	2,551	2,270	2,206	1,889	1,731	1,558	1,499	1,461
771	Conditions of the cord	1,078	937	929	906	810	756	664	537	526	478	439
772	Birth injury without mention of cause	1,024	828	825	750	724	561	490	382	360	351	351
774-775	Haemolytic disease of newborn	734	672	615	525	391	309	242	181	149	139	117
776	Anoxic and hypoxic conditions not elsewhere classified	2,966	3,127	3,190	2,982	2,886	2,694	2,457	2,271	1,994	1,805	1,684
777	Immaturity	1,849	1,548	1,625	1,492	1,179	1,050	960	822	732	646	535
778-779	Other conditions of fetus and newborn	1,514	1,381	1,341	1,164	1,042	978	957	813	756	731	708
780-796	Symptoms and ill-defined conditions	8	6	8	6	14	14	11	11	12	18	12
795	Sudden death cause unknown	0	0	0	3	9	9	8	10	7	15	12
E800-E999	Accidents, poisoning and violence	75	47	42	44	53	34	35	34	17	13	24

Table 18.11 Perinatal deaths by cause, England and Wales, 1968-78-continued

(b) Rates per 1,000 total births

ICD No.	Cause	1968	1969	1970	1971	1972	1973	1974	1975	1976	1977	1978
000-999	All causes	24.70	23.37	23.44	22.23	21.76	21.02	20.33	19.21	17.65	16.91	15.48
000-136	Infective and parasitic diseases	0.04	0.04	0.04	0.06	0.06	0.07	0.07	0.07	0.08	0.09	0.10
460-519	Diseases of the respiratory system	0.28	0.25	0.27	0.21	0.23	0.19	0.20	0.18	0.17	0.13	0.12
480-486	Pneumonia	0.26	0.23	0.25	0.19	0.22	0.17	0.19	0.18	0.17	0.12	0.12
740-759	Congenital anomalies	4.35	4.25	4.24	4.44	4.44	4.23	4.33	4.15	3.79	3.68	3.45
740	Anencephalus	1.69	1.69	1.73	1.79	1.82	1.59	1.61	1.50	1.32	1.21	1.03
741	Spina bifida	0.53	0.48	0.47	0.57	0.56	0.56	0.60	0.61	0.49	0.57	0.46
742	Congenital hydrocephalus	0.45	0.40	0.38	0.39	0.39	0.43	0.35	0.33	0.32	0.28	0.27
743-744	Other congenital anomalies of central nervous system and eye	0.13	0.12	0.12	0.14	0.11	0.11	0.14	0.14	0.16	0.16	0.13
746-747	Congenital anomalies of circulatory system	0.61	0.61	0.59	0.60	0.59	0.57	0.55	0.59	0.52	0.49	0.54
760-779	Certain causes of perinatal morbidity and mortality	19.66	18.51	18.50	17.18	16.66	16.17	15.38	14.46	13.34	12.78	11.51
760-761	Maternal conditions	0.57	0.57	0.59	0.60	0.57	0.57	0.47	0.48	0.41	0.47	0.48
762	Toxaemias of pregnancy	1.66	1.52	1.30	1.29	1.18	1.07	1.10	0.99	0.92	0.90	0.78
763	Maternal ante and post partum infection*	0.04	0.04	0.04	0.03	0.03	0.03	0.03	0.04	0.04	0.05	0.04
764-768	Difficult labour	0.87	0.84	0.76	0.67	0.69	0.59	0.54	0.49	0.43	0.37	0.32
769	Other complications of pregnancy and childbirth	1.71	1.55	1.59	1.52	1.52	1.40	1.40	1.42	1.25	1.16	1.08
769.4	Multiple pregnancy	0.79	0.82	0.81	0.79	0.75	0.72	0.80	0.79	0.72	0.68	0.65
770	Conditions of the placenta	3.78	3.49	3.51	3.22	3.09	3.23	2.92	2.84	2.64	2.61	2.43
771	Conditions of the cord	1.30	1.16	1.17	1.14	1.10	1.11	1.03	0.88	0.89	0.83	0.73
772	Birth injury without mention of cause	1.23	1.02	1.04	0.95	0.99	0.82	0.76	0.63	0.61	0.61	0.58
774-775	Haemolytic disease of newborn	0.88	0.83	0.77	0.66	0.53	0.45	0.37	0.30	0.25	0.24	0.19
776	Anoxic and hypoxic conditions not elsewhere classified	3.57	3.87	4.01	3.76	3.93	3.94	3.80	3.72	3.38	3.14	2.80
777	Immaturity	2.22	1.92	2.04	1.88	1.61	1.54	1.48	1.35	1.24	1.12	0.89
778-779	Other conditions of fetus and newborn	1.82	1.71	1.69	1.47	1.42	1.43	1.48	1.33	1.28	1.27	1.18
780-796	Symptoms and ill-defined conditions	0.01	0.01	0.01	0.01	0.02	0.02	0.02	0.02	0.02	0.03	0.02
795	Sudden death cause unknown	—	—	—	0.00	0.01	0.01	0.01	0.02	0.01	0.03	0.02
E800-E999	Accidents, poisoning and violence	0.09	0.06	0.05	0.06	0.07	0.05	0.05	0.06	0.03	0.02	0.04

*For the years 1968-73 ICD 763 is described as "Maternal ante and intra partum infection".

Source: Derived from data in OPCS Mortality statistics, childhood, Series DH3.

Table A3.12 Neonatal deaths by cause, England and Wales, 1968-78

ICD No.	Cause	1968	1969	1970	1971	1972	1973	1974	1975	1976	1977	1978
		(a) Numbers										
000-999	All causes	10,125	9,599	9,661	9,113	8,375	7,528	7,067	6,408	5,598	5,231	5,140
000-136	Infective and parasitic system	127	117	113	126	124	103	106	94	111	114	140
460-519	Diseases of the respiratory system	517	472	435	411	322	275	261	212	208	158	164
480-486	Pneumonia	454	403	377	343	280	231	221	182	187	136	141
740-759	Congenital anomalies	2,086	1,942	1,940	1,997	1,894	1,724	1,782	1,643	1,441	1,435	1,464
740	Anencephalus	186	160	171	163	154	112	118	80	90	72	69
741	Spina bifida	298	266	286	371	403	383	466	455	350	367	320
742	Congenital hydrocephalus	63	58	44	50	44	60	52	49	42	41	36
743-744	Other congenital anomalies of central nervous system and eye	91	83	81	76	73	58	70	66	71	72	60
746-747	Congenital anomalies of circulatory system	758	732	727	719	649	511	532	521	437	435	469
760-779	Certain causes of perinatal morbidity and mortality	6,887	6,592	6,651	6,105	5,584	5,029	4,553	4,138	3,567	3,290	3,085
760-761	Maternal conditions	45	36	52	41	40	35	26	25	17	20	20
762	Toxaemias of pregnancy	93	117	77	79	77	66	61	41	40	27	32
763	Maternal ante and post partum infection	7	7	8	5	7	8	4	10	3	5	12
764-768	Difficult labour	191	157	128	120	125	105	81	85	66	62	56
769	Other complications of pregnancy and childbirth	713	713	664	620	575	503	495	468	376	319	317
769.4	Multiple pregnancy	537	554	545	473	444	392	423	388	305	255	258
770	Conditions of the placenta	128	119	122	122	99	92	75	58	69	54	57
771	Conditions of the cord	65	53	66	59	55	51	40	32	35	34	39
772	Birth injury without mention of cause	966	768	782	711	692	564	485	376	355	344	363
774-775	Haemolytic disease of newborn	249	238	208	195	124	106	75	60	43	48	38
776	Anoxic and hypoxic conditions not elsewhere classified	2,407	2,675	2,702	2,511	2,487	2,316	2,108	1,990	1,691	1,581	1,446
777	Immaturity	1,776	1,476	1,570	1,428	1,136	1,000	914	797	695	628	522
778-779	Other conditions of fetus and newborn	247	233	272	214	167	183	189	196	177	168	183
780-796	Symptoms and ill-defined diseases	9	7	14	25	33	44	38	40	49	59	47
795	Sudden death, cause unknown	0	0	2	17	26	38	33	39	44	55	46
E800-E999	Accidents, poisoning and violence	105	90	83	78	78	48	50	41	31	23	34

Table A3.12 Neonatal deaths by cause, England and Wales, 1968-78-continued

(b) Rates per 1,000 live births

ICD No.	Cause	1968	1969	1970	1971	1972	1973	1974	1975	1976	1977	1978
000-999	All causes	12.36	12.04	12.32	11.64	11.54	11.14	11.04	10.62	9.58	9.19	8.62
000-136	Infective and parasitic diseases	0.16	0.15	0.14	0.16	0.17	0.15	0.17	0.16	0.19	0.20	0.23
460-519	Diseases of the respiratory system	0.63	0.59	0.55	0.52	0.44	0.41	0.41	0.35	0.36	0.28	0.27
480-486	Pneumonia	0.55	0.51	0.48	0.44	0.39	0.34	0.35	0.30	0.32	0.24	0.24
740-759	Congenital anomalies	2.55	2.43	2.47	2.55	2.61	2.55	2.78	2.72	2.47	2.52	2.45
740	Anencephalus	0.23	0.20	0.22	0.21	0.21	0.17	0.18	0.13	0.15	0.13	0.12
741	Spina bifida	0.36	0.33	0.36	0.47	0.56	0.57	0.73	0.75	0.60	0.64	0.54
742	Congenital hydrocephalus	0.08	0.07	0.06	0.06	0.06	0.09	0.08	0.08	0.07	0.07	0.06
743-744	Other congenital anomalies of central nervous system and eye	0.11	0.10	0.10	0.10	0.10	0.09	0.11	0.11	0.12	0.13	0.10
746-747	Congenital anomalies of circulatory system	0.93	0.92	0.93	0.92	0.89	0.76	0.83	0.86	0.75	0.76	0.79
760-779	Certain causes of perinatal morbidity and mortality	8.41	8.27	8.48	7.80	7.70	7.44	7.12	6.86	6.11	5.78	5.17
760-761	Maternal conditions	0.05	0.05	0.07	0.05	0.06	0.05	0.04	0.04	0.03	0.04	0.03
762	Toxaemias of pregnancy	0.11	0.15	0.10	0.10	0.11	0.10	0.10	0.07	0.07	0.05	0.05
763	Maternal ante and post partum infection	0.00	0.01	0.01	0.01	0.01	0.01	0.01	0.02	0.01	0.01	0.02
764-768	Difficult labour	0.23	0.20	0.16	0.15	0.17	0.16	0.13	0.14	0.11	0.11	0.09
769	Other complications of pregnancy and childbirth	0.87	0.89	0.85	0.79	0.79	0.74	0.77	0.78	0.64	0.56	0.53
769.4	Multiple pregnancy	0.66	0.69	0.69	0.60	0.61	0.58	0.66	0.64	0.52	0.45	0.43
770	Conditions of the placenta	0.16	0.15	0.16	0.16	0.14	0.14	0.12	0.10	0.12	0.09	0.10
771	Conditions of the cord	0.08	0.07	0.08	0.08	0.08	0.08	0.06	0.05	0.06	0.06	0.07
772	Birth injury without mention of cause	1.18	0.96	1.00	0.91	0.95	0.83	0.76	0.62	0.61	0.60	0.61
774-775	Haemolytic diseases of newborn	0.30	0.30	0.27	0.25	0.17	0.16	0.12	0.10	0.07	0.08	0.06
776	Anoxic and hypoxic conditions not elsewhere classified	2.94	3.35	3.44	3.21	3.43	3.43	3.29	3.30	2.89	2.78	2.42
777	Immaturity	2.17	1.85	2.00	1.82	1.57	1.48	1.43	1.32	1.19	1.10	0.88
778-779	Other conditions of fetus and newborn	0.30	0.29	0.35	0.27	0.23	0.27	0.30	0.32	0.30	0.30	0.31
780-796	Symptoms and ill-defined diseases	0.01	0.01	0.02	0.03	0.05	0.07	0.06	0.07	0.08	0.10	0.08
795	Sudden death, cause unknown	—	—	0.00	0.02	0.04	0.06	0.05	0.06	0.08	0.10	0.08
E800-E999	Accidents, poisoning and violence	0.13	0.11	0.11	0.10	0.11	0.07	0.08	0.07	0.05	0.04	0.06

Source: OPCS unpublished data

25

Table A3.13 Postneonatal deaths by cause, England and Wales, 1968-78

(a) Numbers

ICD No.	Cause	1968	1969	1970	1971	1972	1973	1974	1975	1976	1977	1978
000-999	All Causes	4,857	4,792	4,606	4,607	4,123	3,879	3,392	2,915	2,582	2,480	2,590
000-136	Infective and parasitic diseases	444	473	416	437	345	346	258	219	136	121	149
460-519	Diseases of the respiratory system	2,212	2,208	2,095	2,017	1,583	1,345	1,143	949	824	724	758
460-466	Acute respiratory infections	695	744	683	710	575	460	414	345	308	252	258
480-486	Pneumonia	1,350	1,292	1,220	1,078	814	719	594	490	404	351	394
740-759	Congenital anomalies	1,051	959	976	953	863	828	728	610	535	522	514
740	Anencephalus	1	4	1	2	1	1	0	0	1	2	1
741	Spina bifida	185	148	165	154	183	171	130	121	91	77	90
743-744	Other congenital anomalies of central nervous system and eye	37	39	30	36	26	21	19	24	28	22	23
746-747	Congenital anomalies of heart and circulatory system	571	550	566	541	477	454	398	332	270	274	280
760-779	Certain conditions originating in the perinatal period	49	45	41	54	47	55	54	35	60	46	43
769.4	Multiple pregnancy	0	0	0	0	0	1	0	0	4	0	1
780-796	Symptoms and ill-defined conditions	15	16	87	271	491	559	591	613	590	637	715
795	Sudden death (cause unknown)	1	2	48	225	434	529	545	565	551	610	652
E800-E999	Accidents, poisoning and violence	501	532	432	373	313	291	241	189	191	163	161
E911	Inhalation and ingestion of food causing obstruction of respiratory tract or suffocation	205	231	202	165	128	129	106	81	88	71	76
E913	Accidental mechanical suffocation	151	139	112	89	64	41	47	38	33	33	23

Table A3.13 Postneonatal deaths by cause, England and Wales, 1968-78-*continued*

ICD No.	Cause	1968	1969	1970	1971	1972	1973	1974	1975	1976	1977	1978
	(b) Rates per 1,000 live births											
000-999	All Causes	5.93	6.01	5.87	5.88	5.68	5.74	5.30	4.83	4.42	4.36	4.34
000-136	Infective and parasitic diseases	0.54	0.59	0.53	0.56	0.48	0.51	0.40	0.36	0.23	0.21	0.25
460-519	Diseases of the respiratory system	2.70	2.77	2.67	2.58	2.18	1.99	1.79	1.57	1.41	1.27	1.27
460-466	Acute respiratory infections	0.85	0.93	0.87	0.91	0.79	0.68	0.65	0.57	0.53	0.44	0.43
480-486	Pneumonia	1.65	1.62	1.56	1.38	1.12	1.06	0.93	0.81	0.69	0.62	0.66
740-759	Congenital anomalies	1.28	1.20	1.24	1.22	1.19	1.22	1.14	1.01	0.92	0.92	0.86
740	Anencephalus	0.00	0.01	0.00	0.00	0.00	0.00	—	—	0.00	0.00	0.00
741	Spina bifida	0.23	0.19	0.21	0.20	0.25	0.25	0.20	0.20	0.16	0.14	0.15
743-744	Other congenital anomalies of central nervous system and eye	0.05	0.05	0.04	0.05	0.04	0.03	0.03	0.04	0.05	0.04	0.04
746-747	Congenital anomalies of heart and circulatory system	0.70	0.69	0.72	0.69	0.66	0.67	0.62	0.55	0.46	0.48	0.47
760-779	Certain conditions originating in the perinatal period	0.06	0.06	0.05	0.07	0.06	0.08	0.08	0.06	0.10	0.08	0.07
769.4	Multiple pregnancy	—	—	—	—	—	0.00	—	—	0.01	—	0.00
780-796	Symptoms and ill-defined conditions	0.02	0.02	0.11	0.35	0.68	0.83	0.92	1.02	1.01	1.12	1.20
795	Sudden death (cause unknown)	0.00	0.00	0.06	0.29	0.60	0.78	0.85	0.94	0.94	1.07	1.09
E800-E999	Accidents, poisonings and violence	0.61	0.67	0.55	0.48	0.43	0.43	0.38	0.31	0.33	0.29	0.27
E911	Inhalation and ingestion of food causing obstruction of respiratory tract or suffocation	0.25	0.29	0.26	0.21	0.18	0.19	0.17	0.13	0.15	0.12	0.13
E913	Accidental mechanical suffocation	0.18	0.17	0.14	0.11	0.09	0.06	0.07	0.06	0.06	0.06	0.04

Source: OPCS unpublished data

Table A3.14 Stillbirths by cause, England and Wales, 1979-80

ICD No.	Cause	Numbers		Rates per 1,000 total births	
		1979	1980	1979	1980
000-999	All causes	5,125	4,773	7.97	7.22
460-519	Diseases of the respiratory system	1	0	0.0	—
480-486	Pneumonia	0	0	—	—
740-759	Congenital anomalies	939	809	1.46	1.22
740	Anencephalus and similar anomalies	461	342	0.72	0.52
741	Spina bifida	125	114	0.19	0.17
742	Other congenital anomalies of central nervous system	141	149	0.22	0.23
745-747	Congenital anomalies of the heart and circulatory system	34	27	0.05	0.04
760-779	Certain conditions originating in the perinatal period	4,175	3,952	6.49	5.98
760-761	Maternal conditions	720	629	1.12	0.95
761.5	Multiple pregnancy	99	80	0.15	0.12
762	Conditions of placenta, cord or membrane	2,081	1,955	3.24	2.96
763	Other complications of labour and delivery	122	100	0.19	0.15
764-765	Slow fetal growth, fetal malnutrition and immaturity	74	76	0.12	0.11
767	Birth trauma	23	16	0.04	0.02
768-770	Hypoxia, birth asphyxia and other respiratory conditions	392	412	0.61	0.62
771	Infections specific to perinatal period	8	12	0.01	0.02
773	Haemolytic diseases of fetus or newborn	61	58	0.09	0.09

Source: OPCS *Mortality statistics: perinatal and infant, Series DH3*

Table A3.15   Perinatal deaths by cause, England and Wales, 1979-80

ICD No.	Cause	Numbers		Rates per 1,000 live births	
		1979	1980	1979	1980
000-999	All causes	9,402	8,796	14.62	13.31
000-139	Infectious and parasitic diseases	6	11	0.01	0.02
460-519	Diseases of the respiratory system	57	46	0.09	0.07
480-486	Pneumonia	45	39	0.07	0.06
740-759	Congenital anomalies	2,038	1,940	3.17	2.93
740	Anencephalus and similar anomalies	529	410	0.82	0.62
741	Spina bifida	272	256	0.42	0.39
742	Other congenital anomalies of central nervous system	204	220	0.32	0.33
745-747	Congenital anomalies of heart and circulatory system	314	298	0.49	0.45
760-779	Certain conditions originating in the perinatal period	7,164	6,634	11.14	10.04
760-761	Maternal conditions	894	792	1.39	1.20
761.5	Multiple pregnancy	227	191	0.35	0.29
762	Conditions of placenta, cord or membrane	2,185	2,062	3.40	3.12
763	Other complications of labour and delivery	172	143	0.27	0.22
764-765	Slow fetal growth, fetal malnutrition and immaturity	663	562	1.03	0.85
767	Birth trauma	180	150	0.28	0.23
768-770	Hypoxia, birth asphyxia and other respiratory conditions	1,930	1,774	3.00	2.68
771	Infections specific to perinatal period	56	73	0.09	0.11
773	Haemolytic diseases of fetus or newborn	93	84	0.14	0.13
780-799	Symptoms, signs and ill-defined conditions	12	15	0.02	0.02
798	Sudden death, cause unknown	12	13	0.02	0.02
E800-E999	External causes of injury and poisoning	21	26	0.03	0.04

Source: OPCS *Mortality Statistics: perinatal and infant, Series DH3*

Table A3.16   Neonatal deaths by cause, England and Wales, 1979-80

ICD No.	Cause	Numbers		Rates per 1,000 live births	
		1979	1980	1979	1980
000-999	All causes	5,216	4,987	8.18	7.60
000-139	Infectious and parasitic diseases	21	20	0.03	0.03
460-519	Diseases of the respiratory system	134	118	0.21	0.18
480-486	Pneumonia	107	94	0.17	0.14
740-759	Congenital anomalies	1,530	1,551	2.40	2.36
740	Anencephalus and similar anomalies	69	68	0.11	0.10
741	Spina bifida	312	270	0.49	0.41
742	Other congenital anomalies of central nervous system	97	102	0.15	0.16
745-747	Congenital anomalies of heart and circulatory system	444	452	0.70	0.69
760-779	Certain conditions originating in the perinatal period	3,299	3,011	5.17	4.59
760-761	Maternal conditions	176	170	0.28	0.26
761.5	Multiple pregnancy	128	113	0.20	0.17
762	Conditions of placenta, cord or membrane	105	109	0.16	0.17
763	Other complications of labour and delivery	52	44	0.08	0.07
764-765	Slow fetal growth, fetal malnutrition and immaturity	609	513	0.95	0.78
767	Birth trauma	182	152	0.29	0.23
768-770	Hypoxia, birth asphyxia and other respiratory conditions	1,676	1,506	2.63	2.29
771	Infections specific to perinatal period	80	86	0.13	0.13
773	Haemolytic diseases of fetus or newborn	33	28	0.05	0.04
780-799	Symptoms, signs and ill-defined conditions	49	79	0.08	0.12
798	Sudden death, cause unknown	48	78	0.08	0.12
E800-E999	External causes of injury and poisoning	33	39	0.05	0.06

Source: OPCS *Mortality statistics: perinatal and infant, Series DH3*

Table A3.17 Postneonatal deaths by cause, England and Wales, 1979-80

ICD No.	Cause	Numbers		Rates per 1,000 live births	
		1979	1980	1979	1980
000-999	All causes	2,848	2,803	4.46	4.27
000-139	Infectious and parasitic diseases	128	103	0.20	0.16
460-519	Diseases of the respiratory system	784	677	1.23	1.03
460-466	Acute respiratory infections	271	212	0.42	0.32
480-486	Pneumonia	383	353	0.60	0.54
740-759	Congenital anomalies	508	507	0.80	0.77
740	Anencephalus and similar anomalies	0	1	—	0.00
741	Spina bifida	91	87	0.14	0.13
742-743	Other congenital anomalies of central nervous system and eye	40	37	0.06	0.06
745-747	Congenital anomalies of heart and circulatory system	248	267	0.39	0.41
760-779	Certain conditions originating in the perinatal period	96	110	0.15	0.17
761.5	Multiple pregnancy	0	3	—	0.00
780-799	Symptoms, signs and ill-defined conditions	828	940	1.30	1.43
798	Sudden death, cause unknown	806	929	1.26	1.42
E800-E999	External causes of injury and poisoning	197	145	0.31	0.22
E911	Inhalation and ingestion of food causing obstruction of respiratory tract or suffocation	96	64	0.15	0.10
E913	Accidental mechanical suffocation	25	28	0.04	0.04

Source: OPCS *Mortality statistics: perinatal and infant, Series DH3*

Table A3.18 Bridge coding of 25 per cent sample of infant deaths in England and Wales in 1978: tabulation by ICD chapter

Numbers

8th Revision	9th Revision																	
	I	II	III	IV	V	VI	VII	VIII	IX	X	XI	XII	XIII	XIV	XV	XVI	XVII	Total
I	39	-	-	-	-	-	-	-	-	-	-	-	-	-	23	-	-	62
II	-	8	-	-	-	-	-	-	-	-	-	-	-	-	-	-	-	8
III	-	1	14	-	-	-	-	-	-	-	-	-	-	-	1	-	-	16
IV	-	-	-	3	-	-	-	-	-	-	-	-	-	-	1	-	-	4
V	-	-	-	-	-	-	-	-	-	-	-	-	-	-	-	-	-	-
VI	-	-	-	-	-	44	-	-	-	-	-	-	-	1	-	-	-	45
VII	-	-	-	-	-	1	6	-	-	-	-	-	-	-	-	-	-	7
VIII	2	-	-	-	-	-	1	227	-	-	-	-	-	1	3	-	-	234
IX	-	-	-	-	-	-	-	-	12	-	-	-	-	15	2	-	-	29
X	-	-	-	-	-	-	-	-	-	5	-	-	-	-	-	-	-	5
XI	-	-	-	-	-	-	-	-	-	-	-	-	-	-	-	-	-	-
XII	-	-	-	-	-	-	-	-	-	-	-	1	-	-	-	-	-	1
XIII	-	-	-	-	-	-	-	-	-	-	-	-	1	-	-	-	-	1
XIV	-	-	-	-	-	1	1	-	1	-	-	-	-	462	5	-	-	470
XV	-	-	-	-	-	-	1	1	-	-	-	-	-	2	683	-	-	687
XVI	-	-	1	1	-	-	1	-	-	-	-	-	-	-	-	180	-	183
XVII	-	-	-	-	-	-	-	-	-	-	-	-	-	-	-	-	45	45
Total	**41**	**9**	**15**	**4**	**-**	**46**	**10**	**228**	**13**	**5**	**-**	**1**	**1**	**481**	**718**	**180**	**45**	**1,797**

ICD 8th and 9th Revision chapters by title

8th Revision

I   Infective and parasitic diseases (000–136)
II   Neoplasms (140–239)
III   Endocrine, nutritional and metabolic diseases (240–279)
IV   Diseases of blood and blood-forming organs (280–289)
V   Mental disorders (290–315)
VI   Diseases of the nervous system and sense organs (320–389)
VII   Diseases of the circulatory system (390–458)
VIII   Diseases of the respiratory system (460–519)
IX   Diseases of the digestive system (520–577)
X   Diseases of genito-urinary system (580–629)
XI   Complications of pregnancy, childbirth and the puerperium (630–678)
XII   Diseases of the skin and subcutaneous tissue (680–709)
XIII   Diseases of the musculoskeletal system and connective tissue (710–738)
XIV   Congenital anomalies (740–759)
XV   Certain causes of perinatal morbidity and mortality (760–779)
XVI   Symptoms and ill-defined conditions (780–796)
XVII   Accidents, poisonings and violence (external cause) (E800–E999)

9th Revision

I   Infectious and parasitic diseases (001–139)
II   Neoplasms (140–239)
III   Endocrine, nutritional and metabolic diseases and immunity disorders (240–279)
IV   Diseases of blood and blood-forming organs (280–289)
V   Mental disorders (290–319)
VI   Diseases of the nervous system and sense organs (320–389)
VII   Diseases of the circulatory system (390–459)
VIII   Diseases of the respiratory system (460–519)
IX   Diseases of the digestive system (520–579)
X   Diseases of genito-urinary system (580–629)
XI   Complications of pregnancy, childbirth and the puerperium (630–676)
XII   Diseases of the skin and subcutaneous tissue (680–709)
XIII   Diseases of the musculoskeletal system and connective tissue (710–739)
XIV   Congenital anomalies (740–759)
XV   Certain conditions originating in the perinatal period (760–779)
XVI   Symptoms, signs and ill-defined conditions (780–799)
XVII   Injury and poisoning (800–999)
Supplementary classification of external causes of injury and poisoning (E800–E999)

Source: OPCS unpublished data

Table A3.19 Bridge coding of 25 per cent sample of infant deaths in England and Wales in 1978: tabulation by 3 digit code within ICD chapters

(a) Diseases of the respiratory system

Numbers

8th Revision	9th Revision																Total in chapter	Total outside chapter	Total
	464	465	466	478	480	481	482	485	486	487	490	494	507	516	518	519			
465		5															5		5
466			56														56		56
471										1							1		1
480					13												13		13
481						4								1			5		5
482							5	1									6		6
484													2				2	2	4
485								74	1								75	1	76
486									32					1			33	3	36
490											6						6		6
508	1			3													4		4
517														1			1		1
518												1					1		1
519															1	18	19	1	20
Total in chapter	1	5	56	3	13	4	5	75	33	1	6	1	2	3	1	18	227	7	234
Total outside chapter								1									1		1
Total	1	5	56	3	13	4	5	76	33	1	6	1	2	3	1	18	228	7	235

8th Revision	9th Revision	Description
-	464	Acute laryngitis and tracheitis
465	465	Acute upper respiratory infections of multiple or unspecified sites
466	466	Acute bronchitis and bronchiolitis
471	-	Influenza with pneumonia
-	478	Other diseases of upper respiratory tract
480	480	Viral pneumonia
481	481	Pneumococcal pneumonia
482	482	Other bacterial pneumonia
484	-	Acute interstitial pneumonia
485	485	Bronchopneumonia, organism unspecified

8th Revision	9th Revision	Description
486	486	Pneumonia, organism unspecified
-	487	Influenza
490	490	Bronchitis, not specified as acute or chronic
507	507	Pneumonitis due to solids and liquids
-	516	Other diseases of upper respiratory tract
508	-	Other alveolar and parietoalveolar pneumopathy
517	-	Other chronic interstitial pneumonia
518	494	Bronchiectasis
-	518	Other diseases of lung
519	519	Other diseases of respiratory system

Table A3.19 Bridge coding of 25 per cent sample of infant deaths in England and Wales in 1978: tabulation by 3 digit code within ICD chapters - *continued*

(b) Congenital anomalies (740-759)

8th Revision	9th Revision																	Total in chapter	Total outside chapter	Total
	740	741	742	744	745	746	747	748	749	750	751	753	755	756	757	758	759			
740	13																	13		13
741		92																92		92
742			6															6		6
743			12															12	1	13
745				1														1		1
746					63	73		1										137	1	138
747							39											39		39
748								25										25	5	30
749									2									2		2
750										8								8	1	9
751											17			1				18		18
753												23						23		23
755													4					4		4
756														11				11		11
757															1			1		1
758														2			6	8		8
759	1													2		22	37	62		62
Total in chapter	14	92	18	1	63	73	39	26	2	8	17	23	4	16	1	22	43	462	8	470
Total outside chapter			1			1								17				19		19
Total	**14**	**92**	**19**	**1**	**63**	**74**	**39**	**26**	**2**	**8**	**17**	**23**	**4**	**33**	**1**	**22**	**43**	**481**	**8**	**489**

8th Revision	9th Revision	Description
740	740	Anencephalus and similar anomalies
741	741	Spina bifida
742	-	Congenital hydrocephalus
743	742	Other congenital anomalies of nervous system
745	744	Congenital anomalies of ear, face and neck
-	745	Bulbous cordis anomalies and anomalies of cardiac septal closure
746	746	Other congenital anomalies of heart
747	747	Other congenital anomalies of circulatory system
748	748	Congenital anomalies of respiratory system
749	749	Cleft palate and cleft lip

8th Revision	9th Revision	Description
750	750	Other congenital anomalies of upper alimentary tract
751	751	Other congenital anomalies of digestive system
753	753	Congenital anomalies of urinary system
755	755	Other congenital anomalies of limbs
756	756	Other congenital musculoskeletal anomalies
757	-	Congenital anomalies of skin, hair and nails
-	757	Congenital anomalies of the integument
758	758	Chromosomal anomalies
759	759	Other and unspecified congenital anomalies
-	-	Congenital syndromes affecting multiple systems

Table A3.19 Bridge coding of 25 per cent sample of infant deaths in England and Wales in 1978: tabulation by 3 digit code within ICD chapters - *continued*

(c) Certain conditions originating in the perinatal period (760-779)

8th Revision	9th Revision																	Total in chapter	Total outside chapter	Total
	760	761	762	763	765	767	768	769	770	771	772	773	775	776	777	778	779			
761	1									1	1		1					4		4
762	5									1								8		8
763	1		1															2		2
766				8			1	1										10		10
767				1	1													2		2
768				2	1		1											4		4
769		31	9		1		2	9	9									61		61
770			13				2	2										17		17
771			4															4		4
772			1			40					27							68	1	69
775												5		1				6		6
776							35	179	104					1				341		341
777					122													122	2	124
778									11		3			3	1	3	13	34	1	35
Total in chapter	7	31	28	11	125	40	60	192	128	2	30	5	1	5	1	4	13	683	4	687
Total outside chapter								3	6	10				1	15			35		35
Total	**7**	**31**	**28**	**11**	**125**	**40**	**60**	**195**	**134**	**12**	**30**	**5**	**1**	**6**	**16**	**4**	**13**	**718**	**4**	**722**

Description for 8th Revision

761 Other maternal conditions unrelated to pregnancy
762 Toxaemia of pregnancy
763 Maternal ante - and intrapartum infection
766 Difficult labour with malposition of foetus
767 Difficult labour with abnormality of forces of labour
768 Difficult labour with other and unspecified complication
769 Other complications of pregnancy and childbirth
770 Conditions of placenta
771 Conditions of umbilical cord
772 Birth injury without mention of cause
775 Haemolytic disease of newborn without mention of kernicterus
776 Anoxic and hypoxic conditions not elsewhere classified
777 Immaturity, unqualified
778 Other conditions of foetus or newborn

Description for 9th Revision

760 Foetus or newborn affected by maternal conditions which may be unrelated to present pregnancy
761 Foetus or newborn affected by maternal complications of pregnancy
762 Foetus or newborn affected by complications of placenta, cord and membranes
763 Foetus or newborn affected by other complications of labour and delivery
765 Disorders relating to short gestation and unspecified low birthweight
767 Birth trauma
768 Intrauterine hypoxia and birth asphyxia
769 Respiratory distress syndrome
770 Other respiratory conditions of foetus and newborn
771 Infections specific to the perinatal period
772 Foetal and neonatal haemorrhage
773 Haemolytic disease of foetus or newborn, due to isommunigation
775 Endocrine and metabolic disturbances specific to the foetus and newborn
776 Haematological disorders of foetus and newborn
777 Perinatal disorders of digestive system
778 Conditions involving the integument and temperature regulation of foetus and newborn
779 Other and ill-defined conditions originating in the perinatal period

Table A3.19 Bridge coding of 25 per cent sample of infant deaths in England and Wales in 1978: tabulation by 3 digit code within ICD chapters - *continued*

(d) Sudden death, cause unknown

8th Revision	9th Revision		Total in chapter	Total outside chapter	Total
	798	799			
782	3	3	6	1	7
795	173	1	174	–	174
Total in chapter	176	4	180	1	181
Total outside chapter	–	–	–	–	–
Total	**176**	**4**	**180**	**1**	**181**

8th Revision	9th Revision	Description
782	–	Symptons referable to cardiovascular and lymphatic system
795	798	Sudden death, cause unknown
–	799	Other ill-defined and unknown causes of morbidity and mortality

Source: OPCS unpublished tables

Table A3.20 Ratio of the average number of births on each day of the week to the annual overall daily average, England and Wales, 1966 and 1970-80

Day of week	1966 (sample of year's births)	1970	1971	1972	1973	1974	1975	1976	1977	1978	1979	1980
Sunday	0.92	0.88	0.87	0.84	0.81	0.79	0.78	0.77	0.77	0.78	0.79	0.79
Monday	0.94	0.92	0.92	0.93	0.94	0.96	0.96	0.97	0.97	0.97	0.97	0.97
Tuesday	1.02	1.03	1.04	1.04	1.04	1.06	1.07	1.07	1.06	1.05	1.05	1.05
Wednesday	1.03	1.06	1.06	1.07	1.07	1.08	1.09	1.08	1.09	1.08	1.09	1.08
Thursday	1.04	1.06	1.06	1.06	1.08	1.08	1.08	1.09	1.08	1.09	1.09	1.08
Friday	1.05	1.05	1.07	1.08	1.08	1.09	1.09	1.08	1.10	1.11	1.09	1.08
Saturday	1.02	1.00	0.99	0.98	0.98	0.95	0.93	0.93	0.92	0.93	0.93	0.93
Total number of births	*178,735*	*795,503*	*792,493*	*733,916*	*683,650*	*646,842*	*609,787*	*590,098*	*574,467*	*601,765*	*642,917*	*661,076*

Source: Authors' analysis of OPCS data

Table A3.21 Perinatal mortality by day of the week of birth, England and Wales, 1970-79

Day of birth	Perinatal deaths per 1,000 total births									
	1970	1971	1972	1973	1974	1975	1976	1977	1978	1979
Sunday	25.5	23.5	23.6	22.9	21.9	21.6	20.0	19.6	18.0	16.8
Monday	23.7	22.5	22.0	20.5	19.9	18.3	15.9	16.5	15.1	13.5
Tuesday	22.8	21.3	20.6	20.9	19.5	18.0	17.5	15.3	14.2	14.7
Wednesday	22.8	22.3	21.7	19.9	19.0	18.8	17.1	16.2	15.0	13.6
Thursday	23.1	21.8	21.3	20.5	19.6	19.0	17.4	16.5	14.6	14.0
Friday	22.4	21.6	20.7	21.3	20.8	18.4	17.2	17.0	15.3	14.3
Saturday	24.0	22.8	22.9	21.3	22.3	21.7	19.2	18.8	17.7	16.2
All days	23.4	22.2	21.8	21.0	20.4	19.3	17.6	17.0	15.6	14.6

Source: Authors' analysis of OPCS data

Table A3.22 Percentage distribution of birthweight of live births by day of the week, England and Wales, August-December 1980

Day of birth	Birthweight g									Total live births with known weight	Those with birthweight not known as a percent of all live births
	1,000 or less	1,001-1,500	1,501-2,000	2,001-2,500	All 2,500 or less	2,501-3,000	3001-3,500	3,501-4,000	Over 4,000		
Sunday	0.35	0.71	1.4	5.3	7.8	20.5	39.1	25.5	7.1	30,058	1.3
Monday	0.27	0.63	1.4	5.0	7.3	19.4	39.4	26.4	7.4	36,990	1.3
Tuesday	0.24	0.51	1.3	4.9	7.0	20.0	39.2	26.2	7.6	40,584	1.6
Wednesday	0.26	0.51	1.3	4.8	6.9	19.9	39.4	26.4	7.4	40,820	1.7
Thursday	0.25	0.51	1.2	5.0	6.9	20.2	39.4	25.9	7.6	38,921	1.7
Friday	0.25	0.56	1.3	4.9	7.1	20.0	39.2	26.2	7.6	41,062	1.4
Saturday	0.26	0.57	1.3	5.3	7.5	20.6	38.7	25.9	7.3	35,485	1.3
All days	0.26	0.56	1.3	5.0	7.2	20.1	39.2	26.1	7.4	263,920	1.5

Source: Authors' analysis of OPCS data

Table A3.23 Stillbirths and infant deaths (rates) by area of residence, 1980

Area of residence	Stillbirths*	Perinatal deaths*	Neonatal deaths†		Postneonatal deaths†	Infant deaths†
			Early	Total		
ENGLAND AND WALES	**7.2**	**13.3**	**6.2**	**7.7**	**4.4**	**12.0**
ENGLAND	**7.3**	**13.4**	**6.1**	**7.6**	**4.4**	**12.0**
Northern RHA	**8.3**	**15.0**	**6.7**	**8.4**	**4.0**	**12.4**
Cleveland AHA	9.1	17.6	8.6	10.9	4.0	14.9
Hartlepool HD	15.9	25.0	9.2	11.5	4.6	16.1
North Tees HD	11.0	18.8	7.8	9.3	2.2	11.5
South Tees HD	6.1	14.9	8.9	11.6	4.9	16.5
Cumbria AHA	10.0	14.2	4.2	6.1	4.7	10.8
East Cumbria HD	10.9	16.4	5.5	6.6	4.0	10.7
South West Cumbria HD	8.0	12.1	4.1	5.7	4.9	10.5
West Cumbria HD	10.0	12.2	2.2	5.6	5.6	11.2
Durham AHA	7.8	16.5	8.8	10.8	3.4	14.2
Darlington HD	3.3	17.0	13.8	15.8	3.3	19.1
Durham HD	9.7	16.9	7.3	9.8	4.8	14.6
North West Durham HD	6.1	14.0	7.9	10.6	3.5	14.1
South West Durham HD	9.1	16.8	7.7	8.7	1.5	10.2
Northumberland AHA	5.0	8.9	4.0	5.3	3.7	9.0
Gateshead AHA	7.3	13.6	6.3	7.0	2.6	9.6
Newcastle upon Tyne AHA	8.0	14.1	6.2	8.7	3.4	12.0
North Tyneside AHA	4.9	10.6	5.7	7.4	4.1	11.5
South Tyneside AHA	11.5	15.4	3.9	4.4	4.9	9.2
Sunderland AHA	9.5	17.1	7.7	7.9	4.9	12.8
Yorkshire RHA	**8.3**	**14.9**	**6.6**	**8.2**	**4.7**	**12.9**
Humberside AHA	8.4	13.8	5.5	6.7	3.7	10.4
Hull HD	7.1	11.0	4.0	5.8	3.7	9.5
Beverley HD	8.9	17.0	8.2	9.0	1.6	10.6
Grimsby HD	9.9	15.3	5.4	6.8	5.4	12.3
Scunthorpe HD	8.5	13.7	5.2	5.6	4.1	9.7
North Yorkshire AHA	6.7	11.6	4.9	6.1	4.5	10.7
Northallerton HD	6.0	13.5	7.6	9.8	3.0	12.8
York HD	8.6	13.8	5.2	5.9	5.6	11.5
Scarborough HD	5.7	8.3	2.6	3.8	3.8	7.7
Harrogate HD	4.8	9.0	4.2	4.9	4.9	9.7
Bradford AHA	8.7	15.6	6.9	9.0	7.0	16.0
Bradford HD	9.7	15.8	6.2	8.7	7.7	16.5
Airedale HD	5.8	14.2	8.5	9.4	4.5	13.8

* *Per 1,000 total births*
† *Per 1,000 live births*

Table A3.23 Stillbirths and infant deaths (rates) by area of residence, 1980 - *continued*

Area of residence	Stillbirths*	Perinatal deaths*	Neonatal deaths†		Postneonatal deaths†	Infant deaths†
			Early	Total		
Yorkshire RHA - continued						
Calderdale AHA	7.4	16.7	9.4	11.0	4.7	15.6
Kirklees AHA	9.4	18.2	8.9	11.5	5.4	16.9
Huddersfield HD	8.8	18.0	9.3	13.0	6.9	19.9
Dewsbury HD	10.0	18.4	8.5	9.7	3.6	13.3
Leeds AHA	8.3	14.7	6.4	8.0	3.9	11.8
Western (Leeds) HD	8.5	14.9	6.4	8.2	4.0	12.2
Eastern (Leeds) HD	8.1	14.5	6.4	7.8	3.8	11.5
Wakefield AHA	9.6	17.5	8.0	9.4	3.8	13.2
Western (Wakefield) HD	9.9	18.4	8.5	11.0	1.5	12.5
Eastern (Pontefract) HD	9.2	16.7	7.5	8.0	5.8	13.8
Trent RHA	**7.0**	**13.0**	**6.0**	**7.4**	**3.5**	**10.9**
Derbyshire AHA	8.1	14.6	6.6	7.6	4.5	12.1
Central Derbyshire HD	10.3	15.7	5.4	5.8	2.5	8.3
North Derbyshire HD	7.7	15.1	7.4	8.9	4.2	13.2
South Derbyshire HD	7.7	14.7	7.0	8.0	6.5	14.5
Leicestershire AHA	6.4	12.5	6.1	7.1	2.6	9.7
East Leicestershire HD	7.7	13.9	6.3	7.0	1.8	8.8
North West Leicestershire HD	4.7	11.4	6.7	7.7	2.0	9.7
South West Leicestershire HD	6.9	12.1	5.3	6.5	4.1	10.5
Lincolnshire AHA	6.7	11.9	5.3	6.1	3.5	9.6
Lincolnshire South HD	5.4	9.4	4.0	4.6	3.4	8.0
Lincolnshire North HD	8.0	14.5	6.5	7.7	3.6	11.3
Nottinghamshire AHA	6.1	11.5	5.5	6.6	3.4	9.9
Central Nottinghamshire HD	7.9	14.7	6.9	7.7	1.9	9.6
Worksop & Retford HD	4.0	13.5	9.6	12.0	3.2	15.2
North Nottingham HD	4.7	9.4	4.7	5.9	5.6	11.5
South Nottingham HD	6.1	9.8	3.7	4.6	3.1	7.7
Barnsley AHA	5.8	11.3	5.5	7.9	4.1	12.0
Doncaster AHA	6.7	12.2	5.5	7.0	3.3	10.3
Rotherham AHA	9.0	16.7	7.7	10.8	4.4	15.2
Sheffield AHA	8.3	14.9	6.7	8.7	2.9	11.6
Northern HD	8.1	14.7	6.7	8.5	3.7	12.2
Southern HD	8.4	15.1	6.7	8.8	2.3	11.1

* *Per 1,000 total births*
† *Per 1,000 live births*

Table A3.23 Stillbirths and infant deaths (rates) by area of residence, 1980 - *continued*

Area of residence	Stillbirths*	Perinatal deaths*	Neonatal deaths†		Postneonatal deaths†	Infant deaths†
			Early	Total		
East Anglian RHA	**6.1**	**11.3**	**5.3**	**6.4**	**4.0**	**10.4**
Cambridgeshire AHA	5.8	11.5	5.7	6.2	3.4	9.6
Cambridge HD	3.9	9.3	5.4	5.6	2.9	8.5
Peterborough HD	8.0	14.7	6.7	7.7	4.7	12.4
Norfolk AHA	5.7	10.8	5.1	6.6	4.0	10.6
Norwich HD	5.0	9.3	4.3	6.4	3.6	9.9
Great Yarmouth and Waveney HD	6.0	10.8	4.8	5.2	5.2	10.4
King's Lynn HD	8.6	15.9	7.3	7.8	4.1	11.9
Suffolk AHA	6.7	11.7	5.0	6.4	4.6	11.0
Bury St Edmunds HD	4.9	8.8	3.9	4.6	5.2	9.8
Ipswich HD	8.0	13.6	5.6	7.8	3.7	11.5
North West Thames RHA	**6.1**	**11.0**	**4.9**	**6.4**	**4.5**	**10.9**
Bedfordshire AHA	7.4	12.7	5.4	7.1	4.2	11.2
Northern HD	5.2	11.3	6.1	8.0	4.4	12.4
Southern HD	9.1	13.9	4.8	6.3	3.9	10.3
Hertfordshire AHA	5.6	9.5	3.9	5.1	4.4	9.6
North Hertfordshire HD	5.8	9.2	3.5	4.3	5.4	9.7
East Hertfordshire HD	4.5	9.6	5.1	6.8	4.8	11.6
North West Hertfordshire HD	5.9	10.0	4.1	5.6	2.1	7.7
South West Hertfordshire HD	6.9	9.0	2.2	2.6	5.2	7.8
Barnet AHA	6.9	11.4	4.5	5.6	3.5	9.0
Barnet and Finchley HD	5.5	10.1	4.7	6.3	4.3	10.6
Edgware and Hendon HD	7.5	11.6	4.2	5.0	4.6	9.6
Brent and Harrow AHA	5.0	9.7	4.7	6.1	5.9	12.0
Brent HD	5.0	12.1	7.2	9.7	6.2	15.9
Harrow HD	4.8	7.1	2.2	2.6	5.6	8.2
Ealing, Hammersmith and Hounslow AHA	6.2	11.6	5.4	7.2	3.7	10.9
Hounslow HD	4.4	9.2	4.8	6.8	3.1	9.9
South Hammersmith HD	8.6	13.2	4.6	5.8	2.9	8.7
North Hammersmith HD	7.9	13.6	5.8	7.2	2.2	9.4
Ealing HD	6.0	11.4	5.5	7.2	4.3	11.5
Hillingdon AHA	6.5	11.3	4.9	7.2	3.9	11.1
Kensington, Chelsea and Westminster AHA	5.9	11.7	5.9	8.2	6.7	14.9
North West HD	5.4	10.4	5.0	6.4	4.6	10.9
North East HD	5.3	10.6	5.3	8.9	10.7	19.5
South HD	6.5	13.0	6.5	9.1	7.2	16.3

* *Per 1,000 total births*
† *Per 1,000 live births*

Table A3.23 Stillbirths and infant deaths (rates) by area of residence, 1980 - *continued*

Area of residence	Stillbirths*	Perinatal deaths*	Neonatal deaths†		Postneonatal deaths†	Infant deaths†
			Early	Total		
North East Thames RHA	**7.9**	**13.8**	**6.0**	**7.3**	**4.6**	**12.0**
Essex AHA	7.5	12.9	5.4	6.8	4.9	11.7
Basildon and Thurrock HD	6.3	12.7	6.4	8.3	4.7	13.0
Chelmsford HD	6.6	11.7	5.1	6.8	6.0	12.8
Colchester HD	8.7	12.4	3.8	5.0	4.4	9.3
Harlow HD	9.5	14.1	4.6	5.9	4.0	9.9
Southend HD	7.4	14.0	6.7	7.7	4.9	12.6
Barking and Havering AHA	7.9	14.1	6.2	7.2	4.0	11.2
Barking HD	10.1	14.9	4.9	6.3	3.9	10.2
Havering HD	6.4	13.5	7.2	7.8	4.1	11.9
Camden and Islington AHA	7.6	13.8	6.2	7.7	3.7	11.4
North Camden HD	6.5	10.2	3.7	4.4	2.9	7.3
South Camden HD	4.9	8.5	3.7	7.3	3.7	11.0
Islington HD	9.2	17.6	8.5	9.7	4.2	14.0
City and East London AHA	8.4	15.3	6.9	8.1	4.7	12.8
City and Hackney HD	6.8	15.7	8.9	11.0	5.1	16.1
Newham HD	9.4	15.5	6.1	6.9	3.3	10.2
Tower Hamlets HD	9.0	14.5	5.5	5.9	6.3	12.3
Enfield and Haringey AHA	7.8	12.8	5.1	6.8	4.1	10.9
Enfield HD	7.4	12.7	5.4	6.6	4.8	11.3
Haringey HD	8.2	12.9	4.7	7.0	3.5	10.4
Redbridge and Waltham Forest AHA	8.6	15.3	6.8	8.3	5.2	13.5
East Roding HD	5.9	12.5	6.6	8.7	3.1	11.9
West Roding HD	10.9	17.8	7.0	7.9	7.0	15.0
South East Thames RHA	**7.2**	**12.9**	**5.7**	**7.6**	**4.7**	**12.3**
East Sussex AHA	7.6	13.4	5.9	7.9	4.2	12.2
Brighton HD	7.1	12.7	5.6	7.2	2.5	9.7
Eastbourne HD	6.4	11.3	5.0	7.9	6.0	13.9
Hastings HD	9.8	17.2	7.4	9.3	5.6	14.9
Kent AHA	7.1	12.5	5.5	7.0	4.7	11.7
South East Kent HD	9.0	13.4	4.5	6.8	3.6	10.3
Canterbury and Thanet HD	4.8	10.2	5.4	6.3	3.6	9.9
Dartford and Gravesham HD	8.2	15.8	7.6	9.3	4.3	13.6
Maidstone HD	5.1	10.2	5.1	6.7	4.7	11.5
Medway HD	7.8	12.3	4.6	5.7	5.7	11.5
Tunbridge Wells HD	6.8	13.3	6.5	8.2	6.0	14.2
Greenwich and Bexley AHA	7.1	13.5	6.4	9.0	5.1	14.1
Bexley HD	6.5	13.3	6.9	8.0	3.6	11.6
Greenwich HD	7.6	13.6	6.1	9.9	6.4	16.3
Bromley AHA	4.9	9.7	4.9	6.1	4.0	10.1

* *Per 1,000 total births*
† *Per 1,000 live births*

Table A3.23 Stillbirths and infant deaths (rates) by area of residence, 1980 - *continued*

Area of residence	Stillbirths*	Perinatal deaths*	Neonatal deaths†		Postneonatal deaths†	Infant deaths†
			Early	Total		
South East Thames RHA *- continued*						
Lambeth, Southwark and Lewisham AHA	8.0	13.9	5.9	8.1	5.1	13.2
St Thomas' HD	8.1	14.1	6.1	7.3	6.5	13.8
Kings' HD	8.0	12.8	4.8	6.9	4.5	11.4
Guy's HD	8.9	13.1	4.3	7.1	6.1	13.2
Lewisham HD	7.0	15.8	8.9	11.5	3.5	15.1
South West Thames RHA	**5.6**	**10.8**	**5.2**	**6.3**	**4.6**	**11.0**
Surrey AHA	5.5	11.1	5.6	7.0	4.4	11.4
North Surrey HD	1.8	8.4	6.6	7.2	4.8	12.0
North West Surrey HD	4.9	13.3	8.4	10.3	4.2	14.5
West Surrey and North East Hampshire HD	5.2	9.5	4.4	6.5	4.1	10.6
South West Surrey HD	6.7	9.8	3.1	4.7	2.1	6.7
Mid Surrey HD	5.3	8.3	3.0	3.6	6.5	10.1
East Surrey HD	9.3	14.8	5.6	7.5	5.1	12.6
West Sussex AHA	6.2	11.9	5.6	6.0	4.5	10.5
Chichester HD	8.2	11.8	3.6	3.6	3.6	7.1
Cuckfield and Crawley HD	3.7	9.6	5.9	6.1	5.6	11.7
Worthing HD	8.8	15.6	6.8	7.6	3.4	11.0
Croydon AHA	5.2	9.2	4.1	5.0	6.3	11.3
Kingston and Richmond AHA	3.6	7.6	3.9	5.3	3.9	9.3
Merton, Sutton and Wandsworth AHA	6.2	11.5	5.3	6.9	4.6	11.5
Roehampton HD	3.8	10.3	6.6	8.5	2.8	11.3
Wandsworth and East Merton HD	7.0	12.4	5.4	6.5	5.2	11.7
Sutton and West Merton HD	5.6	10.2	4.5	6.5	4.0	10.5
Wessex RHA	**6.2**	**11.7**	**5.5**	**7.0**	**5.0**	**12.0**
Dorset AHA	6.4	10.8	4.4	6.0	4.4	10.4
East Dorset HD	6.0	10.7	4.7	6.5	4.4	11.0
West Dorset HD	7.1	11.0	3.8	4.8	4.3	9.1
Hampshire AHA	6.1	11.6	5.5	6.9	4.9	11.8
Portsmouth and South East Hampshire HD	5.9	9.9	4.0	5.5	4.8	10.3
Southampton and South West Hampshire HD	4.8	9.9	5.2	5.9	5.2	11.1
Winchester and Central Hampshire HD	7.1	15.0	7.9	8.7	3.8	12.4

* *Per 1,000 total births*
† *Per 1,000 live births*

42

Table A3.23 Stillbirths and infant deaths (rates) by area of residence, 1980 - *continued*

Area of residence	Stillbirths*	Perinatal deaths*	Neonatal deaths†		Postneonatal deaths†	Infant deaths†
			Early	Total		
Wessex RHA - continued						
Basingstoke and North Hampshire HD	7.6	15.5	8.0	10.1	6.2	16.3
Wiltshire AHA	6.0	12.2	6.2	7.7	5.8	13.5
Salisbury HD	5.4	13.4	8.1	10.1	7.4	17.5
Swindon HD	6.7	12.0	5.4	6.7	6.4	13.1
Bath HD	6.7	12.3	5.6	6.7	4.8	11.5
Isle of Wight AHA	8.9	15.3	6.5	10.6	4.1	14.6
Oxford RHA	**6.3**	**12.6**	**6.3**	**7.5**	**3.9**	**11.4**
Berkshire AHA	5.7	12.3	6.6	7.5	5.0	12.5
East Berkshire HD	6.6	14.4	7.9	8.3	4.7	13.0
West Berkshire HD	5.1	11.2	6.2	7.5	5.3	12.7
Buckinghamshire AHA	7.8	14.0	6.3	7.5	3.6	11.1
Aylesbury HD	7.0	12.7	5.7	7.3	4.8	12.1
High Wycombe HD	8.7	15.2	6.5	7.4	2.0	9.4
Northamptonshire AHA	7.4	13.9	6.6	7.9	2.9	10.8
Kettering HD	7.7	15.6	8.0	9.4	3.9	13.2
Northampton HD	7.2	12.4	5.3	6.5	2.0	8.5
Oxfordshire AHA	4.1	9.8	5.7	6.9	4.0	10.9
Oxford HD	4.0	9.2	5.2	6.5	3.9	10.4
South Western RHA	**6.7**	**12.6**	**5.9**	**7.4**	**4.1**	**11.5**
Avon AHA	6.8	13.7	7.0	8.7	4.7	13.5
Bristol and Weston HD	6.6	13.7	7.1	8.8	5.2	14.0
Frenchay HD	5.8	14.5	8.8	10.6	4.0	14.6
Southmead HD	8.2	14.2	6.1	7.9	5.4	13.3
Cornwall (and Scilly) AHA	5.9	12.5	6.6	7.7	2.5	10.2
Devon AHA	6.6	11.7	5.1	6.6	4.2	10.8
Exeter HD	9.0	12.4	3.5	5.0	5.3	10.4
North Devon HD	11.8	17.3	5.6	7.0	4.9	11.9
Plymouth HD	4.2	9.2	5.0	6.1	3.1	9.2
Torbay HD	4.2	11.7	7.5	9.4	4.2	13.7
Gloucestershire AHA	6.6	12.2	5.7	6.9	3.8	10.7
Somerset AHA	7.6	12.3	4.7	6.3	4.7	11.0
West Midlands RHA	**8.2**	**15.1**	**6.9**	**8.7**	**4.5**	**13.1**
Hereford and Worcester AHA	9.1	14.2	5.1	6.3	4.9	11.2
Hereford HD	8.0	13.9	5.9	6.5	7.0	13.5

* *Per 1,000 total births*
† *Per 1,000 live births*

Area of residence	Stillbirths*	Perinatal deaths*	Neonatal deaths†		Postneonatal deaths†	Infant deaths†
			Early	Total		
West Midlands RHA - continued						
Bromsgrove and Redditch HD	9.5	14.5	5.0	5.4	3.3	8.8
Kidderminster HD	9.2	14.6	5.4	7.0	4.7	11.6
Worcester HD	9.3	13.8	4.5	6.6	4.9	11.5
Salop AHA	6.9	13.4	6.5	7.8	3.8	11.6
Staffordshire AHA	7.8	14.8	7.1	8.6	3.7	12.4
Mid Staffordshire HD	6.8	13.9	7.1	8.4	2.7	11.1
North Staffordshire HD	9.1	15.4	6.4	8.3	5.0	13.3
South East Staffordshire HD	6.7	14.7	8.1	9.4	2.9	12.2
Warwickshire AHA	6.1	14.7	8.7	10.8	4.2	15.0
North Warwickshire HD	5.9	15.7	9.8	11.5	3.8	15.3
Rugby HD	8.3	15.7	7.4	10.2	0.9	11.2
South Warwickshire HD	5.4	13.5	8.2	10.5	5.8	16.3
Birmingham AHA	8.7	15.1	6.5	8.6	5.1	13.7
Central HD	7.5	14.7	7.3	8.8	7.3	16.0
East HD	13.2	21.1	8.0	8.9	3.6	12.4
North HD	8.3	14.2	5.9	8.4	3.0	11.3
South HD	9.6	16.4	6.8	9.1	5.4	14.5
West HD	6.6	11.3	4.7	7.8	4.7	12.5
Coventry AHA	7.5	15.9	8.4	9.8	2.4	12.2
Dudley AHA	7.1	12.8	5.7	6.2	4.5	10.7
Sandwell AHA	9.8	18.6	8.9	11.0	4.9	16.0
Solihull AHA	5.9	10.5	4.6	5.5	4.2	9.7
Walsall AHA	10.4	19.2	8.9	11.9	3.6	15.5
Wolverhampton AHA	11.2	17.8	6.7	9.7	7.5	17.2
Mersey RHA	**7.3**	**13.7**	**6.4**	**7.9**	**4.9**	**12.8**
Cheshire AHA	7.5	13.5	6.1	7.5	4.3	11.8
Chester HD	8.3	13.0	4.8	6.1	4.4	10.5
Crewe HD	4.8	13.0	8.3	8.6	5.1	13.7
Halton HD	7.1	13.2	6.2	10.4	3.8	14.2
Macclesfield HD	7.4	12.3	5.0	5.0	5.9	10.9
Warrington HD	9.4	13.4	4.1	5.9	1.8	7.7
Liverpool AHA	8.1	14.8	6.7	8.4	6.2	14.5
St Helens and Knowsley AHA	7.2	13.3	6.2	8.0	4.9	12.9

* *Per 1,000 total births*
† *Per 1,000 live births*

Table A3.23 Stillbirths and infant deaths (rates) by area of residence, 1980 - *continued*

Area of residence	Stillbirths*	Perinatal deaths*	Neonatal deaths†		Postneonatal deaths†	Infant deaths†
			Early	Total		
Mersey RHA - continued						
Sefton AHA	7.2	13.5	6.4	7.5	3.9	11.4
Northern HD	7.4	11.6	4.2	5.0	1.7	6.7
Southern HD	7.0	14.5	7.5	8.8	5.0	13.8
Wirral AHA	5.9	13.2	7.3	8.2	5.5	13.7
Wirral HD	6.7	14.5	7.8	8.7	5.5	14.2
North Western RHA	**8.2**	**15.3**	**7.2**	**8.5**	**4.4**	**12.9**
Lancashire AHA	8.3	15.2	7.0	7.9	4.1	12.0
Lancaster HD	7.9	12.2	4.3	4.3	5.8	10.1
Blackpool HD	9.1	15.7	6.7	7.3	3.2	10.5
Preston HD	8.6	14.8	6.3	6.9	2.9	9.8
Blackburn HD	9.0	16.5	7.6	8.8	5.4	14.2
Burnley HD	9.0	16.6	7.7	9.3	4.7	14.0
Ormskirk HD	2.1	11.2	9.1	9.1	3.5	12.6
Bolton AHA	7.6	14.2	6.6	8.8	3.5	12.2
Bury AHA	8.4	19.0	10.6	11.9	4.2	16.1
Manchester AHA	7.3	15.9	8.6	10.3	6.4	16.8
North HD	6.9	12.9	6.0	6.9	3.7	10.6
Central HD	8.6	18.1	9.6	12.2	10.7	22.9
South HD	6.6	16.7	10.2	12.0	5.3	17.3
Oldham AHA	10.2	17.1	7.0	8.5	4.2	12.7
Rochdale AHA	10.8	18.4	7.6	9.1	5.8	14.9
Salford AHA	7.1	13.7	6.6	8.1	5.9	14.1
Stockport AHA	8.5	16.2	7.8	9.1	4.0	13.2
Tameside AHA	7.7	14.3	6.7	8.4	5.4	13.8
Tameside HD	6.7	12.8	6.2	7.6	5.0	12.6
Trafford AHA	7.6	13.9	6.3	7.4	4.2	11.6
Wigan AHA	6.8	12.5	5.7	6.4	1.6	8.0
WALES	**6.5**	**12.8**	**6.4**	**7.9**	**3.5**	**11.4**
Clwyd AHA	8.4	15.0	6.6	7.7	4.0	11.7
Clwyd North HD	7.5	14.5	7.0	8.7	4.3	13.0
Clwyd South HD	8.9	15.3	6.4	7.1	3.8	10.9
Dyfed AHA	5.5	11.9	6.5	7.2	2.5	9.7
Ceredigion HD	6.3	9.5	3.2	3.2	-	3.2

* *Per 1,000 total births*
† *Per 1,000 live births*

45

Area of residence	Stillbirths*	Perinatal deaths*	Neonatal deaths†		Postneonatal deaths†	Infant deaths†
			Early	Total		
Wales - continued						
Carmarthen/Dinefwr HD	9.7	15.8	6.1	6.1	1.2	7.4
Preseli/South						
Pembrokeshire HD	1.4	10.6	9.2	9.9	4.9	14.8
Llanelli/Dinefwr HD	6.9	12.1	5.2	6.9	1.7	8.7
Gwent AHA	4.5	11.3	6.8	8.3	2.9	11.2
North Gwent HD	3.5	11.3	7.8	7.8	2.1	9.9
South Gwent HD	4.9	11.3	6.4	8.4	3.1	11.6
Gwynedd AHA	7.0	13.3	6.3	7.4	1.8	9.2
Mid Glamorgan AHA	7.2	13.3	6.2	8.3	3.3	11.6
Ogwr HD	6.6	11.6	5.0	6.7	1.7	8.3
Rhymney Valley HD	5.7	9.6	4.0	5.7	2.8	8.5
East Glamorgan HD	8.5	14.7	6.2	9.0	2.7	11.7
Merthyr and						
Cynon Valley HD	7.5	16.7	9.2	11.4	6.0	17.4
Powys AHA	7.4	9.7	2.2	3.0	3.7	6.7
South Glamorgan AHA	5.2	12.2	7.1	8.9	4.8	13.8
West Glamorgan AHA	7.6	13.8	6.3	8.3	4.2	12.5
Neath HD	6.1	13.9	7.9	9.2	3.7	12.8
Swansea HD	8.4	13.8	5.4	7.8	4.5	12.4
SCOTLAND	**6.7**	**13.1**	**6.5**	**7.8**	**4.3**	**12.1**
Highland Region & HBA	**6.9**	**11.7**	**4.9**	**6.6**	**6.2**	**12.8**
Health districts						
Northern	1.7	5.2	3.5	7.0	7.0	14.0
Southern	8.1	13.3	5.2	6.5	6.1	12.5
Orkney Islands Area & HBA	**7.6**	**7.6**	**-**	**3.8**	**-**	**3.8**
Shetland Islands Area & HBA	**7.9**	**15.8**	**8.0**	**10.6**	**2.7**	**13.3**
Western Isles Islands						
Area & HBA	**8.0**	**8.0**	**-**	**-**	**2.7**	**2.7**
Grampian Region & HBA	**5.7**	**8.1**	**2.5**	**4.2**	**4.5**	**8.6**
Health districts						
West Grampian	5.1	8.5	3.4	5.1	3.4	8.5
North Grampian	6.9	9.1	2.2	3.9	4.8	8.7
South Grampian	4.9	7.3	2.3	4.0	4.6	8.6

* *Per 1,000 total births*
† *Per 1,000 live births*

Table A3.23 Stillbirths and infant deaths (rates) by area of residence, 1980 - *continued*

Area of residence	Stillbirths*	Perinatal deaths*	Neonatal deaths†		Postneonatal deaths†	Infant deaths†
			Early	Total		
Scotland - continued						
Tayside Region & HBA	**9.2**	**13.3**	**4.1**	**4.5**	**3.9**	**8.5**
Health districts						
Angus	10.8	18.3	7.6	8.4	2.5	11.0
Dundee	11.2	12.9	1.7	2.2	4.3	6.5
Perth and Kinross	4.4	9.5	5.1	5.1	4.4	19.6
Fife Region & HBA	**6.2**	**12.9**	**6.7**	**8.7**	**2.8**	**11.5**
Health districts						
East Fife	5.0	9.9	5.0	7.5	2.9	10.3
West Fife	8.2	17.5	9.4	10.5	2.8	13.2
Lothian Region & HBA	**5.1**	**11.7**	**6.6**	**8.3**	**4.6**	**12.9**
Health districts						
West Lothian	6.5	14.4	7.9	10.3	5.6	15.9
South Lothian	6.0	11.8	5.8	6.8	5.1	11.9
North Lothian	3.1	9.8	6.8	8.9	3.4	12.3
Borders region & HBA	**7.9**	**17.6**	**9.8**	**10.6**	**1.8**	**12.4**
Central region [Forth Valley HBA]	**6.0**	**12.3**	**6.3**	**6.9**	**4.4**	**11.2**
Health districts						
Stirling	5.4	9.1	3.6	4.2	4.9	9.1
Falkirk	6.5	14.9	8.5	9.0	4.0	13.0
Strathclyde region	**7.1**	**14.5**	**7.5**	**8.7**	**4.3**	**12.9**
Argyll and Clyde HBA	**6.0**	**13.4**	**7.4**	**8.9**	**3.3**	**12.2**
Health districts						
Argyll and Bute	1.1	13.5	12.4	14.6	2.2	16.9
Dumbarton	6.7	12.5	5.9	6.7	5.9	12.6
Renfrew	6.0	11.3	5.3	6.8	3.6	10.3
Inverclyde	8.3	18.1	9.8	11.2	1.4	12.6
Greater Glasgow HBA	**6.5**	**13.8**	**7.3**	**8.6**	**4.6**	**13.2**
Health districts						
Western	4.8	11.8	6.9	9.7	4.2	13.9
Northern	5.1	12.9	7.8	8.6	2.4	11.0
Eastern	6.1	16.8	10.8	11.9	7.3	19.2
South Eastern	5.3	10.9	5.7	6.9	4.4	11.3
South Western	12.9	18.0	5.1	5.6	4.7	10.3

* *Per 1,000 total births*
† *Per 1,000 live births*

Table A3.23 Stillbirths and infant deaths (rates) by area of residence, 1980 - *continued*

Area of residence	Stillbirths*	Perinatal deaths*	Neonatal deaths†		Postneonatal deaths†	Infant deaths†
			Early	Total		
Scotland - continued						
Lanarkshire HBA	**6.9**	**14.0**	**7.2**	**8.3**	**3.5**	**11.8**
Health districts						
Monklands/Cumbernauld	7.9	14.0	6.2	6.5	2.5	9.0
Motherwell/Lanark	4.8	13.8	9.0	11.1	3.8	14.9
Hamilton/East Kilbride	8.0	14.2	6.2	7.3	4.0	11.4
Ayrshire and Arron HBA	**10.3**	**18.7**	**8.5**	**9.0**	**6.1**	**15.1**
Health districts						
North Ayrshire and Arran	9.5	19.0	9.6	9.9	8.0	17.9
South Ayrshire	11.6	18.1	6.6	7.6	3.1	10.7
Dumfries and Galloway Region & HBA	**4.5**	**15.1**	**10.7**	**11.2**	**6.7**	**17.9**
NORTHERN IRELAND	**9.2**	**15.6**	**6.4**	**8.0**	**5.4**	**13.4**
District Council Areas						
Ards	8.3	18.5	10.2	11.2	6.5	17.7
Belfast	10.2	14.1	3.9	5.8	4.9	10.7
Castlereagh	18.1	20.3	2.3	4.6	11.5	16.1
Down	9.4	17.8	8.5	8.5	6.6	15.2
Lisburn	9.1	15.6	6.6	8.5	5.9	14.4
North Down	5.4	12.7	7.3	9.1	4.6	13.7
Antrim	7.0	11.0	4.0	7.0	6.0	13.1
Ballymena	6.5	15.7	9.3	11.1	8.4	19.5
Ballymoney	7.8	15.6	7.9	9.8	5.9	15.7
Carrickfergus	11.5	18.3	7.0	9.3	4.6	13.9
Coleraine	6.5	9-2	2.6	2.6	5.3	7.9
Cookstown	4.4	11.0	6.6	6.6	4.4	11.0
Larne	7.4	7.4	-	5.0	5.0	9.9
Magherafelt	8.1	14.8	6.8	6.8	5.4	12.2
Mayle	10.3	30.9	20.8	26.0	5.2	31.3
Newtownabbey	8.9	14.2	5.3	6.0	4.5	10.5
Armagh	5.8	12.7	7.0	9.3	-	9.3
Banbridge	14.8	29.6	15.0	15.0	8.6	23.6
Craigavon	4.7	8.8	4.1	5.4	2.7	8.2
Dungannon	5.0	15.1	10.1	10.1	3.0	13.2
Newry and Mourne	10.2	15.8	5.7	6.8	3.4	10.3·
Fermanagh	18.0	26.0	8.2	9.1	3.7	12.8
Limavady	14.2	32.5	18.5	24.7	8.2	32.9
Londonderry	10.8	17.1	6.3	8.0	8.4	16.4
Omagh	7.7	13.6	5.9	7.8	5.9	13.7
Strabane	11.9	17.9	6.0	7.5	6.0	13.6

* Per 1,000 total births
† Per 1,000 live births

Table A3.23 Stillbirths and infant deaths (rates) by area of residence, 1980 - *continued*

Area of residence	Stillbirths*	Perinatal deaths*	Neonatal deaths†		Postneonatal deaths†	Infant deaths†
			Early	Total		
GUERNSEY	**8.0**	**14.4**	**6.4**	**8.0**	**4.8**	**12.9**
JERSEY	**6.9**	**14.9**	**8.1**	**8.1**	**2.3**	**10.4**

* *Per 1,000 total births*
† *Per 1,000 live births*

Source: OPCS SD52 tabulations (England and Wales)
           Registrar General, Scotland, *Annual Report* (Scotland)
           Registrar General, Northern Ireland, *Annual Report* (Northern Ireland)
           Medical Officer of Health for the States of Guernsey, *Annual Report*
           Medical Officer of Health for the States of Jersey, *Report*

Table A3.24 Live births, stillbirths and infant deaths (numbers) by area of residence, 1980

Area of residence	Live births	Still-births	Total births	Deaths under 24 hrs	Neonatal deaths			Post-neonatal deaths
					Early	Late	Total	
ENGLAND AND WALES	**656,234**	**4,773**	**661,007**	**2,215**	**4,042**	**981**	**5,023**	**2,876**
ENGLAND	**618,371**	**4,523**	**622,894**	**2,077**	**3,793**	**911**	**4,704**	**2,706**
Northern RHA	**41,191**	**345**	**41,536**	**158**	**277**	**69**	**346**	**163**
Cleveland AHA	8,713	80	8,793	44	75	20	95	35
Hartlepool HD	1,301	21	1,322	6	12	3	15	6
North Tees HD	2,690	30	2,720	12	21	4	25	6
South Tees HD	4,722	29	4,751	26	42	13	55	23
Cumbria AHA	5,737	58	5,795	9	24	11	35	27
East Cumbria HD	2,717	30	2,747	5	15	3	18	11
South West Cumbria HD	1,233	10	1,243	2	5	2	7	6
West Cumbria HD	1,787	18	1,805	2	4	6	10	10
Durham AHA	7,881	62	7,943	43	69	16	85	27
Darlington HD	1,522	5	1,527	14	21	3	24	5
Durham HD	3,155	31	3,186	14	23	8	31	15
North West Durham HD	1,137	7	1,144	6	9	3	12	4
South West Durham HD	2,067	19	2,086	9	16	2	18	3
Northumberland AHA	3,796	19	3,815	9	15	5	20	14
Gateshead AHA	2,703	20	2,723	11	17	2	19	7
Newcastle upon Tyne AHA	3,576	29	3,605	13	22	9	31	12
North Tyneside AHA	2,436	12	2,448	5	14	4	18	10
South Tyneside AHA	2,060	24	2,084	4	8	1	9	10
Sunderland AHA	4,289	41	4,330	20	33	1	34	21

Table A3.24 Livebirths, stillbirths and infant deaths (numbers) by area of residence, 1980 - *continued*

Area of residence	Live births	Still-births	Total births	Deaths under 24 hrs	Neonatal deaths Early	Late	Total	Post-neonatal deaths
Yorkshire RHA	**47,739**	**401**	**48,140**	**175**	**316**	**76**	**392**	**222**
Humberside AHA	11,105	94	11,199	32	61	13	74	41
Hull HD	3,779	27	3,806	6	15	7	22	14
Beverley HD	2,445	22	2,467	11	20	2	22	4
Grimsby HD	2,204	22	2,226	7	12	3	15	12
Scunthorpe HD	2,677	23	2,700	8	14	1	15	11
North Yorkshire AHA	7,696	52	7,748	22	38	9	47	35
Northallerton HD	1,324	8	1,332	4	10	3	13	4
York HD	2,882	25	2,901	10	15	2	17	16
Scarborough HD	1,560	9	1,569	3	4	2	6	6
Harrogate HD	1,441	7	1,448	4	6	1	7	7
Bradford AHA	7,707	68	7,775	30	53	16	69	54
Bradford HD	5,952	58	6,010	25	37	15	52	46
Airedale HD	2,244	13	2,257	6	19	2	21	10
Calderdale AHA	2,556	19	2,575	10	24	4	28	12
Kirklees AHA	5,391	51	5,442	23	48	14	62	29
Huddersfield HD	2,915	26	2,941	11	27	11	38	20
Dewsbury HD	2,476	25	2,501	12	21	3	24	9
Leeds AHA	9,036	76	9,112	36	58	14	72	35
Western (Leeds) HD	4,524	39	4,563	16	29	8	37	18
Eastern (Leeds) HD	4,512	37	4,549	20	29	6	35	17
Wakefield AHA	4,248	41	4,289	22	34	6	40	16
Western (Wakefield) HD	1,996	20	2,016	9	17	5	22	3
Eastern (Pontefract) HD	2,252	21	2,273	13	17	1	18	13
Trent RHA	**60,356**	**427**	**60,783**	**201**	**365**	**80**	**445**	**212**
Derbyshire AHA	11,691	95	11,786	43	77	12	89	53
Central Derbyshire HD	2,781	29	2,810	8	15	1	16	7
North Derbyshire HD	4,483	35	4,518	20	33	7	40	19
South Derbyshire HD	3,996	31	4,027	15	28	4	32	26
Leicestershire AHA	12,194	79	12,273	45	74	12	86	32
East Leicestershire HD	4,000	31	4,031	14	25	3	28	7
North West Leicestershire HD	4,011	19	4,030	14	27	4	31	8
South West Leicestershire HD	4,183	29	4,212	17	22	5	27	17
Lincolnshire AHA	6,843	46	6,889	16	36	6	42	24
Lincolnshire South HD	3,480	19	3,499	5	14	2	16	12
Lincolnshire North HD	3,363	27	3,390	11	22	4	26	12
Nottinghamshire AHA	12,975	79	13,054	37	71	14	85	44
Central Nottingham HD	3,768	30	3,798	16	26	3	29	7
Worksop & Retford HD	1,252	5	1,257	2	12	3	15	4

Table A3.24 Livebirths, stillbirths and infant deaths (numbers) by area of residence, 1980 - *continued*

Area of residence	Live births	Still-births	Total births	Deaths under 24 hrs	Neonatal deaths			Post-neonatal deaths
					Early	Late	Total	
Trent RHA - continued								
North Nottingham HD	3,386	16	3,402	10	16	4	20	19
South Nottingham HD	4,569	28	4,597	9	17	4	21	14
Barnsley AHA	2,908	17	2,925	7	16	7	23	12
Doncaster AHA	4,000	27	4,027	14	22	6	28	13
Rotherham AHA	3,621	33	3,654	15	28	11	39	16
Sheffield AHA	6,124	51	6,175	24	41	12	53	18
Northern HD	2,706	22	2,728	8	18	5	23	10
Southern HD	3,418	29	3,447	16	23	7	30	8
East Anglian RHA	**24,782**	**151**	**24,933**	**63**	**131**	**28**	**159**	**99**
Cambridgeshire AHA	8,220	48	8,268	20	47	4	51	28
Cambridge HD	4,834	19	4,853	10	26	1	27	14
Peterborough HD	2,977	24	3,001	9	20	3	23	14
Norfolk AHA	8,582	49	8,631	23	44	13	57	34
Norwich HD	5,331	27	5,358	10	23	11	34	19
Great Yarmouth and Waveney HD	2,309	14	2,323	4	11	1	12	12
King's Lynn HD	2,187	19	2,206	11	16	1	17	9
Suffolk AHA	7,980	54	8,034	20	40	11	51	37
Bury St Edmunds HD	3,049	15	3,064	6	12	2	14	16
Ipswich HD	4,095	33	4,128	13	23	9	32	15
North West Thames RHA	**47,524**	**293**	**47,817**	**129**	**231**	**75**	**306**	**214**
Bedfordshire AHA	8,191	61	8,252	27	44	14	58	34
Northern HD	3,618	19	3,637	14	22	7	29	16
Southern HD	4,573	42	4,615	13	22	7	29	18
Hertfordshire AHA	12,447	70	12,517	28	49	15	64	55
North Hertfordshire HD	2,587	15	2,602	5	9	2	11	14
East Hertfordshire HD	3,540	16	3,556	11	18	6	24	17
North West Hertfordshire HD	3,392	20	3,412	7	14	5	19	7
South West Hertfordshire HD	2,317	16	2,333	3	5	1	6	12
Barnet AHA	3,761	26	3,787	12	17	4	21	13
Barnet and Finchley HD	2,552	14	2,566	7	12	4	16	11
Edgware and Hendon HD	2,390	18	2,408	8	10	2	12	11
Brent and Harrow AHA	6,564	33	6.597	17	31	9	40	39
Brent HD	3,209	16	3,225	12	23	8	31	20
Harrow HD	2,671	13	2,684	3	6	1	7	15

Table A3.24 Livebirths, stillbirths and infant deaths (numbers) by area of residence, 1980 - *continued*

Area of residence	Live births	Still-births	Total births	Deaths under 24 hrs	Neonatal deaths			Post-neonatal deaths
					Early	Late	Total	
North West Thames RHA								
- continued								
Ealing, Hammersmith								
and Hounslow AHA	9,584	60	9,644	28	52	17	69	35
Hounslow HD	2,926	13	2,939	7	14	6	20	9
South Hammersmith HD	1,733	15	1,748	4	8	2	10	5
North Hammersmith HD	1,388	11	1,399	4	8	2	10	3
Ealing HD	3,481	21	3,502	11	19	6	25	15
Hillingdon AHA	3,073	20	3.093	6	15	7	22	12
Kensington, Chelsea								
and Westminster AHA	3,904	23	3,927	11	23	9	32	26
North West HD	2,193	12	2,205	4	11	3	14	10
North East HD	563	3	566	3	3	2	5	6
South HD	1,531	10	1,541	5	10	4	14	11
North East Thames RHA	**51,598**	**411**	**52,009**	**149**	**308**	**71**	**379**	**238**
Essex AHA	19,607	149	19,756	54	106	28	134	96
Basildon and Thurrock HD	4,225	27	4,252	14	27	8	35	20
Chelmsford HD	4,678	31	4,709	14	24	8	32	28
Colchester HD	3,430	30	3,460	7	13	4	17	15
Harlow HD	3,228	31	3,259	5	15	4	19	13
Southend HD	4,046	30	4,076	14	27	4	31	20
Barking and Havering AHA	4,994	40	5,034	14	31	5	36	20
Barking HD	2,058	21	2,079	6	10	3	13	8
Havering HD	2,936	19	2,955	8	21	2	23	12
Camden and Islington AHA	4,546	35	4,581	17	28	7	35	17
North Camden HD	1,367	9	1,376	4	5	1	6	4
South Camden HD	817	4	821	2	3	3	6	3
Islington HD	2,362	22	2,384	11	20	3	23	10
City and East London AHA	9,799	83	9,882	25	68	11	79	46
City and Hackney HD	3,361	23	3,384	14	30	7	37	17
Newham HD	3,910	37	3,947	7	24	3	27	13
Tower Hamlets HD	2,528	23	2,551	4	14	1	15	16
Enfield and Haringey AHA	6,508	51	6,559	13	33	11	44	27
Enfield HD	3,350	25	3,375	8	18	4	22	16
Haringey HD	3,158	26	3,184	5	15	7	22	11
Redbridge and								
Waltham Forest AHA	6,144	53	6,197	26	42	9	51	32
East Roding HD	2,868	17	2,885	14	19	6	25	9
West Roding HD	3,276	36	3,312	12	23	3	26	23

Area of residence	Live births	Still-births	Total births	Deaths under 24 hrs	Neonatal deaths			Post-neonatal deaths
					Early	Late	Total	
South East Thames RHA	**45,681**	**331**	**46,012**	**142**	**261**	**84**	**345**	**216**
East Sussex AHA	6,829	52	6,881	20	40	14	54	29
Brighton HD	3,197	23	3,220	9	18	5	23	8
Eastbourne HD	2,016	13	2,029	3	10	6	16	12
Hastings HD	1,616	16	1,632	8	12	3	15	9
Kent AHA	19,518	139	19,657	65	107	29	136	92
South East Kent HD	3,095	28	3,123	7	14	7	21	11
Canterbury and Thanet HD	3,328	16	3,344	8	18	3	21	12
Dartford and Gravesham HD	3,013	25	3,038	18	23	5	28	13
Maidstone HD	2,530	13	2,543	5	13	4	17	12
Medway HD	5,231	41	5,272	18	24	6	30	30
Tunbridge Wells HD	2,321	16	2,337	9	15	4	19	14
Greenwich and Bexley AHA	5,894	42	5,936	21	38	15	53	30
Bexley HD	2,758	18	2,776	12	19	3	22	10
Greenwich HD	3,136	24	3,160	9	19	12	31	20
Bromley AHA	3,275	16	3,291	4	16	4	20	13
Lambeth, Southwark and Lewisham AHA	10,165	82	10,247	32	60	22	82	52
St Thomas' HD	2,462	20	2,482	10	15	3	18	16
Kings' HD	3,331	27	3,358	6	16	7	23	15
Guy's HD	2,114	19	2,133	4	9	6	15	13
Lewisham HD	2,258	16	2,274	12	20	6	26	8
South West Thames RHA	**35,288**	**199**	**35,487**	**105**	**183**	**41**	**224**	**164**
Surrey AHA	11,662	65	11,727	36	65	17	82	51
North Surrey HD	1,667	3	1,670	7	11	1	12	8
North West Surrey HD	2,617	13	2,630	10	22	5	27	11
West Surrey and North East Hampshire HD	3,856	20	3,876	8	17	8	25	16
South West Surrey HD	1,931	13	1,944	4	6	3	9	4
Mid Surrey HD	1,683	9	1,692	4	5	1	6	11
East Surrey HD	2,139	20	2,159	9	12	4	16	11
West Sussex AHA	7,793	49	7,842	28	44	3	47	35
Chichester HD	1,687	14	1,701	2	6	0	6	6
Cuckfield and Crawley HD	3,750	14	3,764	13	22	1	23	21
Worthing HD	2,356	21	2,377	13	16	2	18	8
Croydon AHA	4,413	23	4,436	12	18	4	22	28
Kingston and Richmond AHA	3,562	13	3,575	7	14	5	19	14
Merton, Sutton and Wandsworth AHA	7,858	49	7,907	22	42	12	54	36
Roehampton HD	1,059	4	1,063	5	7	2	9	3

Table A3.21 Livebirths, stillbirths and infant deaths (numbers) by area of residence, 1980 - *continued*

Area of residence	Live births	Still-births	Total births	Deaths under 24 hrs	Neonatal deaths			Post-neonatal deaths
					Early	Late	Total	
South West Thames RHA - continued								
Wandsworth and East Merton HD	3,673	26	3,699	11	20	4	24	19
Sutton and West Merton HD	3,522	20	3,542	6	16	7	23	14
Wessex RHA	**34,194**	**214**	**34,408**	**96**	**188**	**52**	**240**	**170**
Dorset AHA	6,365	41	6,406	14	28	10	38	28
East Dorset HD	4,282	26	4,308	10	20	8	28	19
West Dorset HD	2,083	15	2,098	4	8	2	10	9
Hampshire AHA	19,855	121	19,976	56	110	27	137	98
Portsmouth and South East Hampshire HD	6,710	40	6,750	12	27	10	37	32
Southampton and South West Hampshire HD	5,233	25	5,258	16	27	4	31	27
Winchester and Central Hampshire HD	2,656	19	2,675	11	21	2	23	10
Basingstoke and North Hampshire HD	2,885	22	2,907	10	23	6	29	18
Wiltshire AHA	6.743	41	6,784	22	42	10	52	39
Salisbury HD	1.485	8	1,493	6	12	3	15	11
Swindon HD	2,978	20	2,998	10	16	4	20	19
Bath HD	4,604	31	4,635	14	26	5	31	22
Isle of Wight AHA	1,231	11	1,242	4	8	5	13	5
Oxford RHA	**33,016**	**209**	**33,225**	**119**	**208**	**38**	**246**	**130**
Berkshire AHA	9,859	57	9,916	38	65	9	74	49
East Berkshire HD	5,089	34	5,123	20	40	2	42	24
West Berkshire HD	5,493	28	5,521	22	34	7	41	29
Buckinghamshire AHA	8,311	65	8,376	28	52	10	62	30
Aylesbury HD	4,383	31	4,414	14	25	7	32	21
High Wycombe HD	3,518	31	3,549	12	23	3	26	7
Northamptonshire AHA	7,627	57	7,684	32	50	10	60	22
Kettering HD	3,630	28	3,658	18	29	5	34	14
Northampton HD	3,997	29	4,026	14	21	5	26	8
Oxfordshire AHA	7,219	30	7,249	21	41	9	50	29
Oxford HD	6,906	28	6,934	19	36	9	45	27
South Western RHA	**39,159**	**264**	**39,423**	**128**	**231**	**58**	**289**	**162**
Avon AHA	11,581	79	11,660	52	81	20	101	55
Bristol and Weston HD	4,633	31	4,664	22	33	8	41	24
Frenchay HD	2,739	16	2,755	15	24	5	29	11
Southmead HD	2,790	23	2,813	10	17	5	22	15

Table A3.24 Livebirths, stillbirths and infant deaths (numbers) by area of residence, 1980 - *continued*

Area of residence	Live births	Still-births	Total births	Deaths under 24 hrs	Neonatal deaths			Post-neonatal deaths
					Early	Late	Total	
South Western RHA - continued								
Cornwall (and Scilly) AHA	5,188	31	5,219	23	34	6	40	13
Devon AHA	10,959	73	11,032	26	56	16	72	46
Exeter HD	3,184	29	3,213	5	11	5	16	17
North Devon HD	1,424	17	1,441	3	8	2	10	7
Plymouth HD	4,228	18	4,246	8	21	5	26	13
Torbay HD	2,123	9	2,132	10	16	4	20	9
Gloucestershire AHA	6,336	42	6,378	20	36	8	44	24
Somerset AHA	5,095	39	5,134	7	24	8	32	24
Somerset HD	4,423	33	4,456	6	22	8	30	18
West Midlands RHA	**71,186**	**592**	**71,778**	**277**	**493**	**124**	**617**	**317**
Hereford and Worcester AHA	8,403	77	8,480	20	43	10	53	41
Hereford HD	1,850	15	1,865	6	11	1	12	13
Bromsgrove and Redditch HD	2,391	23	2,414	3	12	1	13	8
Kidderminster HD	1,290	12	1,302	2	7	2	9	6
Worcester HD	2,872	27	2,899	9	13	6	19	14
Salop AHA	4,758	33	4,791	23	31	6	37	18
Staffordshire AHA	14,150	111	14,261	59	100	22	122	53
Mid Staffordshire HD	4,066	28	4,094	16	29	5	34	11
North Staffordshire HD	6,235	57	6,292	20	40	12	52	31
South East Staffordshire HD	3,849	26	3,875	23	31	5	36	11
Warwickshire AHA	5,999	37	6,036	33	52	13	65	25
North Warwickshire HD	2,349	14	2,363	12	23	4	27	9
Rugby HD	1,074	9	1,083	5	8	3	11	1
South Warwickshire HD	2,576	14	2,590	16	21	6	27	15
Birmingham AHA	15,380	135	15,515	65	100	32	132	79
Central HD	3,994	30	4,024	17	29	6	35	29
East HD	2,249	30	2,279	13	18	2	20	8
North HD	2,029	17	2,046	6	12	5	17	6
South HD	3,507	34	3,541	15	24	8	32	19
West HD	3,601	24	3,625	14	17	11	28	17
Coventry AHA	4,503	34	4,537	19	38	6	44	11
Dudley AHA	4,028	29	4,057	10	23	2	25	18
Sandwell AHA	4,257	42	4,299	18	38	9	47	21
Solihull AHA	2,376	14	2,390	4	11	2	13	10
Walsall AHA	3,612	38	3,650	15	32	11	43	13

Table A3.24 Livebirths, stillbirths and infant deaths (numbers) by area of residence, 1980 - *continued*

Area of residence	Live births	Still-births	Total births	Deaths under 24 hrs	Neonatal deaths			Post-neonatal deaths
					Early	Late	Total	
West Midlands RHA *- continued*								
Wolverhampton AHA	3,720	42	3,762	11	25	11	36	28
Mersey RHA	**32,265**	**238**	**32,503**	**109**	**208**	**46**	**254**	**158**
Cheshire AHA	11,965	90	12,055	34	73	17	90	51
Chester HD	2,282	19	2,301	5	11	3	14	10
Crewe HD	3,131	15	3,146	13	26	1	27	16
Halton HD	2,111	15	2,126	7	13	9	22	8
Macclesfield HD	2,020	15	2,035	4	10	-	10	12
Warrington HD	2,214	21	2,235	5	9	4	13	4
Liverpool AHA	6,825	56	6,881	24	46	11	57	42
St Helens and Knowsley AHA	5,355	39	5,394	18	33	10	43	26
Sefton AHA	3,599	26	3,625	13	23	4	27	14
Northern HD	1,202	9	1,211	2	5	1	6	2
Southern HD	2,397	17	2,414	11	18	3	21	12
Wirral AHA	4,521	27	4,548	20	33	4	37	25
Wirral HD	4,728	32	4,760	20	37	4	41	26
North Western RHA	**54,392**	**448**	**54,840**	**226**	**393**	**69**	**462**	**241**
Lancashire AHA	18,174	152	18,326	70	127	16	143	75
Lancaster HD	1,388	11	1,399	2	6	-	6	8
Blackpool HD	3,152	29	3,181	13	21	2	23	10
Preston HD	4,477	39	4,516	10	28	3	31	13
Blackburn HD	4,088	37	4,125	22	31	5	36	22
Burnley HD	3,646	33	3,679	15	28	6	34	17
Ormskirk HD	1,423	3	1,426	8	13	-	13	5
Bolton AHA	3,764	29	3,793	15	25	8	33	13
Bury AHA	2,353	20	2,373	11	25	3	28	10
Manchester AHA	6,388	47	6,435	31	55	11	66	41
North HD	2,163	15	2,178	6	13	2	15	8
Central HD	1,969	17	1,986	12	19	5	24	21
South HD	2,256	15	2,271	13	23	4	27	12
Oldham AHA	3,299	34	3,333	15	23	5	28	14
Rochdale AHA	3,285	36	3,321	13	25	5	30	19
Salford AHA	3,195	23	3,218	9	21	5	26	19
Stockport AHA	3,725	32	3,757	18	29	5	34	15

Table A3.24 Livebirths, stillbirths and infant deaths (numbers) by area of residence, 1980 - *continued*

Area of residence	Live births	Still-births	Total births	Deaths under 24 hrs	Neonatal deaths			Post-neonatal deaths
					Early	Late	Total	
North Western RHA - continued								
Tameside AHA	2,977	23	3,000	13	20	5	25	16
Tameside HD	3,408	23	3,431	13	21	5	26	17
Trafford AHA	2,856	22	2,878	12	18	3	21	12
Wigan AHA	4,376	30	4,406	19	25	3	28	7
WALES	**37,357**	**245**	**37,602**	**132**	**238**	**58**	**296**	**130**
Clwyd AHA	4,963	42	5,005	18	33	5	38	20
Clwyd North HD	1,846	14	1,860	10	13	3	16	8
Clwyd South HD	3,117	28	3,145	8	20	2	22	12
Dyfed AHA	4,013	22	4,035	20	26	3	29	10
Ceredigion HD	628	4	632	2	2	-	2	-
Carmarthen/Dinefwr HD	814	8	822	3	5	-	5	1
Preseli/South Pembrokeshire HD	1,419	2	1,421	11	13	1	14	7
Llanelli/Dinefwr HD	1,152	8	1,160	4	6	2	8	2
Gwent AHA	5,915	27	5,942	22	40	9	49	17
North Gwent HD	1,416	5	1,421	8	11	-	11	3
South Gwent HD	4,499	22	4,521	14	29	9	38	14
Gwynedd AHA	2,839	20	2,859	13	18	3	21	5
Mid Glamorgan AHA	7,964	58	8,022	29	49	17	66	26
Ogwr HD	1,801	12	1,813	4	9	3	12	3
Rhymney Valley HD	1,755	10	1,765	5	7	3	10	5
East Glamorgan HD	2,567	22	2,589	9	16	7	23	7
Merthyr and Cynon Valley HD	1,841	14	1,855	11	17	4	21	11
Powys AHA	1,335	10	1,345	1	3	1	4	5
South Glamorgan AHA	5,376	28	5,404	15	38	10	48	26
West Glamorgan AHA	4,952	38	4,990	14	31	10	41	21
Neath HD	1,639	10	1,649	6	13	2	15	6
Swansea HD	3,313	28	3,341	8	18	8	26	15
SCOTLAND	**68,892**	**463**	**69,355**	**267**	**446**	**89**	**535**	**296**
Highland Region & HBA	**2,886**	**20**	**2,906**	**9**	**14**	**5**	**19**	**18**
Health districts								
Northern	573	1	574	2	2	2	4	4
Southern	2,313	19	2,332	7	12	3	15	14
Orkney Islands Area & HBA	**260**	**2**	**262**	**-**	**-**	**1**	**1**	**-**

Area of residence	Live births	Still-births	Total births	Deaths under 24 hrs	Neonatal deaths			Post-neonatal deaths
					Early	Late	Total	
Scotland - continued								
Shetland Islands Area & HBA	376	3	379	3	3	1	4	1
Western Isles Islands Area & HBA	374	3	377	-	-	-	-	1
Grampian Region & HBA	6,491	37	6,528	7	16	11	27	29
Health districts								
West Grampian	1,174	6	1,180	2	4	2	6	4
North Grampian	2,299	16	2,315	2	5	4	9	11
South Grampian	3,018	15	3,033	3	7	5	12	14
Tayside Region & HBA	4,847	45	4,892	12	20	2	22	19
Health districts								
Angus	1,186	13	1,199	4	9	1	10	3
Dundee	2,300	26	2,326	4	4	1	5	10
Perth and Kinross	1,361	6	1,367	4	7	-	7	6
Fife Region & HBA	4,616	29	4,645	14	31	9	40	13
Health districts								
East Fife	2,802	14	2,816	7	14	7	21	8
West Fife	1,814	15	1,829	7	17	2	19	5
Lothian Region & HBA	9,347	48	9,395	35	62	16	78	43
Health districts								
West Lothian	2,141	14	2,155	7	17	5	22	12
South Lothian	3,950	24	3,974	12	23	4	27	20
North Lothian	3,256	10	3,266	16	22	7	29	11
Borders region & HBA	1,127	9	1,136	8	11	1	12	2
Central region [Forth Valley HBA]	3,648	22	3,670	16	23	2	25	16
Health districts								
Stirling	1,648	9	1,657	5	6	1	7	8
Falkirk	2,000	13	2,013	11	17	1	18	8
Strathclyde region	33,136	237	33,373	148	247	40	287	142
Argyll and Clyde HBA	6,313	38	6,351	33	47	9	56	21
Health districts								
Argyll and Bute	889	1	890	8	11	2	13	2
Dumbarton	1,194	8	1,202	6	7	1	8	7
Renfrew	2,804	17	2,821	10	15	4	19	10
Inverclyde	1,426	12	1,438	9	14	2	16	2

Table A3.24 Livebirths, stillbirths and infant deaths (numbers) by area of residence, 1980 - *continued*

Area of residence	Live births	Still-births	Total births	Deaths under 24 hrs	Neonatal deaths			Post-neonatal deaths
					Early	Late	Total	
Scotland - continued								
Greater Glasgow HBA	**13,350**	**88**	**13,438**	**52**	**97**	**18**	**115**	**61**
Health districts								
Western	2,878	14	2,892	10	20	8	28	12
Northern	2,552	13	2,565	11	20	2	22	6
Eastern	2,603	16	2,619	19	28	3	31	19
South Eastern	3,180	17	3,197	7	18	4	22	14
South Western	2,137	28	2,165	5	11	1	12	10
Lanarkshire HBA	**8,385**	**58**	**8,443**	**38**	**60**	**10**	**70**	**29**
Health districts								
Monklands/Cumbernauld	2,764	22	2,786	16	17	1	18	7
Motherwell/Lanark	2,890	14	2,904	17	26	6	32	11
Hamilton/East Kilbride	2,731	22	2,753	5	17	3	20	11
Ayrshire and Arran HBA	**5,088**	**53**	**5,141**	**25**	**43**	**3**	**46**	**31**
Health districts								
North Ayrshire and Arran	3,124	30	3,154	17	30	1	31	25
South Ayrshire	1,964	23	1,987	8	13	2	15	6
Dumfries and Galloway Region & HBA	**1,784**	**8**	**1,792**	**15**	**19**	**1**	**20**	**12**
NORTHERN IRELAND	**28,582**	**266**	**28,848**	**119**	**184**	**45**	**229**	**153**
District Council areas								
Ards	1,075	9	1,084	9	11	1	12	7
Belfast	5,322	55	5,377	8	21	10	31	26
Castlereagn	435	8	443	-	1	1	2	5
Down	1,055	10	1,065	7	9	-	9	7
Lisburn	1,524	14	1,538	7	10	3	13	9
North Down	1,098	6	1,104	7	8	2	10	5
Antrim	995	7	1,002	-	4	3	7	6
Ballymead	1,077	7	1,084	4	10	2	12	9
Ballymoney	508	4	512	3	4	1	5	3
Carrickfergus	431	5	436	2	3	1	4	2
Coleraine	760	5	765	2	2	-	2	4
Cookstown	453	2	455	1	3	-	3	2
Larne	403	3	406	-	-	2	2	2
Magherafelt	736	6	742	5	5	-	5	4
Moyie	192	2	194	2	4	1	5	1
Newtownabbey	1,330	12	1,342	6	7	1	8	6
Armagh	863	5	868	4	6	2	8	-
Banbridge	466	7	473	3	7	-	7	4
Craigavon	1471	7	1,478	4	6	2	8	4

Table A3.24 Livebirths, stillbirths and infant deaths (numbers) by area of residence, 1980 - *continued*

| Area of residence | Live births | Still-births | Total births | Deaths under 24 hrs | Neonatal deaths | | | Post-neonatal deaths |
					Early	Late	Total	
Northern Ireland - continued								
Dungannon	988	5	993	7	10	-	10	3
Newry and Mourne	1,756	18	1,774	9	10	2	12	6
Fermanagh	1,094	20	1,114	8	9	1	10	4
Limavady	486	7	493	2	9	3	12	4
Londonderry	2,376	26	2,402	12	15	4	19	20
Omagh	1,025	8	1,033	5	6	2	8	6
Strabane	663	8	671	2	4	1	5	4
GUERNSEY	**622**	**5**	**627**		**4**	**1**	**5**	**3**
JERSEY	**867**	**6**	**873**		**7**	**-**	**7**	**2**

Source: As Table A3.23

Table A3.25 Fertility rates by area of residence, England and Wales, 1980

| Area of residence | Total births per 1,000 women in each age-group | | | | | | |
	15-19	20-24	25-29	30-34	35-39	40-44	15-44
ENGLAND AND WALES	**31.16**	**114.87**	**136.58**	**71.73**	**22.82**	**4.87**	**65.43**
ENGLAND	**30.84**	**114.28**	**136.72**	**71.92**	**22.85**	**4.92**	**65.33**
Northern RHA	**37.24**	**126.54**	**134.40**	**62.37**	**17.09**	**3.87**	**65.60**
Cleveland AHA	45.70	139.33	140.64	62.11	17.54	3.77	71.90
Hartlepool HD	46.98	136.39	120.61	50.00	16.30	4.44	65.77
North Tees HD	43.52	135.42	140.77	67.01	15.85	3.00	72.34
South Tees HD	46.42	142.54	146.92	62.97	18.90	4.00	73.54
Cumbria AHA	29.67	112.98	136.71	66.11	17.46	4.09	62.38
East Cumbria HD	25.96	105.77	136.81	67.14	17.27	4.38	60.64
South West Cumbria HD	34.21	109.71	131.88	64.32	18.44	3.45	61.23
West Cumbria HD	32.55	127.08	140.00	65.65	17.00	4.10	66.12
Durham AHA	35.06	122.12	127.20	62.78	18.56	4.69	63.44
Darlington HD	30.43	111.59	122.25	78.50	19.19	5.43	62.84
Durham HD	33.50	120.78	131.39	59.24	18.44	5.57	62.72
North West Durham HD	33.61	139.33	141.54	57.10	19.63	2.59	64.63
South West Durham HD	41.94	123.28	118.00	60.67	17.61	3.95	64.38
Northumberland AHA	31.80	122.65	138.69	65.70	15.64	3.25	65.21
Gateshead AHA	36.78	136.90	129.55	58.55	14.69	3.93	63.92
Northern Tyneside AHA	33.06	134.58	160.00	66.72	15.52	2.63	66.70
Southern Tyneside AHA	39.53	143.77	136.88	57.45	17.66	2.71	66.16

Table A3.25 Fertility rates by area of residence, England and Wales, 1980 - *continued*

Area of residence	Total births per 1,000 women in each age-group						
	15-19	20-24	25-29	30-34	35-39	40-44	15-44
Northern RHA - continued							
Sunderland AHA	40.38	129.25	123.86	56.90	16.70	4.59	62.11
Newcastle upon Tyne AHA	38.15	109.81	128.40	60.89	16.95	3.33	62.16
Yorkshire RHA	**35.34**	**127.39**	**133.55**	**64.82**	**20.30**	**5.88**	**66.48**
Humberside AHA	34.02	121.49	126.87	59.74	17.28	4.43	63.16
Hull HD	42.16	135.00	134.22	59.58	17.76	3.47	68.95
Beverley HD	20.21	83.76	102.76	61.28	15.83	4.62	50.45
Grimsby HD	40.42	140.17	128.55	51.86	14.38	3.56	65.86
Scunthorpe HD	32.75	131.74	148.55	64.71	20.86	6.18	68.53
North Yorkshire AHA	22.23	100.09	126.63	73.59	21.60	3.99	59.92
Northallerton HD	24.39	107.89	134.86	71.32	23.79	3.45	63.43
York HD	21.35	92.42	122.02	71.21	20.80	4.64	57.45
Scarborough HD	25.00	114.50	130.24	79.56	23.08	3.89	63.52
Harrogate HD	19.35	95.95	125.48	74.35	20.00	3.24	58.39
Bradford AHA	45.07	165.43	150.98	69.78	24.69	12.86	80.73
Bradford HD	52.36	186.89	156.35	68.56	26.04	15.91	87.35
Airedale HD	29.38	119.82	140.34	72.30	22.04	6.81	67.17
Calderdale AHA	43.61	145.25	130.85	69.52	23.58	8.00	71.93
Kirklees AHA	38.13	139.62	147.50	65.59	20.96	7.57	71.42
Huddersfield HD	35.06	133.56	141.01	69.07	22.81	6.23	69.20
Dewsbury HD	41.94	147.24	155.64	61.31	18.60	9.35	74.21
Leeds AHA	35.03	120.92	129.40	62.90	20.75	4.12	62.88
Western (Leeds) HD	31.20	124.92	127.14	61.57	20.37	3.80	62.42
Eastern (Leeds) HD	38.87	116.92	131.77	64.32	21.13	4.42	63.36
Wakefield AHA	39.84	126.00	131.10	55.00	15.80	3.15	64.59
Western (Wakefield) HD	34.73	120.74	144.49	68.55	16.30	3.25	67.42
Eastern (Pontefract) HD	43.80	130.30	120.17	43.54	15.37	3.06	62.27
Trent RHA	**33.56**	**119.66**	**134.29**	**64.50**	**20.23**	**4.03**	**64.62**
Derbyshire AHA	32.43	116.86	134.28	65.94	21.54	3.97	64.19
Central Derbyshire HD	28.26	110.79	129.60	67.47	20.27	2.32	60.17
North Derbyshire HD	31.38	116.39	134.91	65.37	23.21	2.98	63.46
South Derbyshire HD	36.81	121.53	137.07	65.38	20.48	6.71	68.25
Leicestershire AHA	31.96	119.38	146.16	69.85	22.98	4.19	68.79
East Leicestershire HD	38.29	144.15	146.09	69.30	26.36	4.72	74.65
North West Leicestershire HD	31.38	122.48	159.78	74.60	24.50	5.14	72.35
South West Leicestershire HD	27.27	97.98	135.78	66.56	19.21	3.00	61.31

Table A3.25 Fertility rates by area of residence, England and Wales, 1980 - *continued*

Area of residence	Total births per 1,000 women in each age-group						
	15-19	20-24	25-29	30-34	35-39	40-44	15-44
Trent RHA - continued							
Lincolnshire AHA	27.83	106.37	132.46	65.17	20.74	3.93	61.95
Lincolnshire South HD	27.59	106.76	128.84	64.90	19.16	4.67	61.60
Lincolnshire North HD	28.08	105.96	136.36	65.45	22.41	3.20	62.32
Nottinghamshire AHA	37.18	123.95	131.89	65.85	19.77	3.67	65.14
Mansfield and Newark HD	40.29	134.33	129.47	61.54	21.74	4.20	67.70
Worksop & Retford HD	32.50	130.59	130.97	60.59	19.68	3.45	63.17
North Nottingham HD	43.13	133.33	129.64	65.16	17.63	1.71	67.23
South Nottingham HD	32.67	107.70	135.74	71.36	19.72	4.66	62.29
Barnsley AHA	36.67	147.40	132.43	55.31	17.35	4.10	65.58
Doncaster AHA	39.27	139.53	130.10	54.44	15.40	2.93	66.23
Rotherham AHA	43.37	141.12	148.50	67.69	17.09	4.66	71.65
Sheffield AHA	28.13	100.15	116.99	57.82	19.37	4.93	55.78
Northern HD	32.76	121.54	128.68	56.71	18.13	6.07	61.30
Southern HD	24.82	86.36	109.43	58.55	20.21	4.14	52.07
East Anglian RHA	**26.04**	**113.16**	**138.24**	**69.96**	**21.48**	**3.99**	**64.74**
Cambridgeshire AHA	26.00	109.59	139.71	70.90	21.70	4.49	65.40
Cambridge HD	21.06	96.78	137.20	71.96	21.83	4.46	62.22
Peterborough HD	34.29	133.68	144.31	68.77	21.48	4.55	71.28
Norfolk AHA	26.24	109.11	133.65	64.74	21.28	3.88	61.95
Norwich HD	20.70	98.63	134.19	68.04	22.34	3.61	60.20
Great Yarmouth and Waveney HD	35.76	128.98	132.67	58.36	19.82	4.91	64.17
King's Lynn HD	31.23	117.38	133.28	63.02	20.20	3.40	64.13
Suffolk AHA	25.79	123.42	143.45	76.97	21.54	3.62	68.24
Bury St Edmunds HD	29.25	123.75	139.61	71.81	21.32	3.87	68.09
Ipswich HD	23.42	123.18	146.40	81.05	21.70	3.45	68.34
North West Thames RHA	**23.64**	**96.93**	**140.70**	**82.40**	**28.31**	**5.30**	**64.10**
Bedfordshire AHA	30.14	123.28	174.37	84.59	25.71	6.05	75.99
Northern HD	26.46	120.68	172.15	82.89	24.13	4.86	73.03
Southern HD	33.30	125.26	176.21	86.21	27.05	7.07	78.49
Hertfordshire AHA	19.21	92.26	142.30	83.46	24.27	4.05	62.09
North Hertfordshire HD	25.75	112.08	145.08	72.68	20.17	2.00	64.73
East Hertfordshire HD	17.41	86.27	137.80	80.47	23.67	4.11	59.27
North West Hertfordshire HD	18.75	88.22	135.22	92.33	29.49	5.14	64.38
South West Hertfordshire HD	15.58	85.08	157.93	85.86	22.33	4.56	60.60

Table A3.25 Fertility rates by area of residence, England and Wales, 1980 - *continued*

Area of residence	Total births per 1,000 women in each age-group						
	15-19	20-24	25-29	30-34	35-39	40-44	15-44
North West Thames RHA - continued							
Barnet AHA	17.22	88.50	135.15	90.87	30.16	4.62	62.02
Barnet and Finchley HD	14.34	77.36	129.15	90.37	30.71	4.09	58.72
Edgware and Hendon HD	20.44	101.64	142.37	91.49	29.47	5.28	65.97
Brent and Harrow AHA	28.27	99.58	159.85	94.67	33.97	7.02	70.94
Brent HD	41.16	118.05	150.74	93.20	29.70	6.89	74.48
Harrow HD	13.68	78.03	169.68	96.13	38.67	7.17	67.10
Ealing, Hammersmith and Hounslow AHA	29.73	106.02	140.40	88.27	34.26	5.84	69.48
Hounslow HD	23.20	117.12	175.33	96.53	33.06	6.67	74.41
South Hammersmith HD	30.00	66.79	103.02	75.85	35.31	5.00	55.67
North Hammersmith HD	34.68	94.55	110.00	76.67	34.19	6.79	62.18
Ealing HD	32.72	128.89	153.29	96.71	34.63	5.16	78.52
Hillingdon AHA	25.82	99.19	156.13	76.55	25.71	4.33	66.37
Kensington, Chelsea and Westminster AHA	16.80	63.07	82.22	57.84	25.56	7.33	42.74
North West HD	24.57	88.82	108.98	73.00	30.00	8.15	54.85
North East HD	9.64	44.81	76.96	53.44	18.62	6.40	34.51
South HD	9.86	44.56	63.03	48.35	24.72	6.96	34.79
North East Thames RHA	**29.02**	**117.32**	**142.29**	**77.76**	**25.12**	**3.69**	**67.63**
Essex AHA	21.42	101.96	144.61	77.76	22.07	3.69	64.63
Basildon and Thurrock HD	28.24	125.41	151.70	64.73	17.80	3.82	69.14
Chelmsford HD	13.61	86.12	155.79	90.37	24.73	3.85	64.33
Colchester HD	24.04	98.70	130.00	77.05	20.13	2.97	62.57
Harlow HD	21.60	99.25	129.34	72.97	23.83	3.51	61.03
Southend HD	20.88	102.34	151.17	80.55	23.13	4.16	65.43
Barking and Havering AHA	29.30	125.20	142.13	66.88	16.94	4.52	64.79
Barking HD	42.96	163.33	149.13	59.39	15.35	4.88	73.99
Havering HD	21.01	102.03	138.15	70.74	17.82	4.32	59.58
Camden and Islington AHA	27.73	87.77	92.81	68.57	27.44	7.57	54.34
North Camden HD	19.58	73.17	83.20	67.14	23.96	7.37	47.78
South Camden HD	23.75	71.33	75.63	52.63	24.14	7.60	44.14
Islington HD	35.14	103.82	108.91	78.96	32.50	7.71	64.61
City and East London AHA	57.47	184.85	150.16	72.66	30.94	11.97	87.84
City and Hackney HD	54.25	173.48	162.24	89.22	37.50	8.49	88.13
Newham HD	49.89	187.00	156.58	71.33	25.78	8.33	86.93
Tower Hamlets HD	75.09	195.96	126.40	54.42	30.00	22.31	88.89
Enfield and Haringey AHA	23.49	107.04	145.43	82.02	30.00	5.14	64.18
Enfield HD	19.25	106.90	161.56	86.48	24.94	3.70	64.41
Haringey HD	27.86	107.18	128.65	77.61	35.58	6.87	63.94

Area of residence	Total births per 1,000 women in each age-group						
	15-19	20-24	25-29	30-34	35-39	40-44	15-44
North East Thames RHA - continued							
Redbridge and Waltham Forest AHA	23.06	116.99	174.00	88.97	27.71	7.30	71.56
East Roding HD	14.52	96.57	188.50	97.22	24.86	6.94	68.36
West Roding HD	31.12	136.81	161.57	81.40	30.57	7.67	74.59
South East Thames RHA	**30.46**	**110.84**	**134.77**	**75.24**	**23.60**	**4.57**	**64.86**
East Sussex AHA	20.13	93.75	120.29	67.47	23.60	4.38	56.63
Brighton HD	20.17	97.98	120.74	64.30	21.00	4.76	55.04
Eastbourne HD	14.63	79.10	120.48	70.43	25.47	4.04	54.69
Hastings HD	27.87	106.17	119.13	70.20	27.43	4.00	63.01
Kent AHA	29.00	110.00	141.26	77.57	21.49	4.18	66.41
South East Kent HD	33.41	123.88	136.05	72.67	20.14	5.59	66.73
Canterbury and Thanet HD	32.08	107.16	128.05	69.80	23.51	3.19	63.09
Dartford and Gravesham HD	24.59	106.83	144.56	78.54	20.00	3.62	64.91
Maidstone HD	23.29	85.06	140.43	83.29	22.83	4.83	62.18
Medway HD	34.57	141.27	163.10	76.72	17.94	4.22	76.63
Tunbridge Wells HD	20.67	74.38	124.48	89.01	27.32	3.64	58.87
Greenwich and Bexley AHA	31.69	119.67	155.52	72.53	21.04	3.84	67.92
Bexley HD	17.86	91.25	149.07	73.90	21.13	3.28	60.48
Greenwich HD	45.85	151.25	163.73	71.13	20.94	4.48	76.14
Bromley AHA	17.67	77.09	125.81	86.90	28.91	3.26	57.43
Lambeth, Southwark and Lewisham AHA	44.42	132.40	125.22	73.79	27.21	6.47	69.61
St Thomas' HD	43.07	124.75	119.33	67.92	26.67	6.00	64.80
Kings' HD	47.13	146.20	134.14	77.50	30.47	6.07	75.63
Guy's HD	54.43	166.47	122.56	63.62	25.90	6.41	76.18
Lewisham HD	34.62	97.16	122.36	83.93	24.81	7.50	62.30
South West Thames RHA	**20.33**	**87.78**	**136.86**	**88.96**	**27.96**	**4.44**	**62.29**
Surrey AHA	17.95	80.96	135.05	88.57	28.16	4.32	60.25
North Surrey HD	21.48	85.40	143.02	77.69	20.68	3.95	58.39
North West Surrey HD	18.78	89.42	141.21	92.99	31.61	4.69	63.83
West Surrey and North East Hampshire HD	22.17	94.49	146.80	94.26	25.73	3.13	66.83
South West Surrey HD	17.94	67.58	110.33	83.08	32.20	6.04	54.92
Mid Surrey HD	9.83	58.60	127.08	89.68	29.42	4.20	52.55
East Surrey HD	14.78	75.61	135.08	87.71	29.30	4.53	59.15
West Sussex AHA	17.92	93.55	136.98	85.71	25.96	4.65	63.40
Chichester HD	17.89	87.41	102.63	76.48	24.89	3.95	54.87
Cuckfield and Crawley HD	16.95	101.96	165.23	100.64	27.27	4.93	71.83
Worthing HD	19.19	86.52	130.14	73.82	25.08	4.81	58.98
Croydon AHA	28.32	102.11	143.64	83.90	29.42	4.39	66.11

Table A3.25 Fertility rates by area of residence, England and Wales, 1980 - *continued*

Area of residence	Total births per 1,000 women in each age-group						
	15-19	20-24	25-29	30-34	35-39	40-44	15-44
South West Thames RHA - continued							
Kingston and Richmond AHA	12.05	64.50	131.52	94.48	35.06	4.21	57.86
Merton, Sutton and Wandsworth AHA	25.80	95.54	138.57	93.11	26.01	4.59	64.62
Roehampton HD	14.32	49.25	82.89	79.13	29.21	3.82	44.29
Wandsworth and East Merton HD	41.41	131.56	172.65	101.51	29.10	4.70	79.21
Sutton and West Merton HD	16.67	85.94	136.49	92.36	22.07	4.82	61.28
Wessex RHA	**26.48**	**109.95**	**132.87**	**70.72**	**21.05**	**3.12**	**62.84**
Dorset AHA	21.53	94.20	121.41	75.28	23.66	4.84	58.50
East Dorset HD	21.96	90.48	125.87	77.74	22.09	4.73	57.67
West Dorset HD	20.61	101.59	112.97	70.16	27.61	5.11	60.29
Hampshire AHA	29.13	117.08	139.27	70.99	20.78	3.44	65.66
Portsmouth and South East Hampshire HD	32.43	123.82	140.19	63.91	21.08	3.38	66.18
Southampton and South West Hampshire HD	26.65	122.86	138.27	69.73	18.15	2.59	64.75
Winchester and Central Hampshire HD	26.28	104.86	145.37	83.52	20.79	3.09	65.89
Basingstoke and North Hampshire HD	28.41	102.47	133.68	78.40	25.16	5.61	65.92
Wiltshire AHA	25.22	108.51	129.71	67.06	19.54	3.61	61.08
Salisbury HD	27.08	103.26	110.45	70.45	22.06	4.86	59.48
Swindon HD	31.58	114.84	129.88	57.90	18.03	4.13	62.98
Bath HD	20.60	105.95	136.61	71.18	19.66	2.88	60.43
Isle of Wight AHA	27.37	108.00	135.76	69.43	21.72	2.00	62.10
Oxford RHA	**25.61**	**105.97**	**145.94**	**81.27**	**24.76**	**4.77**	**67.30**
Berkshire AHA	24.21	101.42	141.98	87.08	25.15	4.21	65.70
East Berkshire HD	28.17	120.58	145.49	91.30	27.20	4.33	71.65
West Berkshire HD	21.33	87.14	139.04	83.63	23.51	4.11	61.01
Buckinghamshire AHA	25.54	110.41	154.25	95.05	28.42	5.84	72.52
Aylesbury HD	34.32	128.85	153.14	88.42	26.30	4.93	79.53
High Wycombe HD	17.76	89.78	155.68	102.26	30.48	6.59	65.36
Northamptonshire AHA	30.73	114.39	145.23	69.19	21.41	4.33	67.94
Kettering HD	34.44	123.65	146.74	64.75	21.60	3.28	70.08
Northampton HD	27.47	106.24	143.94	73.15	21.25	5.19	66.11
Oxfordshire AHA	22.39	99.51	143.94	72.27	23.78	4.93	63.73

Table A3.25 Fertility rates by area of residence, England and Wales, 1980 - *continued*

Area of residence	Total births per 1,000 women in each age-group						
	15-19	20-24	25-29	30-34	35-39	40-44	15-44
South Western RHA	**25.30**	**108.43**	**132.76**	**68.05**	**21.15**	**4.04**	**61.81**
Avon AHA	23.58	105.82	134.82	68.13	19.31	3.50	61.05
Bristol and Weston HD	28.87	111.39	126.72	62.66	18.57	4.12	60.97
Frenchay HD	16.86	117.73	148.19	66.79	18.24	2.38	62.33
Southmead HD	21.35	86.78	135.45	78.66	21.67	3.61	59.98
Cornwall (and Scilly) AHA	27.47	102.47	131.82	71.38	23.44	4.81	63.41
Devon AHA	26.11	118.16	124.41	64.69	20.97	3.52	61.39
Exeter HD	23.06	106.09	131.38	70.00	22.25	3.03	59.83
North Devon HD	22.50	116.51	115.25	61.28	20.30	5.16	59.55
Plymouth HD	31.76	133.62	125.36	63.04	17.92	2.71	65.63
Torbay HD	23.24	107.80	118.87	62.75	24.66	4.55	57.47
Gloucestershire AHA	26.67	101.64	135.87	71.47	21.90	4.41	62.29
Somerset AHA	22.98	107.79	146.67	67.48	22.09	5.26	62.15
West Midlands RHA	**36.30**	**123.09**	**139.46**	**68.88**	**23.51**	**6.11**	**67.75**
Hereford and Worcester AHA	27.36	106.75	135.76	72.82	24.90	3.99	64.58
Hereford HD	28.91	107.55	121.37	69.45	27.86	4.50	63.01
Bromsgrove and Redditch HD	30.00	111.54	148.50	77.83	25.40	3.49	70.79
Kidderminster HD	24.74	100.00	125.56	74.88	23.71	3.79	60.56
Worcester HD	25.58	105.13	140.13	70.46	23.33	4.09	62.89
Salop AHA	27.11	100.63	129.05	73.33	24.36	6.21	62.55
Staffordshire AHA	33.63	120.98	141.92	67.53	21.21	4.31	66.86
Mid Staffordshire HD	25.56	100.88	145.19	74.46	21.41	3.60	63.67
North Staffordshire HD	40.61	137.00	129.74	58.81	19.31	4.38	66.16
South East Staffordshire HD	30.59	118.21	159.77	74.84	24.49	5.07	71.89
Warwickshire AHA	27.04	95.05	131.52	70.45	23.51	4.23	60.79
North Warwickshire HD	35.00	109.29	128.10	62.66	20.36	5.20	63.18
Rugby HD	30.00	113.10	163.04	81.43	23.20	2.92	68.54
South Warwickshire HD	19.29	76.75	125.00	72.74	26.18	3.97	56.18
Birmingham AHA	47.80	144.61	144.28	71.02	25.30	11.08	76.02
Central HD	51.34	167.88	154.87	78.84	30.28	17.38	84.72
East HD	47.30	148.70	139.58	66.54	24.63	16.05	76.99
North HD	29.71	102.07	124.15	77.07	23.53	4.20	60.18
South HD	44.40	121.81	132.18	63.16	19.87	4.35	67.45
West HD	62.36	180.71	168.73	70.71	28.45	14.91	89.51
Coventry AHA	33.61	123.20	133.19	61.59	20.99	6.06	64.81
Dudley AHA	33.27	117.77	144.69	69.65	23.71	4.53	65.86
Sandwell AHA	47.19	170.67	147.73	61.08	24.09	6.48	74.51

Table A3.25 Fertility rates by area of residence, England and Wales, 1980 - *continued*

Area of residence	Total births per 1,000 women in each age-group						
	15-19	20-24	25-29	30-34	35-39	40-44	15-44
West Midlands RHA *- continued*							
Solihull AHA	28.37	83.10	117.01	75.19	23.64	3.61	55.58
Walsall AHA	39.12	128.11	144.88	62.75	21.95	6.58	67.34
Wolverhampton AHA	48.38	173.60	160.97	64.37	25.41	6.43	77.89
Mersey RHA	**32.78**	**115.94**	**129.00**	**68.14**	**22.10**	**4.55**	**68.94**
Cheshire AHA	28.70	107.55	124.69	68.23	22.36	3.81	61.01
Chester HD	26.99	115.00	125.97	66.34	18.50	4.91	59.77
Crewe HD	27.24	106.93	126.05	69.46	24.47	3.10	61.45
Halton HD	36.56	123.10	130.19	65.09	27.07	4.25	68.80
Macclesfield HD	20.00	70.00	118.23	81.21	25.45	3.33	54.12
Warrington HD	35.31	128.39	123.23	58.71	17.14	3.73	62.26
Liverpool AHA	37.25	127.55	134.15	65.90	21.54	5.56	66.94
St Helens and Knowsley AHA	42.42	151.09	132.32	62.44	19.55	4.40	69.87
Sefton AHA	27.72	96.64	120.67	67.61	21.70	5.84	58.37
Northern HD	17.25	80.00	117.44	72.62	21.43	7.27	54.06
Southern HD	33.38	104.72	122.62	64.65	21.86	5.00	60.81
Wirral AHA	28.80	102.27	137.46	77.18	25.14	4.27	64.59
North Western RHA	**38.04**	**122.45**	**137.30**	**68.98**	**22.17**	**5.66**	**67.69**
Lancashire AHA	35.73	134.70	137.97	70.06	21.39	5.45	68.79
Lancaster HD	30.93	116.32	136.36	71.75	24.38	2.73	63.88
Blackpool HD	28.39	110.33	112.78	60.10	18.75	4.46	55.81
Preston HD	34.88	132.18	149.04	71.29	21.51	4.77	70.78
Blackburn HD	45.28	155.96	145.86	72.45	22.44	7.30	77.39
Burnley HD	42.81	165.77	152.50	77.28	19.71	7.88	78.78
Ormskirk HD	23.83	105.37	122.05	70.70	26.00	3.44	60.17
Bolton AHA	43.75	131.38	146.21	65.10	22.37	5.22	72.11
Bury AHA	32.08	104.60	137.42	72.39	20.86	4.63	63.11
Manchester AHA	46.87	101.49	121.45	67.34	26.81	7.60	66.00
North HD	50.26	131.77	129.53	79.46	27.06	8.16	74.85
Central HD	58.75	127.14	134.87	73.24	31.29	7.65	76.98
South HD	35.76	69.32	107.62	57.79	23.92	7.14	53.31
Oldham AHA	45.67	136.10	142.88	62.50	26.29	8.31	71.83
Rochdale AHA	50.26	156.62	146.25	70.65	20.97	8.28	79.07
Salford AHA	45.00	132.65	119.61	59.77	21.92	5.65	65.01

Table A3.25 Fertility rates by area of residence, England and Wales, 1980 - *continued*

Area of residence	Total births per 1,000 women in each age-group						
	15-19	20-24	25-29	30-34	35-39	40-44	15-44
North Western RHA *- continued*							
Stockport AHA	24.71	91.43	142.35	78.65	21.58	3.49	61.19
Tameside AHA	36.04	130.94	145.19	63.19	19.47	5.59	68.08
Trafford AHA	28.28	88.41	129.13	76.10	21.27	4.46	60.08
Wigan AHA	32.66	126.15	147.33	68.58	21.80	4.22	67.99
Wales	**36.39**	**124.98**	**134.19**	**68.42**	**22.25**	**4.09**	**67.15**
Clwyd AHA	28.93	113.61	134.42	70.98	23.05	4.12	64.66
Rhyl (North) HD	27.19	96.21	111.61	62.17	21.00	5.81	56.19
Wrexham (South) HD	30.24	127.07	151.92	77.35	24.56	2.88	70.99
Dyfed AHA	33.17	114.63	124.53	67.33	24.42	4.53	63.54
Ceredigion HD	15.00	79.47	105.45	55.00	23.68	7.33	48.99
Carmarthen/Dinefwr HD	34.76	126.32	140.00	74.35	25.00	4.44	67.93
Preseli/South Pembrokeshire HD	36.67	112.50	131.18	85.14	24.83	4.29	69.32
Llanelli/Dinefwr HD	42.06	132.33	120.67	54.41	24.07	3.20	64.44
Gwent AHA	39.32	129.68	129.05	63.50	19.62	4.96	66.24
North (Abergavenny) HD	40.00	115.81	104.36	61.19	18.24	5.48	60.73
South (Newport) HD	39.09	135.05	137.89	64.32	20.10	4.79	68.19
Gwynedd AHA	32.86	122.50	121.08	75.57	28.10	5.44	66.64
Mid Glamorgan AHA	47.75	146.33	142.35	64.68	19.88	3.05	73.33
Ogwr HD	40.39	140.00	146.43	65.22	19.23	4.05	70.27
Rhymney Valley HD	44.44	151.90	146.75	57.61	20.00	2.19	73.85
East Glamorgan HD	50.77	133.87	140.16	67.34	21.13	3.54	73.14
Merthyr and Cynon Valley HD	54.58	166.10	136.92	67.56	18.61	2.06	76.34
Powys AHA	26.67	111.62	132.35	78.33	31.11	4.29	66.92
South Glamorgan AHA	34.13	106.49	139.61	75.00	23.30	4.81	65.74
West Glamorgan AHA	34.35	136.02	139.09	64.33	19.55	2.64	66.71
Neath HD	40.20	130.45	139.25	54.32	18.38	2.86	65.96
Swansea HD	31.54	139.11	139.01	69.22	20.14	2.54	67.09

Numbers of live and stillbirths are given in Table A3.24
Source: OPCS unpublished data

Table A3.26 Incidence of low birthweight by area of residence, England and Wales, 1978-1980

Area of residence	Percentage of total births with birthweights									Total births notified* 1978-80
	1,000 g and under	1,001-1,500 g	1,501-2,000 g	2,000 g or less	2,001-2,250 g	2,251-2,500 g	2,001-2,500 g	2,500 g and under	Over 2,500 g	
ENGLAND AND WALES	0.4	0.7	1.4	2.4	1.5	3.2	4.8	7.2	92.8	1,906,779
Northern RHA	0.4	0.6	1.4	2.4	1.5	3.0	4.5	6.9	93.1	
Cleveland AHA	0.4	0.6	1.4	2.5	1.6	3.3	4.9	7.4	92.6	25,647
Cumbria AHA	0.3	0.7	1.4	2.4	1.5	2.8	4.3	6.6	93.4	16,719
Durham AHA	0.3	0.7	1.3	2.4	1.5	2.7	4.2	6.6	93.4	23,449
Northumberland AHA	0.3	0.4	1.1	1.8	1.4	2.5	3.9	5.7	94.3	11,463
Gateshead AHA	0.3	0.6	1.5	2.5	1.7	3.6	5.3	7.8	92.2	8,245
Newcastle upon Tyne AHA	0.3	0.6	1.4	2.3	1.7	2.8	4.5	6.8	93.2	10,558
North Tyneside AHA	0.4	0.5	1.6	2.7	1.3	3.3	4.6	7.2	92.8	7,335
South Tyneside AHA	0.4	0.9	1.4	2.6	1.6	3.3	4.9	7.6	92.4	6,024
Sunderland AHA	0.4	0.5	1.2	2.2	1.4	3.0	4.4	6.7	93.3	12,804
Yorkshire RHA	0.4	0.7	1.5	2.6	1.6	3.7	5.3	7.9	92.1	139,093
Humberside AHA	0.4	0.7	1.4	2.4	1.5	3.2	4.7	7.2	92.8	32,649
North Yorkshire AHA	0.4	0.6	1.2	2.2	1.1	2.9	4.1	6.2	93.8	21,056
Bradford AHA	0.4	0.8	1.9	3.1	2.2	4.6	6.8	9.9	90.1	23,337
Calderdale AHA	0.4	0.9	1.6	2.9	1.8	4.2	6.0	8.9	91.1	7,557
Kirklees AHA	0.3	0.7	1.6	2.7	1.8	4.2	6.0	8.7	91.3	15,779
Leeds AHA	0.4	0.7	1.4	2.6	1.7	3.6	5.2	7.8	92.2	26,665
Wakefield AHA	0.4	0.7	1.2	2.4	1.3	3.4	4.7	7.1	92.9	12,050
Trent RHA	0.4	0.7	1.4	2.5	1.6	3.3	4.9	7.3	92.7	173,068
Derbyshire AHA	0.3	0.7	1.3	2.3	1.5	3.0	4.6	6.8	93.2	32,548
Leicestershire AHA	0.4	0.7	1.6	2.7	1.7	3.7	5.4	8.0	92.0	34,893
Lincolnshire AHA	0.2	0.6	1.2	2.0	1.4	2.8	4.2	6.3	93.7	20,435
Nottinghamshire AHA	0.5	0.7	1.5	2.7	1.7	3.6	5.3	8.0	92.0	37,032
Barnsley AHA	0.5	0.6	1.3	2.5	1.6	3.2	4.7	7.2	92.8	8,384
Doncaster AHA	0.3	0.5	1.4	2.2	1.8	3.9	5.7	7.9	92.1	11,612
Rotherham AHA	0.5	0.6	1.3	2.5	1.5	2.9	4.4	6.9	93.1	10,265
Sheffield AHA	0.3	0.8	1.3	2.5	1.4	2.9	4.2	6.7	93.3	17,899
East Anglian RHA	0.3	0.6	1.3	2.2	1.5	2.9	4.3	6.6	93.4	70,889
Cambridgeshire AHA	0.3	0.7	1.4	2.3	1.6	2.9	4.5	6.9	93.1	22,425
Norfolk AHA	0.3	0.6	1.3	2.3	1.5	2.8	4.2	6.5	93.5	28,078
Suffolk AHA	0.3	0.6	1.2	2.1	1.4	2.9	4.3	6.4	93.6	20,386

* These totals are derived from birth notification and may therefore differ from the numbers of births registered

Table A3.26 Incidence of low birthweight by area of residence, England and Wales, 1978-1980-continued

Area of residence	Percentage of total births with birthweights									Total births notified* 1978-80
	1,000 g and under	1,001-1,500 g	1,501-2,000 g	2,000 g and under	2,001-2,250 g	2,251-2,500 g	2,001-2,500 g	2,500 g and under	Over 2,500 g	
North West Thames RHA	0.4	0.7	1.4	2.4	1.6	3.4	5.0	7.4	92.6	140,724
Bedfordshire AHA	0.4	0.6	1.1	2.1	1.4	3.0	4.3	6.4	93.6	23,898
Hertfordshire AHA	0.3	0.6	1.3	2.1	1.5	3.0	4.5	6.6	93.4	36,214
Barnet AHA	0.3	0.7	1.3	2.3	1.7	3.7	5.4	7.7	92.3	11,931
Brent and Harrow AHA	0.3	0.7	1.6	2.6	1.9	4.5	6.4	9.0	91.0	19,537
Ealing, Hammersmith and Hounslow AHA	0.4	0.8	1.6	2.9	1.9	3.5	5.4	8.3	91.7	27,473
Hillingdon AHA	0.3	0.6	1.2	2.1	1.4	3.1	4.5	6.6	93.4	9,002
Kensington, Chelsea and Westminster AHA	0.4	0.8	1.3	2.6	1.6	3.1	4.7	7.2	92.8	12,669
North East Thames RHA	0.4	0.7	1.4	2.4	1.6	3.3	4.9	7.3	92.7	149,534
Essex AHA	0.2	0.6	1.1	1.9	1.3	2.6	3.9	5.8	94.2	57,556
Barking and Havering AHA	0.3	0.6	1.4	2.4	1.7	3.2	4.9	7.3	92.7	14,433
Camden and Islington AHA	0.3	0.7	1.6	2.7	1.6	3.3	5.0	7.7	92.3	12,896
City and East London AHA	0.5	1.0	1.7	3.2	2.1	4.5	6.6	9.8	90.2	27,567
Enfield and Haringey AHA	0.4	0.7	1.4	2.5	1.6	3.4	5.0	7.5	92.5	19,191
Redbridge and Waltham Forest AHA	0.5	0.7	1.4	2.6	1.7	3.8	5.5	8.1	91.9	17,891
South East Thames RHA	0.3	0.7	1.4	2.4	1.5	3.2	4.7	7.2	92.8	132,857
East Sussex AHA	0.3	0.6	1.4	2.3	1.5	2.9	4.4	6.8	93.2	19,835
Kent AHA	0.3	0.6	1.4	2.3	1.4	3.0	4.4	6.6	93.4	57,028
Greenwich and Bexley AHA	0.3	0.6	1.4	2.3	1.6	3.1	4.7	7.0	93.0	17,176
Bromley AHA	0.2	0.7	1.1	2.0	1.4	3.1	4.4	6.4	93.6	9,926
Lambeth, Southwark and Lewisham AHA	0.4	0.9	1.7	3.2	1.9	3.8	5.6	8.8	91.2	28,892
South West Thames RHA	0.3	0.6	1.1	2.0	1.3	2.7	4.0	6.1	93.9	108,987
Surrey AHA	0.2	0.4	0.9	1.6	1.1	2.2	3.3	4.9	95.1	40,714
West Sussex AHA	0.3	0.7	1.2	2.2	1.4	3.0	4.4	6.6	93.4	22,484
Croydon AHA	0.3	0.6	1.6	2.5	1.6	3.4	4.9	7.5	92.5	12,913
Kingston and Richmond AHA	0.3	0.4	1.0	1.8	1.2	2.5	3.8	5.6	94.4	8,326
Merton, Sutton and Wandsworth AHA	0.4	0.7	1.2	2.3	1.4	3.1	4.6	6.9	93.1	24,550

* These totals are derived from birth notification and may therefore differ from the numbers of births registered

Table A3.26   Incidence of low birthweight by area of residence, England and Wales, 1978-1980-continued

Area of residence	Percentage of total births with birthweights									Total births notified* 1978-80
	1,000 g and under	1,001-1,500 g	1,501-2,000 g	2,000 g and under	2,001-2,250 g	2,251-2,500 g	2,001-2,500 g	2,500 g and under	Over 2,500 g	
Wessex RHA	0.3	0.6	1.4	2.2	1.5	3.2	4.7	7.0	93.0	98,306
Dorset AHA	0.2	0.5	1.2	2.0	1.5	3.1	4.6	6.5	93.5	18,176
Hampshire AHA	0.3	0.7	1.4	2.3	1.6	3.4	5.0	7.3	92.7	49,705
Wiltshire AHA	0.2	0.5	1.4	2.3	1.4	3.1	4.5	6.8	93.2	26,771
Isle of Wight AHA	0.2	0.7	1.2	2.1	1.1	2.3	3.4	5.5	94.5	3,654
Oxford RHA	0.3	0.6	1.3	2.2	1.4	3.0	4.4	6.6	93.4	95,528
Berkshire AHA	0.3	0.6	1.3	2.2	1.2	3.0	4.2	6.4	93.6	30,710
Buckinghamshire AHA	0.3	0.6	1.3	2.2	1.5	2.9	4.4	6.6	93.4	22,865
Northamptonshire AHA	0.3	0.6	1.4	2.3	1.5	3.3	4.9	7.2	92.8	22,063
Oxfordshire AHA	0.3	0.5	1.1	2.0	1.4	2.7	4.0	6.0	94.0	19,890
South Western RHA	0.3	0.6	1.3	2.2	1.4	2.8	4.2	6.4	93.6	107,284
Avon AHA	0.4	0.8	1.4	2.6	1.4	3.0	4.4	6.9	93.1	29,479
Cornwall and Scilly Isles AHA	0.4	0.6	1.3	2.3	1.2	2.7	3.9	6.2	93.8	14,982
Devon AHA	0.3	0.5	1.1	1.9	1.3	2.6	3.9	5.8	94.2	31,778
Gloucestershire AHA	0.2	0.6	1.4	2.2	1.7	3.1	4.9	7.0	93.0	18,262
Somerset AHA	0.3	0.5	1.3	2.2	1.2	2.4	3.6	5.8	94.2	12,783
West Midlands RHA	0.4	0.8	1.4	2.6	1.7	3.6	5.3	7.9	92.1	205,076
Hereford and Worcester AHA	0.3	0.5	1.1	1.9	1.4	2.8	4.2	6.1	93.9	24,350
Shropshire AHA	0.4	0.8	1.3	2.5	1.4	3.1	4.5	7.0	93.0	14,241
Staffordshire AHA	0.3	0.7	1.3	2.4	1.4	3.2	4.6	7.0	93.0	39,887
Warwickshire AHA	0.3	0.6	1.4	2.4	1.6	3.6	5.2	7.6	92.4	17,602
Birmingham AHA	0.4	0.9	1.8	3.0	2.0	4.3	6.3	9.4	90.6	44,072
Coventry AHA	0.5	0.7	1.4	2.9	1.8	3.6	5.4	8.2	91.8	12,991
Dudley AHA	0.4	0.7	1.3	2.4	1.6	3.2	4.8	7.1	92.9	11,498
Sandwell AHA	0.5	0.9	1.8	3.2	2.0	4.3	6.3	9.6	90.4	12,178
Solihull AHA	0.2	0.5	1.2	1.9	1.5	2.9	4.4	6.2	93.8	7,025
Walsall AHA	0.4	0.9	1.5	2.8	1.9	4.4	6.3	9.1	90.9	10,561
Wolverhampton AHA	0.5	1.1	1.8	3.4	2.4	4.3	6.6	10.0	90.0	10,671

* These totals are derived from birth notification and may therefore differ from the numbers of births registered

Table A3.26 Incidence of low birthweight by area of residence, England and Wales, 1978-1980-*continued*

Area of residence	Percentage of total births with birthweights									Total births notified* 1978-80
	1,000 g and under	1,001-1,500 g	1,501-2,000 g	2,000 g and under	2,001-2,250 g	2,251-2,500 g	2,001-2,500 g	2,500 g and under	Over 2,500 g	
Mersey RHA	0.3	0.6	1.2	2.3	1.4	3.0	4.4	6.7	93.3	95,717
Cheshire AHA	0.3	0.6	1.1	2.0	1.1	2.6	3.7	5.7	94.3	34,994
Liverpool AHA	0.4	0.6	1.4	2.5	1.6	3.8	5.4	7.9	92.1	20,255
St Helens and Knowsley AHA	0.4	0.6	1.5	2.5	1.8	3.5	5.2	7.8	92.2	16,147
Sefton AHA	0.3	0.6	1.3	2.5	1.7	2.9	4.6	7.1	92.9	10,492
Wirral AHA	0.3	0.8	1.0	2.2	1.1	2.4	3.5	5.6	94.4	13,829
North Western RHA	0.4	0.7	1.5	2.6	1.7	3.7	5.4	8.0	92.0	159,711
Lancashire AHA	0.4	0.8	1.4	2.6	1.6	3.5	5.1	7.7	92.3	52,491
Bolton AHA	0.5	0.6	1.4	2.4	1.9	3.8	5.7	8.1	91.9	10,993
Bury AHA	0.5	0.8	1.4	2.7	1.6	3.4	5.0	7.6	92.4	7,126
Manchester AHA	0.6	0.9	1.9	3.5	2.1	4.4	6.4	9.9	90.1	18,632
Oldham AHA	0.3	0.5	1.5	2.2	2.0	4.3	6.3	8.5	91.5	9,585
Rochdale AHA	0.5	0.9	1.5	2.9	2.0	4.7	6.7	9.7	90.3	9,678
Salford AHA	0.5	0.8	1.5	2.7	1.7	3.8	5.5	8.2	91.8	9,268
Stockport AHA	0.3	0.7	1.4	2.4	1.4	3.0	4.4	6.8	93.2	11,018
Tameside AHA	0.3	0.5	1.5	2.3	1.6	3.8	5.4	7.6	92.4	9,809
Trafford AHA	0.2	0.7	1.2	2.3	1.4	3.1	4.4	6.7	93.3	8,289
Wigan AHA	0.3	0.7	1.2	2.2	1.5	3.0	4.5	6.7	93.3	12,822
Wales	0.3	0.6	1.3	2.3	1.4	3.0	4.4	6.7	93.3	107,761
Clwyd AHA	0.3	0.7	1.3	2.3	1.3	2.7	4.0	6.2	93.8	14,631
Dyfed AHA	0.2	0.4	1.0	1.7	1.1	2.7	3.8	5.5	94.5	11,946
Gwent AHA	0.4	0.7	1.3	2.5	1.6	3.3	4.8	7.3	92.7	17,017
Gwynedd AHA	0.2	0.5	1.1	1.9	1.3	2.3	3.7	5.6	94.4	8,324
Mid Glamorgan AHA	0.3	0.7	1.3	2.4	1.5	3.3	4.8	7.2	92.8	22,461
Powys AHA	0.4	0.4	1.4	2.2	1.3	2.2	3.5	5.7	94.3	3,816
South Glamorgan AHA	0.4	0.5	1.4	2.6	1.5	3.1	4.6	7.2	92.8	15,392
West Glamorgan AHA	0.4	0.7	1.3	2.4	1.5	2.9	4.4	6.8	93.2	14,174

* These totals are derived from birth notification and may therefore differ from the numbers of births registered

Source: Authors' analysis of DHSS LHS 27/1 returns.

Table A3.27 Perinatal mortality by area of residence, Regional Health Authorities, Wales, Scotland, Northern Ireland, 1970-81

Numbers and rates per 1,000 total births

Area or residence		1970	1971	1972	1973	1974	1975	1976	1977	1978	1979	1980	1981
		All causes											
ENGLAND AND WALES	Number	18,671	17,649	15,943	14,374	13,169	11,769	10,472	9,757	9,350	9,432	8,815	7,563
	Rate	23.5	22.3	21.7	21.0	20.4	19.3	17.7	17.0	15.5	14.7	13.3	11.8
ENGLAND	Number	17,572	16,583	15,039	13,557	12,391	11,091	9,830	9,182	8,784	8,863	8,332	7,044
	Rate	23.4	22.1	21.7	21.0	20.3	19.3	17.7	16.9	15.5	14.6	13.4	11.7
Regional Health Authorities													
Northern	Number	1,203	1,147	1,060	906	910	765	710	695	679	687	622	531
	Rate	24.3	23.0	23.5	21.8	22.5	19.9	19.1	19.1	17.6	16.4	15.0	13.2
Yorkshire	Number	1,344	1,201	1,192	1,039	1,059	973	797	754	718	775	717	653
	Rate	24.7	22.4	24.2	22.9	22.2	21.6	18.4	18.1	16.3	16.6	14.9	13.9
Trent	Number	1,849	1,790	1,618	1,405	1,257	1,044	1,047	882	837	856	792	660
	Rate	23.5	22.8	22.5	21.0	21.0	18.6	19.3	16.7	15.3	14.6	13.0	11.3
East Anglian	Number	574	565	534	464	399	360	310	282	296	311	282	243
	Rate	20.8	19.9	19.5	17.4	16.6	15.8	14.0	13.0	13.3	13.0	11.3	10.2
North West Thames	Number	1,511	1,324	1,163	1,092	799	791	714	623	622	624	524	499
	Rate	22.2	19.8	18.7	19.2	17.5	18.4	17.0	14.8	14.1	13.2	11.0	10.7
North East Thames	Number	1,142	1,174	1,042	955	970	857	768	728	708	675	719	556
	Rate	21.5	21.9	20.9	20.4	19.2	18.0	16.6	16.1	15.1	13.5	13.8	11.0
South East Thames	Number	1,080	1,025	895	871	869	816	717	675	636	629	592	539
	Rate	21.0	20.1	19.0	19.6	19.5	19.2	17.4	16.8	15.0	14.1	12.9	12.0
South West Thames	Number	1,097	982	895	787	619	580	462	454	444	467	382	372
	Rate	22.3	20.1	19.7	18.8	18.1	18.0	14.9	14.6	13.5	13.3	10.8	10.7
Wessex	Number	657	681	573	585	616	553	471	462	411	425	402	331
	Rate	20.8	21.4	19.3	20.6	17.8	17.1	15.1	15.5	13.2	12.8	11.7	9.9
Oxford	Number	679	685	585	536	483	455	399	427	400	371	417	299
	Rate	19.6	19.7	17.7	17.0	15.7	15.6	13.8	15.0	13.4	11.6	12.6	9.4
South Western	Number	1,000	957	896	822	739	611	564	560	543	505	495	429
	Rate	21.0	19.9	19.9	19.0	19.0	16.9	16.1	16.2	15.1	13.3	12.6	11.3
West Midlands	Number	2,318	2,123	1,956	1,793	1,597	1,446	1,341	1,193	1,109	1,155	1,085	875
	Rate	25.6	23.7	23.9	23.6	22.5	21.8	21.1	19.4	17.2	16.8	15.1	12.9

Table A3.27 Perinatal mortality by area of residence, Regional Health Authorities, Wales, Scotland, Northern Ireland, 1970-81 - *continued*

Numbers and rates per 1,000 total births

Area of residence		1970	1971	1972	1973	1974	1975	1976	1977	1978	1979	1980	1981
All causes - continued													
Mersey	Number	1,045	997	844	775	778	699	586	539	459	506	446	397
	Rate	26.8	26.2	24.2	24.6	23.6	22.1	19.5	18.8	15.2	15.6	13.7	12.4
North Western	Number	2,073	1,932	1,751	1,504	1,271	1,122	921	883	904	853	841	660
	Rate	27.1	25.3	25.0	23.4	23.1	21.9	18.7	18.5	18.1	15.9	15.3	12.4
WALES	Number	1,099	1,066	904	817	778	678	642	575	566	569	483	508
	Rate	**25.5**	**24.4**	**22.3**	**21.4**	**21.2**	**19.7**	**19.0**	**17.9**	**16.8**	**15.6**	**12.8**	**14.1**
SCOTLAND	Number	2,200	2,151	1,888	1,690	1,617	1,448	1,199	1,150	999	973	909	808
	Rate	**24.8**	**24.5**	**23.7**	**22.5**	**22.8**	**21.1**	**18.3**	**18.3**	**15.4**	**14.1**	**13.1**	**11.6**
NORTHERN IRELAND	Number	900	877	790	757	696	677	593	544	480	472	450	..
	Rate	**27.6**	**27.2**	**26.0**	**25.6**	**25.3**	**25.5**	**22.3**	**21.1**	**18.1**	**16.6**	**15.6**	**..**
Congenital malformations ICD 740-759													
ENGLAND AND WALES	Number	3,376	3,522	3,263	2,893	2,806	2,538	2,245	2,121	2,085	2,041	1,944	..
	Rate	**4.2**	**4.4**	**4.4**	**4.2**	**4.3**	**4.2**	**3.8**	**3.7**	**3.5**	**3.2**	**2.9**	**..**
ENGLAND	Number	3,159	3,261	3,051	2,720	2,624	2,379	2,121	1,993	1,963	1,919	1,863	..
	Rate	**4.2**	**4.4**	**4.4**	**4.2**	**4.3**	**4.1**	**3.8**	**3.7**	**3.5**	**3.2**	**3.0**	**..**
Regional Health Authorities													
Northern	Number	218	249	220	174	181	158	155	151	157	168	109	..
	Rate	4.4	5.0	4.9	4.2	4.5	4.1	4.2	4.2	4.1	4.0	2.6	..
Yorkshire	Number	207	205	208	186	215	219	173	141	144	158	170	..
	Rate	3.8	3.8	4.2	4.1	4.5	4.9	4.0	3.4	3.3	3.4	3.5	..
Trent	Number	345	352	354	334	302	252	236	208	192	170	173	..
	Rate	4.4	4.5	4.9	5.0	5.1	4.5	4.3	3.9	3.5	2.9	2.8	..
East Anglian	Number	101	120	118	86	83	85	85	69	84	91	74	..
	Rate	3.9	4.2	4.3	3.2	3.5	3.7	3.8	3.2	3.8	3.8	3.0	..

Table A3.27 Perinatal mortality by area of residence, Regional Health Authorities, Wales, Scotland, Northern Ireland, 1970-81 - *continued*

Numbers and rates per 1,000 total births

Area of residence		1970	1971	1972	1973	1974	1975	1976	1977	1978	1979	1980	1981
Congenital malformations ICD 740-759 - continued													
North West Thames	Number	272	234	242	222	151	151	150	120	135	104	115	..
	Rate	4.0	3.5	3.9	3.9	3.3	3.5	3.6	2.8	3.0	2.2	2.4	..
North East Thames	Number	182	216	189	172	199	189	139	148	135	127	121	..
	Rate	3.4	4.0	3.8	3.7	3.9	4.0	3.0	3.3	2.9	2.5	2.3	..
South East Thames	Number	192	196	175	187	175	150	137	147	132	125	141	..
	Rate	3.7	3.8	3.7	4.2	3.9	3.5	3.3	3.6	3.1	2.8	3.1	..
South West Thames	Number	153	181	168	152	125	93	102	101	103	108	90	..
	Rate	3.1	3.7	3.7	3.6	3.7	2.9	3.3	3.3	3.1	3.1	2.5	..
Wessex	Number	118	157	126	139	144	134	127	127	88	104	109	..
	Rate	3.7	4.9	4.2	4.9	4.2	4.1	4.1	4.2	2.8	3.1	3.2	..
Oxford	Number	126	143	141	122	128	110	93	109	105	85	87	..
	Rate	3.6	4.1	4.3	3.9	4.2	3.8	3.2	3.8	3.5	2.7	2.6	..
South Western	Number	202	221	215	196	184	144	141	151	145	127	138	..
	Rate	4.2	4.6	4.8	4.5	4.7	4.0	4.0	4.4	4.0	3.3	3.5	..
West Midlands	Number	421	427	369	324	314	311	269	238	249	298	266	..
	Rate	4.6	4.8	4.5	4.3	4.4	4.7	4.2	3.9	3.9	4.3	3.7	..
Mersey	Number	203	214	188	161	176	150	127	119	99	99	106	..
	Rate	5.2	5.6	5.4	5.1	5.3	4.7	4.2	4.1	3.3	3.0	3.3	..
North Western	Number	413	346	332	259	239	228	178	157	194	154	160	..
	Rate	5.4	4.5	4.7	4.0	4.3	4.4	3.6	3.3	3.9	2.9	2.9	..
WALES	**Number**	**217**	**261**	**212**	**173**	**182**	**159**	**124**	**128**	**122**	**122**	**81**	**..**
	Rate	**5.0**	**6.0**	**5.2**	**4.5**	**5.0**	**4.6**	**3.7**	**4.0**	**3.6**	**3.3**	**2.2**	**..**
SCOTLAND	**Number**	**481**	**544**	**428**	**416**	**401**	**350**	**292**	**269**	**238**	**223**	**192**	**163**
	Rate	**5.4**	**6.2**	**5.4**	**5.5**	**5.7**	**5.1**	**4.5**	**4.3**	**3.7**	**3.2**	**2.8**	**2.3**
NORTHERN IRELAND	**Number**	230	232	220	167	175	153	130	129	115	126	126	..
	Rate	7.1	7.2	7.2	5.6	6.4	5.8	4.9	5.0	4.3	4.4	4.4	..

Table A3.27 Perinatal mortality by area of residence, Regional Health Authorities, Wales, Scotland, Northern Ireland, 1970-81 - *continued*

Numbers and rates per 1,000 total births

Area of residence		1970	1971	1972	1973	1974	1975	1976	1977	1978	1979	1980	1981
All other causes													
ENGLAND AND WALES	Number	**15,295**	**14,127**	**12,680**	**11,481**	**10,363**	**9,231**	**8,227**	**7,636**	**7,265**	**7,391**	**6,871**	..
	Rate	**19.2**	**17.8**	**17.3**	**16.8**	**16.0**	**15.1**	**13.9**	**13.3**	**12.1**	**11.5**	**10.4**	..
ENGLAND	Number	**14,413**	**13,322**	**11,988**	**10,837**	**9,767**	**8,712**	**7,709**	**7,189**	**6,821**	**6,944**	**6,469**	..
	Rate	**19.2**	**17.8**	**17.3**	**16.8**	**16.0**	**15.1**	**13.9**	**13.2**	**12.0**	**11.4**	**10.4**	..
Regional Health Authorities													
Northern	Number	985	898	840	732	729	607	555	544	522	519	513	..
	Rate	19.9	18.0	18.6	17.6	18.1	15.8	14.9	15.0	13.5	12.4	12.4	..
Yorkshire	Number	1,137	996	984	853	844	754	624	613	574	617	547	..
	Rate	20.9	18.5	20.0	18.8	17.7	16.7	14.4	14.7	13.0	13.2	11.4	..
Trent	Number	1,504	1,438	1,264	1,071	955	792	811	674	645	686	619	..
	Rate	19.1	18.3	17.6	16.0	16.0	14.1	14.9	12.8	11.8	11.7	10.2	..
East Anglian	Number	467	445	416	378	316	275	225	213	212	220	208	..
	Rate	16.9	15.7	15.2	14.1	13.1	12.1	10.1	9.8	9.5	9.2	8.3	..
North West Thames	Number	1,239	1,090	921	870	648	640	564	503	487	520	409	..
	Rate	18.2	16.3	14.8	15.3	14.2	14.9	13.4	11.9	11.0	11.0	8.6	..
North East Thames	Number	960	958	853	783	771	668	629	580	573	548	598	..
	Rate	18.1	17.9	17.1	16.7	15.3	14.0	13.6	12.8	12.2	11.0	11.5	..
South East Thames	Number	888	829	719	684	694	666	580	528	504	504	451	..
	Rate	17.3	16.2	15.2	15.4	15.6	15.7	14.1	13.1	11.9	11.3	9.8	..
South West Thames	Number	944	801	727	635	494	487	360	353	341	359	292	..
	Rate	19.2	16.4	16.0	15.2	14.5	15.1	11.6	11.4	10.4	10.2	8.2	..
Wessex	Number	539	524	447	446	472	419	344	335	323	321	293	..
	Rate	17.0	16.5	15.1	15.7	13.7	12.9	11.1	11.2	10.4	9.7	8.5	..
Oxford	Number	553	542	444	414	355	345	306	318	295	286	330	..
	Rate	16.0	15.6	13.4	13.2	11.5	11.8	10.6	11.2	9.9	8.9	9.9	..
South Western	Number	798	736	681	626	555	467	423	409	398	378	357	..
	Rate	16.8	15.3	15.1	14.5	14.3	12.9	12.1	11.8	11.1	9.9	9.1	..
West Midlands	Number	1,897	1,696	1,587	1,469	1,283	1,135	1,072	955	860	857	819	..
	Rate	20.9	19.0	19.4	19.4	18.1	17.1	16.9	15.5	13.3	12.5	11.4	..

Table A3.27 Perinatal mortality by area of residence, Regional Health Authorities, Wales, Scotland, Northern Ireland, 1970-81 - *continued*

Numbers and rates per 1,000 total births

Area of residence		1970	1971	1972	1973	1974	1975	1976	1977	1978	1979	1980	1981
		All other causes - continued											
Mersey	Number	842	783	656	614	602	549	459	420	360	407	340	..
	Rate	21.6	20.5	18.8	19.5	18.3	17.4	15.3	14.6	11.9	12.5	10.5	..
North Western	Number	1,660	1,586	1,419	1,245	1,032	894	743	726	710	699	681	..
	Rate	21.7	20.8	20.2	19.4	18.7	17.4	15.1	15.2	14.2	13.1	12.4	..
WALES	**Number**	**882**	**805**	**692**	**644**	**596**	**519**	**518**	**447**	**444**	**447**	**402**	..
	Rate	**20.5**	**18.4**	**17.1**	**16.9**	**16.3**	**15.1**	**15.4**	**13.9**	**13.2**	**12.3**	**10.7**	..
SCOTLAND	**Number**	**1,719**	**1,607**	**1,460**	**1,274**	**1,216**	**1,098**	**907**	**881**	**761**	**750**	**717**	**645**
	Rate	**19.4**	**18.3**	**18.3**	**16.9**	**17.1**	**16.0**	**13.8**	**14.0**	**11.7**	**10.9**	**10.3**	**9.3**
NORTHERN IRELAND	**Number**	**670**	**645**	**570**	**590**	**521**	**524**	**463**	**415**	**365**	**346**		..
	Rate	**20.6**	**20.0**	**18.7**	**19.9**	**18.9**	**19.8**	**17.4**	**16.1**	**13.8**	**12.2**		..

Source: OPCS *mortality statistics: childhood, Series DH3* (England and Wales)
Registrar General, Scotland, *Annual Report* (Scotland)
Registrar General, Northern Ireland, *Annual Report* (Northern Ireland)

Table A3.28 Infant mortality by area of residence, Regional Health Authorities, Wales, Scotland, Northern Ireland, 1970-80

Numbers and rates per 1,000 live births

Area of residence		1970	1971	1972	1973	1974	1975	1976	1977	1978	1979	1980	1981
		All causes											
ENGLAND AND WALES	Number	**14,267**	**13,120**	**12,498**	**11,407**	**10,459**	**9,488**	**8,334**	**7,841**	**7,881**	**8,178**	**7,899**	**7,021**
	Rate	**18.19**	**17.52**	**17.23**	**16.88**	**16.35**	**15.72**	**14.26**	**13.77**	**13.21**	**12.82**	**12.04**	**11.07**
ENGLAND	Number	**13,473**	**12,926**	**11,859**	**10,792**	**9,842**	**8,995**	**7,877**	**7,411**	**7,441**	**7,731**	**7,473**	**6,502**
	Rate	**18.16**	**17.47**	**17.30**	**16.91**	**16.32**	**15.81**	**14.31**	**13.80**	**13.23**	**12.86**	**12.08**	**10.87**
Regional Health Authorities													
Northern	Number	919	928	867	729	690	568	558	536	532	553	509	426
	Rate	18.82	18.87	19.45	17.72	17.31	14.94	15.13	14.92	13.90	13.28	12.36	10.69
Yorkshire	Number	1,093	1,049	932	895	920	800	646	638	597	660	614	586
	Rate	20.37	19.77	19.18	19.95	19.48	17.93	15.08	15.47	13.68	14.25	12.86	12.62
Trent	Number	1,464	1,460	1,296	1,058	927	867	796	729	720	726	657	632
	Rate	18.89	18.80	18.27	16.05	15.70	15.59	14.80	13.94	13.24	12.51	10.89	10.88
East Anglian	Number	431	421	412	356	335	332	258	241	238	301	258	232
	Rate	15.77	15.03	15.21	13.46	14.07	14.67	11.73	11.22	10.18	12.65	10.41	9.79
North West Thames	Number	1,147	1,115	913	862	640	647	581	493	534	548	520	476
	Rate	17.04	16.87	14.87	15.31	14.18	15.21	13.92	11.79	12.16	11.71	10.94	10.26
North East Thames	Number	857	875	800	767	785	701	616	626	625	592	617	519
	Rate	16.35	16.53	16.20	16.57	15.74	14.87	13.41	13.98	13.41	11.94	11.96	10.37
South East Thames	Number	853	732	723	662	672	664	602	524	556	580	561	506
	Rate	16.81	14.50	15.47	15.02	15.22	15.81	14.75	13.14	13.25	13.06	12.28	11.37
South West Thames	Number	838	763	713	670	476	467	394	356	421	385	388	358
	Rate	17.25	15.80	15.86	16.17	14.08	14.59	12.77	11.57	12.92	11.07	11.00	10.38
Wessex	Number	478	515	465	408	511	496	392	388	380	423	410	378
	Rate	15.29	16.39	15.83	14.58	14.94	15.43	12.71	13.09	12.31	12.84	11.99	11.38
Oxford	Number	578	534	491	428	420	367	370	358	365	358	376	259
	Rate	15.12	15.50	14.98	13.74	13.77	12.68	12.90	12.69	12.35	11.26	11.39	8.18
South Western	Number	797	742	725	644	564	518	448	427	441	452	451	392
	Rate	16.96	15.62	16.26	15.04	14.65	14.46	12.91	12.48	12.41	11.97	11.52	10.43
West Midlands	Number	1,689	1,565	1,487	1,434	1,185	1,109	986	917	871	942	934	788
	Rate	18.91	17.73	18.39	19.14	16.90	16.94	15.73	15.05	13.65	13.82	13.12	11.68

Table A3.28 Infant mortality by area of residence, Regional Health Authorities, Wales, Scotland, Northern Ireland, 1970-81

Numbers and rates per 1,000 live births

Area of residence		1970	1971	1972	1973	1974	1975	1976	1977	1978	1979	1980	1981
All causes – continued													
Mersey	Number	811	794	622	624	600	513	422	409	364	420	412	361
	Rate	21.11	21.13	18.07	20.05	18.45	16.42	14.18	14.39	12.16	13.05	12.77	11.34
North Western	Number	1,578	1,433	1,361	1,215	1,077	901	765	703	726	731	703	589
	Rate	20.93	19.06	19.68	19.18	19.79	17.77	15.65	14.85	14.67	13.77	12.92	11.14
WALES	Number	794	794	639	615	617	493	457	430	440	447	426	452
	Rate	18.69	18.44	15.99	16.36	17.04	14.51	13.69	13.54	13.21	12.36	11.40	12.61
SCOTLAND	Number	1,714	1,722	1,477	1,412	1,326	1,168	959	1,004	830	878	831	780
	Rate	19.63	19.86	18.80	18.98	18.92	17.19	14.78	16.10	12.91	12.84	12.06	11.30
NORTHERN IRELAND	Number	734	722	616	610	567	534	483	438	417	417	382	..
	Rate	22.88	22.73	20.54	20.89	20.88	20.44	18.32	17.22	15.89	14.80	13.37	..
Congenital malformations ICD 740-759													
ENGLAND AND WALES	Number	2,916	2,950	2,757	2,552	2,510	2,303	2,014	2,009	2,033	2,083	2,113	1,914
	Rate	3.72	3.77	3.80	3.78	3.92	3.82	3.45	3.53	3.41	3.26	3.22	3.02
ENGLAND	Number	2,756	2,753	2,619	2,424	2,354	2,176	1,899	1,895	1,924	1,957	1,999	1,752
	Rate	3.71	3.72	3.82	3.80	3.90	3.82	3.45	3.53	3.42	3.25	3.23	2.93
Regional Health Authorities													
Northern	Number	194	185	218	163	160	123	143	135	145	145	140	125
	Rate	3.97	3.76	4.89	3.96	4.02	3.23	3.88	3.76	3.79	3.48	3.40	3.14
Yorkshire	Number	198	176	183	181	214	195	156	149	137	139	149	161
	Rate	3.69	3.32	3.77	4.03	4.53	4.37	3.64	3.61	3.14	3.00	3.12	3.47
Trent	Number	299	316	302	271	243	229	204	208	210	200	203	197
	Rate	3.86	4.07	4.26	4.11	4.12	4.12	3.79	3.98	3.86	3.45	3.36	3.39
East Anglian	Number	102	95	105	81	89	96	78	67	58	81	79	65
	Rate	3.73	3.39	3.88	3.06	3.74	4.24	3.55	3.12	2.63	3.40	3.19	2.74

Table A3.28 Infant mortality by area of residence, Regional Health Authorities, Wales, Scotland, Northern Ireland, 1970-81 - *continued*

Numbers and rates per 1,000 live births

Area of residence		1970	1971	1972	1973	1974	1975	1976	1977	1978	1979	1980	1981
Congenital malformations ICD 740-759 - continued													
North West Thames	Number	244	256	195	172	160	150	138	125	142	128	152	139
	Rate	3.63	3.87	3.18	3.06	3.54	3.53	3.31	2.99	3.23	2.73	3.20	3.00
North East Thames	Number	180	203	168	167	200	172	140	154	147	153	132	119
	Rate	3.43	3.83	3.40	3.61	4.01	3.65	3.05	3.44	3.15	3.09	2.56	2.38
South East Thames	Number	182	133	138	134	148	128	135	134	124	142	146	119
	Rate	3.59	2.63	2.95	3.04	3.35	3.05	3.31	3.36	2.96	3.20	3.20	2.68
South West Thames	Number	164	163	166	153	115	103	90	91	112	93	105	92
	Rate	3.38	3.38	3.69	3.69	3.40	3.22	2.92	2.96	3.44	2.67	2.98	2.67
Wessex	Number	87	140	109	93	140	130	99	105	92	99	119	92
	Rate	2.78	4.45	3.71	3.32	4.09	4.04	3.21	3.54	2.98	3.00	3.48	2.77
Oxford	Number	96	127	125	124	111	99	104	102	109	92	95	76
	Rate	2.80	3.69	3.81	3.98	3.64	3.42	3.63	3.62	3.69	2.89	2.88	2.40
South Western	Number	188	187	180	177	140	146	121	117	121	128	140	122
	Rate	4.00	3.94	4.04	4.13	3.64	4.08	3.49	3.42	3.41	3.39	3.58	3.25
West Midlands	Number	356	350	303	310	277	249	213	231	226	280	254	208
	Rate	3.98	3.96	3.75	4.14	3.95	3.80	3.40	3.79	3.54	4.11	3.57	3.08
Mersey	Number	164	149	124	129	116	110	86	82	77	94	98	90
	Rate	4.27	3.97	3.60	4.15	3.57	3.52	2.89	2.88	2.57	2.92	3.04	2.83
North Western	Number	302	273	285	249	220	217	169	156	184	153	146	147
	Rate	4.01	3.63	4.12	3.93	4.04	4.28	3.46	3.29	3.72	2.88	2.68	2.78
WALES	Number	**160**	**197**	**138**	**128**	**156**	**127**	**115**	**114**	**109**	**126**	**114**	**121**
	Rate	**3.77**	**4.58**	**3.45**	**3.40**	**4.31**	**3.74**	**3.45**	**3.59**	**3.27**	**3.48**	**3.05**	**3.38**
SCOTLAND	Number	**391**	**459**	**334**	**360**	**349**	**287**	**242**	**287**	**239**	**241**	**225**	**200**
	Rate	**4.48**	**5.29**	**4.25**	**4.84**	**4.98**	**4.22**	**3.73**	**4.60**	**3.72**	**3.53**	**3.27**	**2.90**
NORTHERN IRELAND	Number	**177**	**183**	**146**	**133**	**131**	**138**	**108**	**126**	**115**	**133**	**125**	**..**
	Rate	**5.52**	**5.76**	**4.87**	**4.55**	**4.82**	**5.28**	**4.10**	**4.95**	**4.38**	**4.72**	**4.37**	**..**

Table A3.28 Infant mortality by area of residence, Regional Health Authorities, Wales, Scotland, Northern Ireland, 1970-81 - continued

Numbers and rates per 1,000 live births

Area of residence		1970	1971	1972	1973	1974	1975	1976	1977	1978	1979	1980	1981
		All other causes											
ENGLAND AND WALES	Number	**11,351**	**10,770**	**9,741**	**8,855**	**7,949**	**7,185**	**6,320**	**5,832**	**5,848**	**6,095**	**5,786**	**5,107**
	Rate	**14.47**	**13.75**	**13.43**	**13.10**	**12.42**	**11.91**	**10.82**	**10.24**	**9.81**	**9.55**	**8.82**	**8.05**
ENGLAND	Number	**10,717**	**10,173**	**9,240**	**8,368**	**7,488**	**6,819**	**5,978**	**5,516**	**5,517**	**5,774**	**5,474**	**4,750**
	Rate	**14.44**	**13.75**	**13.48**	**13.11**	**12.41**	**11.99**	**10.86**	**10.27**	**9.81**	**9.60**	**8.85**	**7.94**
Regional Health Authorities													
Northern	Number	725	743	649	566	530	445	415	401	387	408	369	301
	Rate	14.85	15.11	14.56	13.76	13.30	11.70	11.25	11.17	10.11	9.80	8.96	7.56
Yorkshire	Number	895	873	749	714	706	605	490	489	460	521	465	425
	Rate	16.68	16.46	15.41	15.91	14.95	13.56	11.44	11.86	10.54	11.25	9.74	9.15
Trent	Number	1,165	1,144	994	787	684	638	592	521	510	526	454	435
	Rate	15.03	14.73	14.01	11.94	11.59	11.47	11.00	9.96	9.38	9.07	7.52	7.49
East Anglian	Number	329	326	307	275	246	236	180	174	180	220	179	167
	Rate	12.04	11.64	11.34	10.40	10.33	10.43	8.19	8.10	8.16	9.24	7.22	7.05
North West Thames	Number	903	859	718	690	480	497	443	368	392	420	368	337
	Rate	13.42	13.00	11.69	12.26	10.63	11.68	10.62	8.80	8.92	8.97	7.74	7.27
North East Thames	Number	677	672	632	600	585	529	476	472	478	439	485	400
	Rate	12.91	12.69	12.80	12.96	11.73	11.22	10.37	10.54	10.26	8.86	9.40	7.99
South East Thames	Number	671	599	585	528	524	536	467	390	432	438	415	387
	Rate	13.22	11.86	12.51	11.98	11.87	12.76	11.44	9.78	10.30	9.86	9.08	8.70
South West Thames	Number	674	600	547	517	361	364	304	265	309	292	283	266
	Rate	13.88	12.42	12.17	12.47	10.68	11.38	9.85	8.62	9.48	8.40	8.02	7.71
Wessex	Number	391	375	356	315	371	366	293	283	288	324	291	286
	Rate	12.51	11.93	12.12	11.26	10.85	11.39	9.50	9.54	9.33	9.83	8.51	8.61
Oxford	Number	422	407	366	304	309	268	266	256	256	266	281	183
	Rate	12.32	11.82	11.17	9.76	10.13	9.26	9.27	9.08	8.66	8.37	8.51	5.78
South Western	Number	609	555	545	467	424	372	327	310	320	324	311	270
	Rate	12.96	11.69	12.22	10.91	11.01	10.39	9.42	9.06	9.01	8.58	7.94	7.18
West Midlands	Number	1,333	1,215	1,184	1,124	908	860	773	686	645	662	680	580
	Rate	14.92	13.76	14.64	15.00	12.95	13.14	12.33	11.26	10.11	9.71	9.55	8.60

81

Table A3.28 Infant mortality by area of residence, Regional Health Authorities, Wales, Scotland, Northern Ireland, 1970-81 - *continued*

Numbers and rates per 1,000 live births

Area of residence		1970	1971	1972	1973	1974	1975	1976	1977	1978	1979	1980	1981
		All other causes - continued											
Mersey	Number	647	645	498	495	484	403	336	327	287	326	314	271
	Rate	16.84	17.17	14.47	15.91	14.89	12.90	11.29	11.50	9.59	10.13	9.73	8.51
North Western	Number	1,276	1,160	1,076	966	857	684	596	547	542	578	557	442
	Rate	16.93	15.43	15.56	15.25	15.75	13.49	12.19	11.55	10.95	10.88	10.24	8.36
WALES	**Number**	**634**	**597**	**501**	**487**	**461**	**366**	**342**	**316**	**331**	**321**	**312**	**331**
	Rate	**14.92**	**13.87**	**12.54**	**12.95**	**12.73**	**10.77**	**10.25**	**9.95**	**9.94**	**8.87**	**8.35**	**9.23**
SCOTLAND	**Number**	**1,323**	**1,263**	**1,145**	**1,052**	**977**	**881**	**717**	**717**	**591**	**637**	**606**	**580**
	Rate	**15.15**	**14.56**	**14.58**	**14.14**	**13.94**	**12.97**	**11.05**	**11.50**	**9.19**	**9.32**	**8.80**	**8.40**
NORTHERN IRELAND	**Number**	**557**	**539**	**470**	**477**	**436**	**396**	**375**	**312**	**302**	**284**	**257**	**. .**
	Rate	**17.36**	**16.97**	**15.67**	**16.34**	**16.05**	**15.15**	**14.23**	**12.27**	**11.51**	**10.08**	**8.99**	**. .**

Source: As for Table A3.27

Table A3.29   Infant and perinatal mortality, England and Wales, England, Wales, Standard Regions, 1970-80

Area			1970	1971	1972	1973	1974	1975	1976	1977	1978	1979	1980
ENGLAND AND WALES	Perinatal	Number*	18,671	17,649	15,943	14,374	13,169	11,769	10,472	9,757	9,350	9,432	8,815
		Rate*	23.5	22.3	21.7	21.0	20.4	19.3	17.7	17.0	15.5	14.7	13.3
	Infant	Number†	14,267	13,720	12,498	11,407	10,459	9,488	8,334	7,841	7,881	8,178	7,899
		Rate†	18.2	17.5	17.2	16.9	16.3	15.7	14.3	13.8	13.2	12.8	12.0
ENGLAND	Perinatal	Number	17,572	16,583	15,039	13,557	12,366	11,072	9,807	9,157	8,766	8,839	8,316
		Rate	23.4	22.1	21.7	21.0	20.3	19.3	17.6	16.9	15.4	14.6	13.4
	Infant	Number	13,473	12,926	11,859	10,792	9,802	8,950	7,834	7,345	7,370	7,671	7,410
		Rate	18.2	17.5	17.3	16.9	16.3	15.7	14.2	13.7	13.1	12.8	12.0
Standard Regions													
North	Perinatal	Number	1,291	1,228	1,136	969	910	765	710	695	679	687	622
		Rate	24.4	23.0	23.4	21.7	22.5	19.9	19.1	19.1	17.6	16.4	15.0
	Infant	Number	978	988	925	779	690	568	558	536	532	553	509
		Rate	18.7	18.7	19.3	17.7	17.3	14.9	15.1	14.9	13.9	13.3	12.4
Yorkshire and Humberside	Perinatal	Number	2,060	1,842	1,751	1,511	1,405	1,268	1,090	979	932	1,011	952
		Rate	25.0	22.7	23.7	22.3	21.8	20.9	18.7	17.5	15.7	16.1	14.7
	Infant	Number	1,675	1,585	1,376	1,251	1,189	1,038	854	848	781	868	816
		Rate	20.6	19.8	18.9	18.7	18.7	17.3	14.8	15.3	13.3	13.9	12.7
North West	Perinatal	Number	3,100	2,912	2,580	2,265	2,049	1,821	1,507	1,422	1,363	1,359	1,287
		Rate	27.0	25.6	24.7	23.8	23.3	22.0	19.0	18.6	17.0	15.8	14.7
	Infant	Number	2,375	2,218	1,973	1,827	1,677	1,414	1,187	1,112	1,090	1,151	1,115
		Rate	21.0	19.8	19.2	19.5	19.3	17.3	15.1	14.7	13.7	13.5	12.9
East Midlands	Perinatal	Number	1,245	1,260	1,143	1,028	1,040	863	860	764	728	719	664
		Rate	22.0	22.0	21.5	20.4	20.5	18.1	18.6	17.0	15.6	14.5	12.8
	Infant	Number	981	1,023	929	793	770	713	675	614	620	608	537
		Rate	17.6	18.0	17.7	15.9	15.4	15.1	14.7	13.8	13.4	12.4	10.5

* Per 1,000 total births
† Per 1,000 live births

83

Table A3.29 Infant and perinatal mortality, England and Wales, England, Wales, Standard Regions, 1970-80-*continued*

Area			1970	1971	1972	1973	1974	1975	1976	1977	1978	1979	1980
Standard Regions-*continued*													
West Midlands	Perinatal	Number	2,318	2,123	1,956	1,793	1,597	1,446	1,341	1,193	1,109	1,155	1,085
		Rate	25.6	23.7	23.9	23.6	22.5	21.8	21.1	19.4	17.2	16.8	15.1
	Infant	Number	1,689	1,565	1,487	1,434	1,185	1,109	986	917	871	942	934
		Rate	18.9	17.7	18.4	19.1	16.9	16.9	15.7	15.0	13.7	13.8	13.1
East Anglia	Perinatal	Number	547	541	512	449	399	360	310	282	296	311	282
		Rate	20.8	20.1	19.7	17.7	16.6	15.8	14.0	13.0	13.3	13.0	11.3
	Infant	Number	415	406	401	346	335	332	258	241	238	301	258
		Rate	16.0	15.2	15.6	13.8	14.1	14.7	11.7	11.2	10.8	12.6	10.4
South East	Perinatal	Number	5,783	5,513	4,822	4,520	3,993	3,727	3,235	3,074	2,963	2,913	2,777
		Rate	21.4	20.5	19.2	19.3	18.2	18.0	16.0	15.5	14.2	13.1	12.2
	Infant	Number	4,401	4,233	3,804	3,549	3,201	3,081	2,717	2,485	2,650	2,616	2,633
		Rate	16.5	15.9	15.3	15.3	14.8	15.0	13.6	12.6	12.8	11.9	11.6
South West	Perinatal	Number	1,228	1,164	1,104	999	973	822	754	748	696	684	647
		Rate	21.4	20.1	20.2	19.1	18.5	16.9	16.0	16.2	14.6	13.5	12.3
	Infant	Number	959	908	912	773	755	695	599	592	588	632	608
		Rate	16.9	15.9	16.9	14.9	14.5	14.4	12.9	13.0	12.4	12.5	11.6
WALES	Perinatal	Number	1,099	1,066	904	817	778	678	642	575	566	569	483
		Rate	25.5	24.4	22.3	21.4	21.2	19.7	19.0	17.9	16.8	15.6	12.8
	Infant	Number	794	794	639	615	617	493	457	430	440	447	426
		Rate	18.7	18.4	16.0	16.4	17.0	14.5	13.7	13.5	13.2	12.4	11.4

* *Per 1,000 total births*
† *Per 1,000 live births*

Source: *Registrar General's Statistical Reviews 1970-73.* OPCS, *Local authority vital statistics, Series VS*

Table A3.30 Birthweight-specific mortality by area of residence, England and Wales, 1978-80

Area of residence	Birthweight							Over 2,500 g
	2,500 g or under							
	Live births (number)	Stillbirths		Mortality rates				Perinatal mortality rate*φ
		Number	Rate*	Perinatal*	Under 24 hours†	Early neonatal†	Neonatal†	
ENGLAND AND WALES	126,941	9,769	71.5	131.8	42.0	64.8	73.9	5.3
Northern RHA	7,699	701	83.5	157.4	51.2	80.7	87.8	5.7
Cleveland AHA	1,726	162	85.8	153.6	30.1	74.2	78.2	6.3
Cumbria AHA	1,016	95	85.5	157.5	56.1	78.7	88.6	5.8
Durham AHA	1,425	123	79.5	177.0	80.0	106.0	111.6	5.3
Northumberland AHA	599	54	82.7	153.1	46.7	76.8	88.5	4.6
Gateshead AHA	596	45	70.2	131.0	45.3	65.4	73.8	5.1
Newcastle upon Tyne AHA	662	60	83.1	128.8	22.7	49.8	63.4	6.1
North Tyneside AHA	485	44	83.2	162.6	47.4	86.6	92.8	6.2
South Tyneside AHA	412	43	94.5	149.5	46.1	60.7	70.4	5.2
Sunderland AHA	778	75	87.9	178.2	75.8	99.0	101.5	6.0
Yorkshire RHA	10,130	821	75.0	139.0	43.8	69.2	78.8	5.4
Humberside AHA	2,153	183	78.3	137.4	41.8	64.1	77.1	5.9
North Yorkshire AHA	1,208	101	77.2	142.9	48.0	71.2	77.0	4.7
Bradford AHA	2,170	147	63.4	116.1	34.1	56.2	63.1	5.5
Calderdale AHA	631	43	63.8	149.9	50.7	91.9	107.8	5.4
Kirklees AHA	1,297	83	50.1	120.3	34.7	64.0	72.5	6.4
Leeds AHA	1,901	177	35.2	150.6	46.3	71.5	81.5	4.9
Wakefield AHA	770	87	101.5	192.5	74.0	101.3	110.4	4.6
Trent RHA	11,803	901	70.9	134.1	45.6	68.0	76.3	4.8
Derbyshire AHA	2,058	170	76.3	129.3	39.8	57.3	65.1	6.0
Leicestershire AHA	2,605	195	69.6	124.3	39.5	58.7	67.6	5.3
Lincolnshire AHA	1,168	113	88.2	144.4	44.5	61.6	65.9	5.3
Nottinghamshire AHA	2,778	185	62.4	136.0	51.1	78.5	83.5	3.4
Barnsley AHA	559	45	74.5	162.3	76.9	94.8	112.7	4.1
Doncaster AHA	865	53	57.7	115.5	37.0	61.3	74.0	3.4
Rotherham AHA	655	52	73.6	138.6	32.1	70.2	84.0	6.3
Sheffield AHA	1,115	88	73.2	148.0	56.5	80.7	89.7	4.0

* Per 1,000 total births

† Per 1,000 live births

φ Estimated using OPCS death registration data

85

Table A3.30 Birthweight-specific mortality by area of residence, England and Wales, 1978-80-*continued*

Area of residence	Birthweight							Over 2,500 g
	2,500 g or under							
	Live births (number)	Stillbirths		Mortality rates				Perinatal mortality rate* φ
		Number	Rate*	Perinatal*	Under 24 hours†	Early neonatal†	Neonatal†	
East Anglian RHA	4,340	319	68.5	121.1	38.0	56.5	63.6	4.8
Cambridgeshire AHA	1,446	92	59.8	107.3	28.4	50.5	58.1	5.4
Norfolk AHA	1,693	133	72.8	133.6	42.5	65.6	73.2	4.6
Suffolk AHA	1,201	94	72.6	119.7	43.3	50.8	56.6	4.6
North West Thames RHA	9,710	652	62.9	111.9	33.6	52.2	62.5	4.7
Bedfordshire AHA	1,375	147	96.6	148.5	40.7	57.5	63.3	5.1
Hertfordshire AHA	2,237	152	63.6	121.8	39.3	62.1	72.9	4.0
Barnet AHA	862	58	63.0	110.9	36.0	51.0	60.3	4.6
Brent and Harrow AHA	1,671	79	45.1	81.7	20.3	38.3	46.7	5.1
Ealing, Hammersmith and Hounslow AHA	2,137	130	57.3	100.6	29.5	45.9	58.0	4.6
Hillingdon AHA	561	37	61.9	112.0	39.2	53.5	74.9	5.3
Kensington, Chelsea and Westminster AHA	867	49	53.5	111.4	36.9	61.1	70.4	5.3
North East Thames RHA	10,210	773	70.4	122.1	33.8	55.6	66.9	5.4
Essex AHA	3,081	263	78.6	128.0	34.7	53.6	64.9	5.4
Barking and Havering AHA	966	84	80.0	145.7	42.4	71.4	84.9	4.4
Camden and Islington AHA	932	55	55.7	92.2	24.7	38.6	51.5	7.1
City and East London AHA	2,518	189	69.8	120.1	31.4	54.0	63.9	5.9
Enfield and Haringey AHA	1,373	68	47.2	99.2	29.9	54.6	66.3	5.1
Redbridge and Waltham Forest AHA	1,340	114	78.4	138.2	40.3	64.9	75.4	4.3
South East Thames RHA	8,837	657	69.2	128.7	42.4	63.9	73.2	4.9
East Sussex AHA	1,236	104	77.6	147.8	45.3	76.1	85.0	3.7
Kent AHA	3,502	279	73.8	128.8	42.0	59.4	67.1	5.0
Greenwich and Bexley AHA	1,124	70	58.6	118.1	43.6	63.2	68.5	6.4
Bromley AHA	584	55	86.1	136.2	34.2	54.8	58.2	4.9
Lambeth, Southwark and Lewisham AHA	2,391	149	58.7	121.7	43.1	66.9	82.0	4.7

* *Per 1,000 total births*

† *Per 1,000 live births*

φ *Estimated using OPCS death registration data*

Table A3.30 **Birthweight-specific mortality by area of residence, England and Wales, 1978-80**-*continued*

Area of residence	Birthweight							Over 2,500 g
	2,500 g or under							
	Live births (number)	Stillbirths		Mortality rates				Perinatal mortality rate* φ
		Number	Rate*	Perinatal*	Under 24 hours†	Early neonatal†	Neonatal†	
South West Thames RHA	6,131	473	71.6	131.9	42.1	64.9	73.1	4.8
Surrey AHA	1,874	130	64.9	131.2	51.8	71.0	79.0	5.2
West Sussex AHA	1,349	137	92.2	158.8	39.3	73.4	78.6	4.5
Croydon AHA	892	72	74.7	121.4	37.0	50.4	60.5	4.9
Kingston and Richmond AHA	445	22	47.1	122.1	36.0	78.7	89.9	2.8
Merton, Sutton and Wandsworth AHA	1,571	112	66.5	117.6	37.6	54.7	63.7	5.0
Wessex RHA	6,425	419	61.2	115.0	34.4	57.3	70.2	5.2
Dorset AHA	1,116	71	59.8	120.5	41.2	64.5	70.8	4.0
Hampshire AHA	3,417	208	57.4	102.9	25.5	48.3	66.1	5.0
Wiltshire AHA	1,710	121	66.1	127.3	43.9	65.5	72.5	6.2
Isle of Wight AHA	182	19	94.5	189.1	71.4	104.4	120.9	6.4
Oxford RHA	5,881	391	62.3	118.9	41.7	60.4	67.8	4.8
Berkshire AHA	1,857	123	62.1	124.2	49.5	66.2	71.6	4.5
Buckinghamshire AHA	1,396	115	76.1	135.0	39.4	63.8	70.2	4.8
Northamptonshire AHA	1,482	99	62.6	117.0	41.2	58.0	64.8	6.0
Oxfordshire AHA	1,146	54	45.0	92.5	32.3	49.7	62.8	4.1
South Western RHA	6,348	511	74.5	130.5	39.7	60.5	68.2	5.4
Avon AHA	1,896	148	72.4	137.5	40.1	70.1	74.9	4.8
Cornwall AHA	869	66	70.6	140.1	54.1	74.8	90.9	5.7
Devon AHA	1,707	151	81.3	134.6	38.7	58.0	66.8	5.2
Gloucestershire AHA	1,203	80	62.4	88.9	24.1	28.3	31.6	5.9
Somerset AHA	673	66	89.3	161.0	50.5	78.8	89.2	5.7

* *Per 1,000 total births*

† *Per 1,000 live births*

φ *Estimated using OPCS death registration data*

Table A3.30 Birthweight-specific mortality by area of residence, England and Wales, 1978-80-*continued*

Area of residence	Birthweight 2,500 g or under							Over 2,500 g
	Live births (number)	Stillbirths		Mortality rates				Perinatal mortality rate* φ
		Number	Rate*	Perinatal*	Under 24 hours†	Early neonatal†	Neonatal†	
West Midlands RHA	15,051	1,214	74.6	136.6	42.3	67.0	76.5	5.9
Hereford and Worcester AHA	1,376	117	78.4	131.9	32.0	58.1	64.7	5.3
Shropshire AHA	919	77	77.3	149.6	60.9	78.3	92.5	6.0
Staffordshire AHA	2,563	229	82.0	152.6	51.5	76.9	86.2	4.9
Warwickshire AHA	1,259	73	54.8	121.6	43.7	70.7	77.8	7.0
Birmingham AHA	3,856	278	67.2	130.1	42.5	67.4	77.5	5.5
Coventry AHA	1,009	61	57.0	105.6	36.7	51.5	57.5	8.7
Dudley AHA	742	80	97.3	155.7	40.4	64.7	68.7	7.5
Sandwell AHA	1,065	98	84.3	147.0	46.9	68.5	77.9	6.6
Walsall AHA	888	72	75.0	129.2	24.8	58.6	74.3	6.3
Wolverhampton AHA	967	99	92.9	145.4	33.1	57.9	72.4	5.2
Solihull AHA	407	30	68.6	135.0	34.4	71.3	78.6	3.7
Mersey RHA	5,895	477	74.9	131.7	38.8	61.4	70.6	6.2
Cheshire AHA	1,836	163	81.5	144.6	35.4	68.6	76.8	7.0
Liverpool AHA	1,478	119	74.5	119.0	29.1	48.0	56.8	5.9
St Helens and Knowlsey AHA	1,168	87	69.3	114.7	36.8	48.8	63.4	8.1
Sefton AHA	695	47	63.3	121.3	36.0	61.9	67.6	4.3
Wirral AHA	718	61	78.3	161.7	73.8	90.5	97.5	4.0
North Western RHA	11,831	919	72.1	138.5	48.3	71.6	80.4	5.7
Lancashire AHA	3,733	304	75.3	144.9	49.6	75.3	83.3	5.4
Bolton AHA	834	60	67.1	128.6	42.0	65.9	71.9	7.2
Bury AHA	506	39	71.6	145.0	49.4	79.1	92.9	4.7
Manchester AHA	1,760	93	50.2	111.7	44.3	64.8	80.1	5.5
Oldham AHA	761	53	65.1	109.3	34.2	47.3	55.2	9.0

* Per 1,000 total births
† Per 1,000 live births
φ Estimated using OPCS death registration data

Table A3.30 Birthweight-specific mortality by area of residence, England and Wales, 1978-80-*continued*

Area of residence	Birthweight							Over 2,500 g
	2,500 g or under							
	Live births (number)	Stillbirths		Mortality rates				Perinatal mortality rate* φ
		Number	Rate*	Perinatal*	Under 24 hours†	Early neonatal†	Neonatal†	
North Western RHA-continued								
Rochdale AHA	882	54	57.7	141.0	69.2	88.4	94.1	5.0
Salford AHA	705	56	73.6	141.9	48.2	73.8	83.7	5.9
Stockport AHA	678	68	91.2	162.2	48.7	78.2	85.5	5.4
Tameside AHA	689	59	78.9	136.4	37.7	62.4	68.2	6.7
Trafford AHA	514	41	73.9	133.3	42.8	64.2	72.0	5.4
Wigan AHA	769	92	106.9	178.9	61.1	80.6	85.8	4.7
Wales RHA	6,650	541	75.2	144.5	49.5	74.9	82.1	5.8
Clwyd AHA	834	77	84.5	167.9	50.4	91.1	94.7	4.8
Dyfed AHA	608	49	74.6	140.0	52.6	70.7	80.6	6.3
Gwent AHA	1,154	89	71.6	129.5	47.7	62.4	71.1	6.2
Gwynedd AHA	425	39	84.1	146.6	47.1	68.2	80.0	6.2
Mid Glamorgan AHA	1,527	101	62.0	124.7	44.5	66.8	74.0	6.7
Powys AHA	197	21	96.3	156.0	45.7	66.0	66.0	4.9
South Glamorgan AHA	1,036	72	65.0	139.0	46.3	79.2	91.7	6.0
West Glamorgan AHA	869	93	96.7	180.9	63.3	93.2	93.2	4.4

* Per 1,000 total births

† Per 1,000 live births

φ Estimated using OPCS death registration data

Source: Authors' analysis of DHSS LHS 27/1 returns

Table A4.1 Women's use of birth control services, 1975-81

	1975	1976	1977	1978	1979	1980	1981
England and Wales							
Numbers of women (thousands) using:							
Family planning clinics	1,481.2	1,524.7	1,610.1	1,585.0	1,553.2	1,553.8	1,533.7
Domiciliary services	20.9	19.5	18.4	16.6	16.5	17.3	16.1
General practitioners	1,224.6	2,001.6	2,142.6	2,060.2	2,018.6	2,127.0	2,195.2
Total	2,726.7	3,545.8	3,771.1	3,661.8	3,588.3	3,698.1	3,745.0
Per cent of women aged 15-44	28.6	37.0	38.9	37.3	36.0	36.6	36.5
Scotland							
Numbers of women (thousands) using:							
Family planning clinics	126.6	125.6	133.3	130.5	134.0	137.9	..
Domiciliary services	0.6	1.1	1.3	1.2	3.4	3.4	..
General practitioners	171.4	224.5	238.8	227.5	222.1	222.1	..
Total	298.6	351.1	373.4	359.2	359.4	358.5	..
Per cent of women aged 15-44	29.0	33.8	35.6	33.9	33.6	33.2	..
Northern Ireland							
Numbers of women (thousands) using:							
Family planning clinics	..	..	..	..	..	..	..
Domiciliary services	0	0	0	0	0	0	0
General practitioners	30.8	44.4	37.7	38.8	30.3	32.3	31.7
Per cent of women aged 15-44 using general practitioners	38.3	38.7	39.1	39.5	40.0	40.4	40.8

Sources: Department of Health and Social Security, Information Services Division, Department of Health and Social
Services

Table A4.2   Primary method of birth control chosen by couples attending family planning clinics, 1975-80

Method	1975	1976	1977	1978	1979	1980
England and Wales	%	%	%	%	%	%
Oral contraceptives	68.5	65.6	63.0	57.5	53.8	53.7
IUD	14.3	15.6	16.6	19.4	21.1	20.5
Cap/diaphragm	6.3	6.7	6.5	7.5	7.8	8.1
Sheath	5.7	6.4	7.1	8.7	9.7	9.8
Chemicals	1.0	0.9	0.9	1.0	0.9	0.7
Rhythm	0.0	0.0	0.0	0.0	0.0	0.0
Female sterilisation	0.0	0.1	0.1	0.1	0.1	0.1
Vasectomy	0.9	1.1	1.0	1.1	1.0	1.0
Other	0.8	0.5	0.5	0.6	0.7	0.7
None	2.6	3.2	3.6	4.3	4.9	5.4
Total men and women attending (thousands)	1,489.3	1,545.4	1,630.8	1,607.7	1,570.4	1,568.1
Scotland						
Oral contraceptives	75	68	70	61	57	55
IUD	10	11	13	16	17	17
Cap/diaphragm	4	5	5	6	6	6
Sheath	5	6	5	8	8	10
Chemicals	1	1	1	1	1	1
Rhythm	0	0	0	0	0	0
Female sterilisation	0	0	0	0	0	0
Vasectomy	1	2	1	3	3	3
Other	1	3	1	1	1	1
None	4	4	5	5	8	8
Total mcn and women attending (thousands)	127.8	127.5	134.3	135.3	137.3	141.5

Source: DHSS, SBL708 return, *Scottish Health Statistics*

Table A4.3   General practitioners' claims for providing contraceptive services, 1975-81

	1975	1976	1977	1978	1979	1980	1981
General practitioners registered for providing contraceptive services							
England	18,809	19,515	19,869	20,140	20,512	21,018	..
Wales	1,219	1,235	1,256	1,274	1,299	1,342	..
Scotland	7,689	2,732	2,767	2,800	2,858	2,899	..
Northern Ireland	587	614	616	645	648	698	723
Women registered with a GP for contraceptive services							
England Total	1,157,254	1,898,306	2,038,039	1,959,008	1,921,825	2,023,893	2,091,519
IUD fitting	13,577	53,802	67,718	97,522	109,976	106,880	102,906
Other services	1,143,677	1,844,504	1,970,321	1,861,486	1,811,849	1,917,013	1,988,613
Wales Total	67,398	103,302	104,546	101,181	96,862	103,026	103,664
IUD fitting	435	1,576	2,201	3,730	3,932	3,913	4,145
Other services	66,963	101,726	102,345	97,451	92,870	99,113	99,519
Scotland Total	171,396	224,464	238,800	227,475	222,065	217,227	..
IUD fitting	919	2,940	4,192	6,028	7,664	9,059	..
Other services	170,477	221,524	234,608	221,447	214,401	208,168	..
Northern Ireland							
Total	31,013	44,812	38,049	39,489	31,457	33,569	32,951
IUD fitting	179	397	324	702	1,160	1,277	1,226
Other services	30,834	44,415	37,727	38,787	30,297	32,292	31,725

Source: Department of Health and Social Security, Welsh Office, Information Services Division, Department of Health and Social Services

Table A4.4 **Estimated numbers of prescriptions for contraceptives by family practitioners** *thousands*

	England and Wales	Scotland	Northern Ireland
Oestrogen-progestogen combinations			
1967	715	. .	. .
1968	820	. .	. .
1969	803	. .	. .
1970	771	. .	. .
1971	876	. .	31
1972	923	. .	36
1973	986	. .	44
1974	1,340	. .	48
1975	3,713	. .	82
1976	. .	. .	138
Oral contraceptives			
1975	3,757	393	. .
1976	5,939	647	136
1977	5,786	627	135
1978	5,188	549	132
1979	5,116	528	114
1980	5,042	550	108
1981	5,288	580	113
Contraceptive appliances			
1975	36	0	. .
1976	85	0	. .
1977	95	0	. .
1978	121	0	. .
1979	158	1	. .
1980	133	4	. .
1981	120	4	. .

Source: DHSS, ISD, Department of Health and Social Services. Based on a 1 in 200 sample in England and Wales and a 1 in 100 sample in Scotland of prescriptions dispensed by chemists and appliance contractors.

Table A4.5   Sales and imports of contraceptive sheaths, United Kingdom, 1974-82

Years ending 31 March	Sales by London Rubber Company Products Ltd in UK		Imported into UK	
	Number of sheaths (thousand gross)	£ (thousands)	Weight of sheaths and packing (thousand kg)	£ (thousands)
1974	840	3,845	na	336
1975	737	3,649	97.3	521
1976	823	4,003	78.7	461
1977	790	4,004	73.3	625
1978	752	4,537	25.2	250
1979	779	5,425	25.0	208
1980	785	6,036	50.8	401
1981	757	7,033	51.6	425
1982	712	7,241	43.2	361

London Rubber Company sales figures were obtained from the company. Import data were obtained from Customs and Excise. Data for 1974 and 1975 include an unknown proportion of rubber items which were not sheaths. As imported sheaths were in packages of different sizes, there is no way of converting the weight, which includes packaging, into numbers of sheaths.
Source: Monopolies and Mergers Commission. *Contraceptive sheaths.* HMSO, 1982.

Table A4.6   Percentage of women using contraception at the earliest stage of marriage

	Year of marriage						
	Before 1910	1910-19	1920-24	1925-29	1930-34	1935-39	1940-42
Percentage of women without pre-nuptial conceptions first using contraception at marriage 1946*	6	11	16	21	26	33	40

	Years in which interval began					
	1946-50	1951-55	1956-60	1961-65	1966-70	1971-75
Percentage of women who ever used contraception in their first inter-pregnancy interval, 1975†	47	50	52	61	72	83

Source: * Lewis-Faning E. *Family Limitation* (Table 68). Women who had been married for less than five years at the time of the interview in 1946 were excluded from the analysis. The survey covered married women in selected hospitals in England and Scotland.

† Bone M. *The family planning services: changes and effects* (Table 7.1).

Table A4.7 Estimated numbers of sterilisations, England and Wales, 1971–78

Year	'Interval'† Estimated number	Rate*	With delivery† Estimated number	Rate*	With legal abortion‡ Number	Rate*	Total Estimated number	Rate*
In-patients								
1971	20,880	224.0	26,650	285.8	14,462	155.1	61,992	664.9
1972	24,420	260.8	22,600	242.0	13,891	148.4	60,911	651.2
1973	28,910	306.6	21,860	234.2	11,918	126.4	62,688	667.1
1974	29,776	314.5	19,219	203.0	10,733	113.4	59,728	630.8
1975	23,680	248.9	17,444	183.3	9,172	96.4	50,296	528.6
1976	35,116	365.9	16,333	170.2	8,909	92.8	60,358	628.9
1977	42,180	435.0	14,641	151.0	8,872	91.5	65,693	677.4
1978	53,260	542.1	14,447	147.0	9,145	93.1	76,852	782.2
1979	..	..	..	..	9,371	94.1	..	..
1980	..	..	..	..	9,426	93.4	..	..
Day cases								
1975	1,020	10.7	0	–	0†	–	1,020	10.7
1976	1,240	12.9	0	–	0†	–	1,240	12.9
1977	2,000	20.6	0	–	0†	–	2,000	20.6
1978	2,560	26.1	0	–	0†	–	2,560	26.1
Total								
1975	24,700	259.6	17,444	183.3	9,172	96.4	51,316	539.4
1976	36,356	378.8	16,333	170.2	8,909	92.8	61,598	641.8
1977	44,180	455.6	14,641	151.0	8,872	91.5	67,693	698.0
1978	55,820	558.1	14,447	147.0	9,145	93.1	79,412	808.3

* Rate per 100,000 women aged 15–44.
† NHS hospitals only.
‡ NHS and private hospitals.
Data about sterilisations done at the time of legal abortion are derived from abortion notifications. Routine tabulations do not distinguish between in-patients and day cases. As the Hospital In-Patient Enquiry sample did not include any instances of sterilisation with legal abortion being done as day cases, it was assessed that all women undergoing sterilisation with legal abortion would have been in-patients.
Source: OPCS, Hospital In-Patient Enquiry and *Abortion Statistics, Series AB*.

Table A4.8 **Interval sterilisation. Estimated numbers of hospital discharges for which sterilisation was recorded, England and Wales, 1971-78**

Year	Division and ligation of oviducts	Endoscopic sterilisation	Method not stated	Total
In-patients				
1971	14,170	1,310	5,400	20,880
1972	12,890	6,150	5,380	24,420
1973	12,780	8,950	7,180	28,910
1974	10,617	8,936	10,223	29,776
1975	7,505	8,670	7,505	23,680
1976	10,057	15,002	10,057	35,116
1977	12,850	23,530	5,800	42,180
1978	14,290	32,660	6,310	53,260
Day cases				
1975	60	960		1,120
1976	120	1,120		1,240
1977	90	1,910		2,000
1978	30	2,530		2,560

Source: OPCS Hospital In-patient Enquiry, reference tables.

Table A4.9 **Estimated numbers of hospital discharges associated with delivery after which sterilisation was performed, England and Wales, 1968, 1971-78**

Year	Estimated numbers of discharges	Percentage of total deliveries in England and Wales	Method of delivery			
			Caesarean section		Other methods	
			Estimated numbers	Percentage of all caesarean sections in NHS hospitals	Estimated numbers	Percentage of all other deliveries in NHS hospitals
1968	10,930	1.3	3,500	10.8	7,430	1.2
1971	26,650	3.4	..	..	..	..
1972	22,600	3.1	..	..	..	..
1973	21,860	3.2	4,640	14.6	17,220	2.9
1974	19,219	3.0	..	..	..	..
1975	17,444	2.9	..	..	..	..
1976	16,333	2.8	..	..	..	..
1977	14,641	2.6	..	..	..	..
1978	14,447	2.4	4,935	11.5	9,912	1.9

Source: OPCS Hospital In-patient Enquiry, unpublished data

Table A4.10 Sterilisation in Scotland, 1975-79

Year	With delivery		With legal abortion		Other in-patient sterilisations		Total	
	Number	Rate*	Number	Rate*	Number	Rate*	Number	Rate*
1975	8,213	798.9	2,610	253.9	1,200	116.7	12,023	1,169.5
1976	9,442	908.7	2,339	225.1	1,002	96.4	12,783	1,230.3
1977	9,464	902.0	1,805	172.0	1,087	103.6	12,356	1,177.6
1978	12,308	1,163.0	1,679	158.7	1,111	105.0	15,098	1,426.7
1979	11,351	1,061.6	1,833	171.4	1,004	93.9	14,188	1,326.9

* Per 100,000 women age 15-44
Source: Information Services Division. *Scottish Health Statistics 1980*

Table A4.11 Sterilisation with legal abortion, England and Wales 1968-80

Year	In NHS hospitals	As a percentage of all NHS abortions	In other approved places	As a percentage of all non-NHS abortions	Total	As a percentage of all abortions
1968	..	..	..	..	5,128	23.0
1969	..	..	..	..	11,126	22.3
1970	13,732	29.0	214	0.7	13,946	18.4
1971	14,193	26.6	269	0.7	14,462	15.3
1972	13,512	23.8	379	0.7	13,891	12.8
1973	11,434	20.6	484	0.9	11,918	10.8
1974	10,250	18.3	483	0.9	10,733	9.8
1975	8,515	16.7	657	1.2	9,172	8.6
1976	8,145	16.1	764	1.5	8,909	8.7
1977	7,889	15.0	983	2.0	8,872	8.6
1978	7,971	14.5	1,174	2.1	9,145	8.2
1979	7,972	14.3	1,399	2.2	9,371	7.8
1980	8,077	13.3	1,349	2.0	9,426	7.3

Source: OPCS, *Abortion Statistics, Series AB*

Table A4.12 Estimated numbers of vasectomies in NHS non-psychiatric hospitals and in family planning clinics, 1975-81

Year	NHS hospitals		Family planning clinics
	In-patients	Day cases	
England and Wales			
1975	2,380	15,080	17,604
1976	2,960	19,280	17,528
1977	3,220	27,130	17,182
1978	4,340	35,880	18,097
1979	3,470	38,760	16,336
1980	..	36,810	14,432
1981	..	..	14,189

Scotland		
	NHS hospitals	Family planning clinics
1975	485	982
1976	844	1,497
1977	1,152	1,737
1978	2,776	2,585
1979	3,615	2,802
1980	..	2,706

Northern Ireland		
	NHS hospitals	Family planning clinics
1975	111	0
1976	136	0
1977	155	0
1978	248	0
1979	235	0
1980	271	0
1981	293	0

Source: OPCS, Hospital In-patient Enquiry
DHSS SBL 708 summary
Scottish Home and Health Department, *Scottish Health Statistics*
Northern Ireland Department of Health and Social Services

Table A4.13 Estimated discharge rates† by age, for selected gynaecological operations, England and Wales, 1970-78

Year	15-44			45-64			65 and over		
	Hysterectomy*	Colporrhaphy	Oophorectomy	Hysterectomy*	Colporrhaphy	Oophorectomy	Hysterectomy*	Colporrhaphy	Oophorectomy
1970	302.3	44.7	..	451.5	181.9	..	128.5	129.1	..
1971	321.4	36.3	57.3	442.1	180.0	19.3	148.6	115.1	17.1
1972	339.0	32.8	46.5	445.5	167.7	21.2	129.2	123.6	13.9
1973	332.9	28.4	47.5	433.0	143.3	22.1	129.3	113.2	16.9
1974	341.5	30.1	45.0	403.9	136.7	23.1	137.0	107.7	15.1
1975	295.9	23.6	47.2	401.3	109.1	21.1	127.7	90.6	12.7
1976	324.5	32.2	49.0	406.9	125.0	18.3	146.6	108.8	13.6
1977	333.2	28.5	39.6	394.6	114.9	14.6	113.3	94.1	13.1
1978	315.3	26.5	41.5	370.1	107.9	17.1	114.7	92.3	12.2

† *Per 100,000 women*
* *Includes hysterectomy with oophorectomy*
Source: OPCS, Hospital In-patient Enquiry

Table A4.14 Percentages of ever-married women who were sterile (or whose husbands were sterile), fecund and at risk by age, 1975

Risk group	Age									
	All ages	20	20-24	25-29	30-34	35-39	40-44	45-49	50-54	55
Fecund	69	95	94	87	76	74	72	61	24	2
- and pregnant/trying	7	17	21	18	8	2	1	0	0	0
- and not pregnant nor trying to conceive = 'at risk'	62	79	73	69	69	72	70	61	24	2
Infecund:										
Sterilisation	11	0	3	9	18	18	13	9	4	2
woman	6	0	1	4	9	10	7	7	3	2
husband	5	0	2	5	9	8	7	2	1	0
Other operation	6	0	0	1	1	3	8	11	15	16
Post-menopausal	10	0	0	0	0	0	2	13	52	74
Other causes	3	0	0	1	3	4	4	4	4	6
Total infecund	30	0	3	10	22	25	27	37	74	98
Not known	2	5	3	3	1	1	2	2	1	0
Base: ever-married women under 56 = 100%	*3,898*	*42*	*372*	*661*	*601*	*558*	*531*	*514*	*568*	*51*

Source: Bone M, *Family planning services: changes and effects*

Table A4.15 Menopausal status by age, 1975

Age (in years)	Percentage of women who are:			Number of women 'at risk'* = 100%
	Pre-menopausal	Menopausal	Post-menopausal	
40	97	1	1	*75*
41	98	1	1	*81*
42	98	2	0	*80*
43	97	0	3	*75*
44	93	0	7	*87*
45	91	0	9	*87*
46	93	3	4	*70*
47	84	1	15	*73*
48	76	3	21	*95*
49	57	6	37	*63*
50	55	4	41	*104*
51	37	6	57	*79*
52	23	7	69	*94*
53	19	4	78	*80*
54	6	0	94	*84*
55	3	0	97	*39*

* *'At risk' here means at risk of being menopausal and excludes those who were otherwise sterile.*
Source: Bone M, *Family Planning services: changes and effects*

Table A4.16 Legal abortions to residents of England and Wales, 1968-80

Year	Abortions as percentage at total births plus abortions	Percentage of married women	Percentage Under NHS	Total aged 15-44	Total per 1,000 women aged 15-44
1968 (8 months)	2.6	45.2	64.9	21,411	3.46
1969	5.8	46.1	67.4	48,051	5.26
1970	8.7	45.2	62.4	73,489	7.97
1971	10.7	43.9	56.5	91,699	10.03
1972	12.9	43.2	52.4	105,511	11.27
1973	13.9	42.3	50.2	107,430	11.39
1974	14.5	41.2	51.2	106,446	11.40
1975	14.8	40.5	48.0	103,022	11.00
1976	14.7	39.6	49.6	98,763	10.46
1977	15.2	38.6	51.2	99,570	10.44
1978	15.7	37.7	49.2	108,678	11.25
1979	15.8	35.9	46.1	117,512	11.97
1980	16.3	34.8	47.0	127,107	12.59

Source: OPCS, *Abortion statistics, Series AB*

Table A4.17 Legal abortions to residents of Scotland, 1970-80

Year	Country of termination		Total	As a percentage of total births and abortions	Abortions per 1,000 women aged 15-44
	Scotland	England and Wales			
1970	5,254	309	5,563	5.9	5.5
1971	6,332	524	6,856	7.2	6.8
1972	7,609	835	8,444	9.6	8.4
1973	7,498	1,068	8,566	10.2	8.4
1974	7,545	1,026	8,571	10.1	8.3
1975	7,300	1,054	8,354	10.8	8.1
1976	7,183	950	8,133	11.0	7.8
1977	7,283	840	8,123	11.4	7.7
1978	7,422	976	8,398	11.5	7.9
1979	7,754	1,028	8,782	11.3	8.2
1980	7,855	1,179	9,034	11.5	8.4

Source: Registrar General, Scotland, *Annual Report.* OPCS, *Abortion Statistics, Series AB*

Table A4.18 Legal abortions to non-residents carried out in England and Wales, 1970-80

Country of usual residence	1970	1971	1972	1973	1974	1975	1976	1977	1978	1979	1980
Scotland	309	524	835	1,068	1,026	1,054	950	840	976	1,028	1,179
Northern Ireland	199	648	775	1,007	1,092	1,115	1,142	1,244	1,311	1,425	1,565
Irish Republic	261	578	974	1,193	1,421	1,573	1,821	2,184	2,548	2,804	3,320
Channel Islands and Isle of Man	165	215	295	306	371	373	336	389	413	457	484
Belgium and Luxembourg*	562	2,111	2,536	1,462	641	403	390	349	338	231	198
Denmark	..	226	86	27	4	3	2	5	3	2	5
France	2,267	11,986	25,189	35,293	36,443	14,056	4,568	4,143	3,187	3,047	4,117
German Federal Republic	3,621	13,560	17,531	11,326	5,991	3,404	2,384	1,705	1,171	722	584
Italy	..	..	480	1,171	1,751	5,647	8,211	7,549	3,911	959	774
Netherlands	816	792	243	101	78	83	97	88	79	38	41
Austria	..	..	257	291	268	87	91	115	103	64	58
Spain	..	..	730	1,763	2,978	4,393	6,397	10,187	14,015	17,061	18,342
Switzerland	115	389	675	719	618	413	308	274	292	234	179
Other European countries†	..	..	185	260	288	277	348	454	480	137	128
Canada	297	67	52	34	24	13	20	11	17	8	6
USA	1,061	187	181	104	63	54	56	57	70	63	68
Other countries	390	924	345	456	438	530	640	733	793	855	928
Total	10,603	32,207	51,319	56,581	53,495	33,478	27,761	30,327	29,707	29,135	31,976
Total as a percentage of all abortions notified	12.2	25.4	32.1	33.9	32.8	24.0	21.4	22.8	21.0	19.5	19.9

* 1970 and 1971 figures are for Belgium only
† Including Norway, Sweden and Portugal
Source: OPCS, Abortion Statistics, Series AB

Table A4.19 Legal abortions by area of residence, 1980

Area of residence	Abortions (percentages)			Total abortions	Total abortions per 1000 women aged 15-44
	As percentage of total births plus abortions	Percentage to married women	Percentage under NHS		
ENGLAND AND WALES	**16.3**	**34.3**	**47.0**	**128,927**	**12.77**
ENGLAND	**16.4**	**34.1**	**46.5**	**122,636**	**12.86**
Northern RHA	**11.9**	**34.8**	**88.2**	**5,619**	**8.87**
Cleveland AHA	9.9	35.3	86.7	969	7.92
Hartlepool HD	7.4	28.3	92.5	106	5.27
North Tees HD	10.3	38.3	93.2	311	8.04
South Tees HD	10.4	35.0	81.9	552	8.54
Cumbria AHA	12.1	36.5	78.2	799	9.60
East Cumbria HD	13.6	34.3	86.4	434	9.58
South West Cumbria HD	10.6	39.9	57.4	148	7.29
West Cumbria HD	10.7	38.7	76.0	217	7.95
Durham AHA	10.4	41.0	89.8	924	7.38
Darlington HD	7.5	41.1	83.1	124	5.10
Durham HD	11.1	43.3	89.9	397	7.81
North West Durham HD	10.4	36.8	91.7	133	7.51
South West Durham HD	11.5	39.6	91.9	270	8.33
Northumberland AHA	11.7	38.3	88.5	504	8.62
Gateshead AHA	10.8	29.6	90.9	331	7.77
Newcastle upon Tyne AHA	16.3	27.1	93.2	704	12.14
North Tyneside AHA	14.4	32.3	93.4	412	11.23
South Tyneside AHA	15.0	29.3	92.4	368	11.68
Sunderland AHA	12.3	36.5	87.7	608	9.28
Yorkshire RHA	**13.6**	**31.7**	**39.2**	**7,574**	**10.46**
Humberside AHA	12.3	36.1	65.0	1,567	8.84
Hull HD	13.8	33.1	51.9	607	11.00
Beverley HD	10.3	33.9	48.4	283	5.79
Grimsby HD	11.0	34.8	79.7	276	8.17
Scunthorpe HD	12.9	43.1	86.3	401	10.18
North Yorkshire AHA	14.1	36.4	50.0	1,267	9.69
Northallerton HD	11.0	46.3	79.3	164	7.81
York HD	14.0	35.8	24.6	472	9.33
Scarborough HD	16.2	30.9	72.4	304	12.31
Harrogate HD	13.6	33.3	36.0	228	9.19
Bradford AHA	11.1	34.5	28.2	972	10.49
Bradford HD	10.8	34.1	16.0	730	10.61
Airedale HD	13.1	38.7	71.3	341	10.15

Table A1.19 Legal abortions by area of residence, 1980 - *continued*

Area of residence	Abortions (percentages)			Total abortions	Total abortions per 1000 women aged 15-44
	As percentage of total births plus abortions	Percentage to married women	Percentage under NHS		
Yorkshire RHA - continued					
Calderdale AHA	12.9	34.7	24.8	383	10.70
Kirklees AHA	12.8	35.8	12.2	802	10.52
Huddersfield HD	13.7	35.0	12.2	466	10.96
Dewsbury HD	11.8	36.9	12.2	336	9.97
Leeds AHA	17.1	30.4	25.5	1,881	12.98
Western (Leeds) HD	17.4	29.3	23.2	961	13.15
Eastern (Leeds) HD	16.8	31.5	27.9	920	12.81
Wakefield AHA	14.1	38.7	52.8	702	10.57
Western (Wakefield) HD	15.2	38.0	37.7	361	12.07
Eastern (Pontefract) HD	13.0	39.6	68.9	341	9.34
Trent RHA	**14.0**	**37.9**	**54.2**	**9,927**	**10.56**
Derbyshire AHA	14.4	42.2	56.3	1,976	10.80
Central Derbyshire HD	15.2	44.2	74.2	504	10.79
North Derbyshire HD	12.6	43.7	28.9	654	9.19
South Derbyshire HD	15.8	39.6	70.5	755	12.80
Leicestershire AHA	13.1	36.0	24.8	1,856	10.40
East Leicestershire HD	14.1	42.6	28.2	664	12.30
North West Leicestershire HD	12.4	31.9	28.2	571	10.25
South West Leicestershire HD	12.8	32.9	18.0	621	9.04
Lincolnshire AHA	11.7	36.3	71.7	909	8.17
Lincolnshire South HD	11.9	39.2	78.6	472	8.31
Lincolnshire North HD	11.4	33.2	64.3	437	8.03
Nottinghamshire AHA	14.3	35.4	71.4	2,181	10.88
Central Nottinghamshire HD	13.4	40.3	64.6	590	10.52
Worksop and Retford HD	13.3	45.8	66.7	192	9.65
North Nottingham HD	14.1	32.0	78.4	560	11.07
South Nottingham HD	15.4	31.7	72.7	839	11.37
Barnsley AHA	14.3	45.2	54.8	487	10.92
Doncaster AHA	15.6	42.7	80.7	745	12.25
Rotherham AHA	11.5	39.5	48.1	474	9.29
Sheffield AHA	17.4	33.7	38.3	1,299	11.73
Northern HD	15.0	38.9	42.4	483	10.85
Southern HD	19.1	30.6	35.9	816	12.33

Table A4.19 Legal abortions by area of residence, 1980 - *continued*

Area of residence	Abortions (percentages)			Total abortions	Total abortions per 1000 women aged 15-44
	As percentage of total births plus abortions	Percentage to married women	Percentage under NHS		
East Anglian RHA	**13.4**	**37.6**	**75.4**	**3,861**	**10.03**
Cambridgeshire AHA	13.4	39.2	80.8	1,284	10.17
Cambridge HD	15.6	37.5	84.0	898	11.51
Peterborough HD	10.0	44.1	73.0	333	7.91
Norfolk AHA	13.9	37.2	78.5	1,394	10.05
Norwich HD	14.2	36.5	79.9	886	9.96
Great Yarmouth and Waveney HD	13.1	33.7	62.3	350	9.67
King's Lynn HD	12.8	39.1	78.8	325	9.45
Suffolk AHA	12.8	36.3	65.8	1,183	9.85
Bury St Edmunds HD	13.0	40.9	83.2	457	10.16
Ipswich HD	12.9	34.6	57.5	612	10.13
North West Thames RHA	**23.7**	**31.8**	**40.1**	**14,845**	**19.91**
Bedfordshire AHA	14.3	39.4	65.2	1,378	12.69
Northern HD	14.9	41.1	78.8	637	12.79
Southern HD	13.8	37.9	53.4	741	12.60
Hertfordshire AHA	16.8	35.4	43.0	2,524	12.48
North Hertfordshire HD	15.3	33.8	40.2	470	11.69
East Hertfordshire HD	17.3	38.0	50.1	743	12.38
North West Hertfordshire HD	16.5	34.5	37.9	672	12.68
South West Hertfordshire HD	17.1	32.2	36.7	482	12.52
Barnet AHA	26.0	34.6	38.6	1,328	22.21
Barnet and Finchley HD	26.2	37.0	41.3	913	20.89
Edgware and Hendon HD	22.3	34.7	38.6	692	18.96
Brent and Harrow AHA	24.8	33.8	23.0	2,172	23.25
Brent HD	28.5	32.3	21.2	1,287	29.72
Harrow HD	20.4	39.6	21.5	687	17.18
Ealing, Hammersmith and Hounslow AHA	25.2	34.8	46.6	3,255	23.33
Hounslow HD	21.7	41.0	57.9	813	20.58
South Hammersmith HD	36.1	23.7	49.4	989	31.50
North Hammersmith HD	25.5	31.5	43.8	479	21.29
Ealing HD	21.5	41.3	38.6	961	21.55
Hillingdon AHA	19.8	39.5	44.6	765	16.42
Kensington, Chelsea and Westminster AHA	46.6	19.1	32.2	3,423	35.92
North West HD	37.9	18.9	42.7	1,344	33.43

Table A4.19 Legal abortions by area of residence, 1980 *continued*

Area of residence	Abortions (percentages)			Total abortions	Total abortions per 1000 women aged 15-44
	As percentage of total births plus abortions	Percentage to married women	Percentage under NHS		
North West Thames RHA - continued					
North East HD	54.8	21.6	32.4	685	41.77
South HD	50.5	18.2	23.3	1,573	35.51
North East Thames RHA	**22.0**	**33.6**	**49.9**	**14,653**	**19.05**
Essex AHA	14.6	40.7	52.7	3,366	11.01
Basildon and Thurrock HD	11.4	40.4	36.8	549	8.93
Chelmsford HD	13.8	41.3	71.3	756	10.33
Colchester HD	14.5	42.9	62.7	587	10.61
Harlow HD	20.2	39.7	47.5	823	15.41
Southend HD	13.8	39.5	41.9	651	10.45
Barking and Havering AHA	19.5	39.1	54.9	1,220	15.70
Barking HD	19.1	38.0	54.1	492	17.51
Havering HD	19.8	39.8	55.5	728	14.68
Camden and Islington AHA	34.6	23.6	41.5	2,425	28.77
North Camden HD	31.3	22.6	35.9	627	21.77
South Camden HD	45.0	19.5	42.8	673	36.18
Islington HD	32.1	26.6	43.8	1,125	30.49
City and East London AHA	25.1	27.6	52.4	3,311	29.43
City and Hackney HD	24.6	25.3	34.6	1,104	28.75
Newham HD	23.6	39.2	53.6	1,219	26.85
Tower Hamlets HD	27.9	15.9	70.9	988	34.43
Enfield and Haringey AHA	25.5	32.3	51.8	2,245	21.97
Enfield HD	21.7	39.3	57.4	937	17.88
Haringey HD	29.1	27.3	47.7	1,308	26.27
Redbridge and Waltham Forest AHA	25.2	41.2	46.5	2,086	24.09
East Roding HD	21.4	42.6	37.2	784	18.58
West Roding HD	28.2	40.4	52.1	1,302	29.32
South East Thames RHA	**19.2**	**31.3**	**48.2**	**10,906**	**15.37**
East Sussex AHA	20.1	31.0	29.5	1,735	14.28
Brighton HD	23.5	30.6	23.3	990	16.92
Eastbourne HD	18.3	32.5	31.1	453	12.21
Hastings HD	15.2	30.1	47.6	292	11.27
Kent AHA	14.2	37.9	49.6	3,241	10.95
South East Kent HD	15.3	40.1	75.6	566	12.09
Canterbury and Thanet HD	16.8	33.4	53.7	674	12.72
Dartford and Gravesham HD	13.2	36.6	37.9	464	9.91
Maidstone HD	12.7	39.6	35.5	369	9.02

Table A4.19 Legal abortions by area of residence, 1980 - *continued*

Area of residence	Abortions (percentages)			Total abortions	Total abortions per 1000 women aged 15-44
	As percentage of total births plus abortions	Percentage to married women	Percentage under NHS		
South East Thames RHA - continued					
Medway HD	12.6	42.2	47.1	763	11.09
Tunbridge Wells HD	14.8	34.1	37.5	405	10.20
Greenwich and Bexley AHA	18.8	35.3	46.3	1,375	15.73
Bexley HD	16.4	40.0	46.4	545	11.87
Greenwich HD	20.8	32.2	46.3	830	20.00
Bromley AHA	18.7	35.6	49.9	756	13.19
Lambeth, Southwark and Lewisham AHA	27.0	23.6	55.9	3,799	25.81
St Thomas' HD	30.7	22.3	47.4	1,098	28.67
Kings' HD	28.5	21.6	62.6	1,336	30.09
Guy's HD	22.1	27.2	57.8	606	21.64
Lewisham HD	25.0	26.0	54.8	759	20.79
South West Thames RHA	**19.3**	**32.6**	**36.5**	**8,505**	**14.84**
Surrey AHA	16.3	33.7	33.0	2,292	11.44
North Surrey HD	17.4	36.1	50.3	352	12.31
North West Surrey HD	14.2	37.2	28.2	436	10.58
West Surrey and North East Hampshire HD	12.9	38.1	38.8	572	9.86
South West Surrey HD	17.9	31.7	25.3	423	11.95
Mid Surrey HD	19.2	30.2	48.4	401	12.45
East Surrey HD	16.3	32.5	16.7	419	11.48
West Sussex AHA	15.7	35.9	24.0	1,456	11.77
Chichester HD	15.2	35.1	41.0	305	9.84
Cuckfield and Crawley HD	14.8	37.3	12.1	652	12.44
Worthing HD	17.4	34.7	29.1	499	12.38
Croydon AHA	20.8	34.9	28.1	1,168	17.41
Kingston and Richmond AHA	19.6	32.5	54.3	871	14.37
Merton, Sutton and Wandsworth AHA	25.6	28.8	44.2	2,718	22.37
Roehampton HD	28.3	29.6	50.4	419	17.46
Wandsworth and East Merton HD	30.0	27.1	48.9	1,582	33.88
Sutton and West Merton HD	18.9	32.8	33.5	827	14.31
Wessex RHA	**13.9**	**35.2**	**50.6**	**5,546**	**10.20**
Dorset AHA	16.6	32.2	29.7	1,276	11.65
East Dorset HD	18.3	32.3	20.7	965	12.92

Table A4.19 Legal abortions by area of residence, 1980 - *continued*

Area of residence	Abortions (percentages)			Total abortions	Total abortions per 1000 women aged 15-44
	As percentage of total births plus abortions	Percentage to married women	Percentage under NHS		
Wessex RHA - continued					
West Dorset HD	12.9	31.8	57.6	311	8.94
Hampshire AHA	13.2	35.3	57.3	3,040	10.04
Portsmouth and South East Hampshire HD	14.0	32.5	57.3	1,103	10.81
Southampton and South West Hampshire HD	13.8	32.4	77.2	842	10.37
Winchester and Central Hampshire HD	13.1	42.7	42.9	403	9.93
Basingstoke and North Hampshire HD	10.8	39.1	35.1	353	8.00
Wiltshire AHA	13.0	39.2	58.6	1,010	9.08
Salisbury HD	15.7	44.4	71.3	279	11.12
Swindon HD	13.0	37.7	46.6	446	9.37
Bath HD	13.5	33.8	67.1	721	9.40
Isle of Wight AHA	15.0	33.2	43.6	220	11.00
Oxford RHA	**14.7**	**37.4**	**50.9**	**5,703**	**11.55**
Berkshire AHA	14.6	37.4	26.5	1,693	11.42
East Berkshire HD	15.7	38.7	23.3	954	13.34
West Berkshire HD	13.8	36.5	31.3	882	9.75
Buckinghamshire AHA	14.3	42.8	48.1	1,401	12.12
Aylesbury HD	13.4	44.5	64.6	681	12.27
High Wycombe HD	15.3	41.4	33.9	643	11.84
Northamptonshire AHA	12.9	37.5	50.4	1,136	10.04
Kettering HD	11.5	42.3	47.2	477	9.14
Northampton HD	14.1	34.0	52.7	659	10.82
Oxfordshire AHA	16.9	32.0	82.1	1,473	12.62
South Western RHA	**14.1**	**33.6**	**74.6**	**6,497**	**10.18**
Avon AHA	15.6	30.8	75.0	2,161	11.25
Bristol and Weston HD	16.6	30.0	77.0	926	12.10
Frenchay HD	12.5	34.5	75.1	394	8.91
Southmead HD	16.1	31.0	76.4	538	11.47
Cornwall (and Scilly) AHA	14.2	40.8	87.9	861	10.46
Devon AHA	13.9	33.3	83.9	1,784	9.93
Exeter HD	14.1	32.7	72.0	529	9.85
North Devon HD	8.2	35.7	87.6	129	5.33
Plymouth HD	13.9	33.9	90.2	687	10.62
Torbay HD	17.1	32.3	87.2	439	11.83

Table A4.19 Legal abortions by area of residence, 1980 - *continued*

Area of residence	Abortions (percentages)			Total abortions	Total abortions per 1000 women aged 15-44
	As percentage of total births plus abortions	Percentage to married women	Percentage under NHS		
South Western RHA - continued					
Gloucestershire AHA	15.3	34.4	54.5	1,153	11.26
Somerset AHA	9.5	32.5	64.1	538	6.58
West Midlands RHA	**16.4**	**36.8**	**22.1**	**14,050**	**13.26**
Hereford and Worcester AHA	16.1	40.9	43.9	1,631	12.42
Hereford HD	16.3	38.7	24.5	364	12.30
Bromsgrove and Redditch HD	13.7	42.9	36.1	382	11.20
Kidderminster HD	14.2	41.2	37.0	216	10.05
Worcester HD	18.8	40.8	61.1	669	14.51
Shropshire AHA	15.8	41.9	35.9	896	11.70
Staffordshire AHA	13.9	39.3	41.2	2,301	10.79
Mid Staffordshire HD	16.3	42.3	23.6	795	12.36
North Staffordshire HD	12.8	34.8	70.7	927	9.75
South East Staffordshire HD	13.0	42.5	18.1	579	10.74
Warwickshire AHA	15.4	38.0	11.8	1,097	11.05
North Warwickshire HD	14.1	39.0	14.2	387	10.35
Rugby HD	16.5	38.8	8.4	214	13.54
South Warwickshire HD	16.1	36.9	11.3	496	10.76
Birmingham AHA	18.0	30.3	10.6	3,408	16.70
Central HD	17.0	31.0	9.8	823	17.33
East HD	15.2	30.0	12.9	410	13.85
North HD	21.7	30.2	7.4	566	16.65
South HD	18.9	26.5	7.5	825	15.71
West HD	17.8	33.8	15.7	784	19.36
Coventry AHA	19.0	37.5	15.4	1,062	15.17
Dudley AHA	15.0	42.9	4.8	715	11.61
Sandwell AHA	16.6	38.1	9.8	855	14.82
Solihull AHA	19.3	33.2	20.8	572	13.30
Walsall AHA	15.8	35.0	22.6	686	12.66
Wolverhampton AHA	18.0	37.0	8.7	827	17.12
Mersey RHA	**14.9**	**29.7**	**27.4**	**5,692**	**11.16**
Cheshire AHA	13.8	34.2	39.2	1,937	9.77
Chester HD	18.2	26.5	19.7	513	13.32

Table A4.19 Legal abortions by area of residence, 1980 - *continued*

Area of residence	Abortions (percentages)			Total abortions	Total abortions per 1000 women aged 15-44
	As percentage of total births plus abortions	Percentage to married women	Percentage under NHS		
Mersey RHA - continued					
Crewe HD	11.9	36.8	62.3	424	8.28
Halton HD	11.6	35.8	32.3	279	9.03
Macclesfield HD	14.1	40.0	54.9	335	8.91
Warrington HD	13.8	35.3	31.9	357	9.94
Liverpool AHA	18.9	22.3	21.3	1,604	15.60
St Helens and Knowsley AHA	11.4	34.2	26.0	696	9.02
Sefton AHA	14.7	27.5	18.9	625	10.06
Northern HD	16.5	26.4	20.5	239	10.67
Southern HD	13.8	28.2	17.9	386	9.72
Wirral AHA	15.4	31.6	18.9	830	11.93
North Western RHA	**14.4**	**32.7**	**42.1**	**9,258**	**11.42**
Lancashire AHA	14.2	37.3	50.1	3,024	11.35
Lancaster HD	16.2	33.9	63.5	271	12.37
Blackpool HD	18.2	32.4	28.2	709	12.44
Preston HD	12.1	36.5	13.9	624	9.78
Blackburn HD	12.4	44.9	67.9	586	10.99
Burnley HD	14.9	39.4	87.9	642	18.72
Ormskirk HD	11.9	32.8	49.5	192	8.10
Bolton AHA	12.8	34.5	30.8	556	10.57
Bury AHA	14.2	33.8	45.8	393	10.45
Manchester AHA	19.1	23.0	41.5	1,522	15.61
North HD	14.9	25.4	28.0	382	13.13
Central HD	20.6	23.2	49.8	514	19.92
South HD	21.6	21.4	43.0	626	14.69
Oldham AHA	11.0	35.4	26.9	413	8.90
Rochdale AHA	12.5	35.4	53.0	474	11.29
Salford AHA	14.2	25.8	32.4	534	10.79
Stockport AHA	15.6	32.4	37.0	697	11.35
Tameside AHA	14.4	35.7	40.7	504	11.35
Trafford AHA	15.4	22.6	31.4	522	10.90
Wigan AHA	12.3	40.2	38.1	619	9.55

Table A4.19 Legal abortions by area of residence, 1980 - *continued*

Area of residence	Abortions (percentages)			Total abortions†	Total abortions per 1000 women aged 15-44†
	As percentage of total births plus abortions†	Percentage to married women†	Percentage under NHS*		
WALES	**14.3**	**39.3**	**57.7**	**6,291**	**11.23**
Clwyd AHA	14.4	38.1	32.9	840	10.85
Clwyd North HD	14.2	33.9	23.8	307	9.27
Clwyd South HD	14.5	40.5	38.1	533	12.03
Dyfed AHA	14.9	42.1	77.4	707	11.13
Ceredigion HD	17.1	36.2	70.8	130	10.08
Carmarthen/Dinefwr HD	13.8	43.2	82.6	132	10.91
Preseli/South Pembrokeshire HD	15.0	41.8	67.3	251	12.24
Llanelli/Dinefwr HD	14.3	45.9	91.2	194	10.78
Gwent AHA	14.3	41.1	53.4	990	11.04
North Gwent HD	18.1	47.0	72.4	315	13.46
South Gwent HD	13.0	38.4	44.6	675	10.18
Gwynedd AHA	14.2	38.2	55.9	474	11.05
Mid Glamorgan AHA	12.7	44.6	55.7	1,164	10.64
Ogwr HD	14.6	45.0	71.1	311	12.05
Rhymney Valley HD	12.1	37.4	67.1	243	10.17
East Glamorgan HD	12.4	48.6	38.5	366	10.34
Merthyr and Cynon Valley HD	11.6	45.1	50.4	244	10.04
Powys AHA	15.1	44.2	54.2	240	11.94
South Glamorgan AHA	14.2	28.3	35.4	898	10.92
West Glamorgan AHA	16.4	39.8	93.6	978	13.07
Neath HD	16.5	45.2	91.7	325	13.00
Swansea HD	16.3	37.1	94.5	653	13.11
SCOTLAND[a]	**10.2**	**34.9**	**97.7**	**7,855**	**7.3**
Argyll and Clyde	7.5	44.2	100.0	516	5.3
Ayrshire and Arran	10.8	47.6	100.0	622	7.9
Borders	12.1	36.3	-	157	8.2
Dumfries and Galloway	10.3	35.4	93.4	206	7.3
Fife	11.6	35.7	100.0	608	8.6
Forth Valley [Central region]	9.0	39.6	98.7	364	6.3
Grampian	11.2	33.2	95.4	825	8.2

Table A4.19 Legal abortions by area of residence, 1980 - *continued*

Area of residence	Abortions (percentages)			Total abortions	Total abortions per 1000 women aged 15-44
	As percentage of total births plus abortions	Percentage to married women	Percentage under NHS		
Scotland - continued					
Greater Glasgow	7.7	30.6	94.5	1,126	5.5
Highland	8.5	38.5	100.0	270	6.7
Islands**	4.9	35.8	100.0	53	4.0
Lanarkshire	6.7	45.1	100.0	605	4.8
Lothian	14.0	36.6	98.0	1,530	9.4
Tayside	15.9	31.3	98.8	926	11.4

*   *In Scotland, abortions by health board of treatment*
†   *In Scotland, abortions by health board of residence*
ø   *Includes some abortions outside Scotland and not known, but not abortions in England and Wales to residents of Scotland, which are included in Table A4.18*
** *Consists of Orkney, Shetland and Western Isles Health Boards*
Source: OPCS, *Abortion statistics, 1980*
        Registrar General, Scotland, *Annual Report 1980*

Table A4.20 Legal abortions to residents of England and Wales by gestational age, method used and category of premises, 1980

Gestational age and method used	NHS hospital Number	NHS hospital Percentage of stated methods	Non-NHS hospital Number	Non-NHS hospital Percentage of stated methods	Total Number	Total Percentage of stated methods
Under 9 weeks						
Hysterotomy (with other)	5	0.05	3	0.01	8	0.03
Vacuum aspiration	9,424	87.61	13,553	67.56	22,977	74.56
Dilation and evacuation	567	5.27	691	3.44	1,258	4.08
Vacuum aspiration with D&C	503	4.68	5,758	28.70	6,261	20.32
Other methods	258	2.40	56	0.28	314	1.02
Not stated	22	—	11	—	33	—
Total	10,779	100	20,072	100	30,851	100
9-12 weeks						
Hysterotomy (with other)	8	0.02	2	0.01	10	0.01
Vacuum aspiration	31,064	86.16	26,293	74.35	57,357	80.31
Dilation and evacuation	1,986	5.51	842	2.38	2,828	3.96
Vacuum aspiration with D&C	1,420	3.94	7,975	22.55	9,395	13.16
Other methods	1,574	4.37	253	0.72	1,827	2.56
Not stated	66	—	33	—	99	—
Total	36,118	100	35,398	100	71,516	100
13-16 weeks						
Hysterotomy (with other)	6	0.07	0	—	6	0.04
Vacuum aspiration	4,530	52.49	4,169	54.49	8,699	53.43
Dilation and evacuation	427	4.95	641	8.38	1,068	6.56
Vacuum aspiration with D&C	260	3.01	1,868	24.42	2,128	13.07
Other methods	3,407	39.48	973	12.72	4,380	26.90
Not stated	23	—	12	—	35	—
Total	8,653	100	7,663	100	16,316	100
17-19 weeks						
Hysterotomy (with other)	1	0.06	0	—	1	0.03
Vacuum aspiration	310	19.68	296	13.44	606	16.04
Dilation and evacuation	35	2.22	281	12.76	316	8.36
Vacuum aspiration with D&C	22	1.40	235	10.67	257	6.80
Other methods	1,207	76.63	1,391	63.14	2,598	68.77
Not stated	9	—	3	—	12	—
Total	1,584	100	2,206	100	3,790	100
20-23 weeks						
Hysterotomy (with other)	0	—	0	—	0	—
Vacuum aspiration	127	18.14	84	7.36	211	11.45
Dilation and evacuation	17	2.43	171	14.97	188	10.21
Vacuum aspiration with D&C	6	0.86	59	5.17	65	3.53
Other methods	550	78.57	828	72.50	1,378	74.81
Not stated	4	—	7	—	11	—
Total	704	100	1,149	100	1,853	100

Table A4.20 Legal abortions to residents of England and Wales by gestational age, method used and category of premises, 1980 - *continued*

Gestational age and method used		NHS hospital		Non-NHS hospital		Total	
		Number	Percentage of stated methods	Number	Percentage of stated methods	Number	Percentage of stated methods
24 and over	Hysterotomy (with other)	0	—	0	—	0	—
	Vacuum aspiration	41	25.79	32	14.61	73	19.31
	Dilation and evacuation	5	3.14	31	14.16	36	9.52
	Vacuum aspiration with D&C	2	1.26	17	7.76	19	5.03
	Other methods	111	69.81	139	63.47	250	66.14
	Not stated	0	—	3	—	3	—
	Total	159	100	222	100	381	100
Not stated	Hysterotomy (with other)	0	—	0	—	0	—
	Vacuum aspiration	1,958	75.57	944	58.27	2,902	68.91
	Dilation and evacuation	124	4.79	92	5.68	216	5.13
	Vacuum aspiration with D&C	125	4.82	376	23.21	501	11.90
	Other methods	384	14.82	208	12.84	592	14.06
	Not stated	6	—	3	—	9	—
	Total	2,597	100	1,623	100	4,220	100
Total	Hysterotomy (with other)	20	0.03	5	0.01	25	0.02
	Vacuum aspiration	47,454	78.48	45,371	66.47	92,825	72.11
	Dilation and evacuation	3,161	5.23	2,749	4.03	5,910	4.59
	Vacuum aspiration with D&C	2,338	3.87	16,288	23.86	18,626	14.47
	Other methods	7,491	12.39	3,848	5.64	11,339	8.81
	Not stated	130	—	72	—	202	—
	Total	60,594	100	68,333	100	128,927	100

Source: OPCS, *Abortion Statistics, Series AB*

Table A4.21 Legal abortions to residents of England and Wales by age and category of premises, 1980

Age	NHS hospitals		Non-NHS hospitals		Total	
	Number	Percentage with stated age	Number	Percentage with stated age	Number	Percentage with stated age
Under 15	680	72.88	253	27.12	933	100
15	1,762	64.85	955	35.15	2,717	100
16-19	14,360	45.05	17,518	54.95	31,878	100
20-24	13,616	41.24	19,398	58.76	33,014	100
25-29	10,281	46.64	11,761	53.36	22,042	100
30-34	9,474	48.79	9,945	51.21	19,419	100
35-39	6,736	52.91	5,994	47.09	12,730	100
40-44	3,162	59.58	2,145	40.42	5,307	100
45 and over	366	66.91	181	33.09	547	100
Not stated	157	46.18	183	53.82	340	100
Total	60,594	47.00	68,333	53.00	128,927	100

Source: OPCS, *Abortion statistics, Series AB*

Table A4.22 Legal abortions to residents of England and Wales by marital status and category of premises, 1980

Marital status	NHS hospitals		Non-NHS hospitals		Total	
	Number	Percentage of known status	Number	Percentage of known status	Number	Percentage of known status
Single	28,063	47.03	40,693	59.83	68,756	53.85
Married	24,213	40.58	20,040	29.46	44,253	34.66
Widowed/divorced/ separated	7,392	12.39	7,283	10.71	14,675	11.49
Unknown	926	—	317	—	1,243	—
Total	60,594	100	68,333	100	128,927	100

Source: *Abortion Statistics, Series AB*

Table A4.23 **Legal abortions to residents of England and Wales by marital status and number of previous liveborn children, 1980**

Marital status	Number of previous live born children									
	0		1		2		3		4 or more	
	Number	Per cent	Number	Per cent	Number	Per cent	Number	Per cent	Number	Per cent
Single	61,140	88.92	5,469	7.95	1,411	2.05	377	0.55	169	0.25
Married	5,723	12.93	7,137	16.13	17,630	39.84	8,767	19.81	4,893	11.06
Other	3,369	21.16	4,058	25.49	4,886	30.69	2,282	14.34	1,291	8.11
Total	70,232	54.47	16,664	12.93	23,927	18.56	11,426	8.86	6,353	4.93

Source: *Abortion Statistics, Series AB.*

Table A4.24 **Legal abortions to residents of England and Wales by gestational age and category of premises, 1980**

Gestational age weeks	NHS hospitals		Non-NHS hospitals		Total	
	Number	Percentage of stated gestational age	Number	Percentage of stated gestational age	Number	Percentage of stated gestational age
Under 9	10,779	18.59	20,072	30.09	30,851	24.74
9-12	36,118	62.28	35,398	53.06	71,516	57.35
13-16	8,653	14.92	7,663	11.49	16,316	13.08
17-19	1,584	2.73	2,206	3.31	3,790	3.04
20-23	704	1.21	1,149	1.72	1,853	1.49
24 and over	159	0.27	222	0.33	381	0.31
Not stated	2,597	—	1,623	—	4,220	—
Total	60,594	100	68,333	100	128,927	100

Source: *Abortion Statistics, Series AB*

Table A4.25 Legal abortions to residents of England and Wales by marital status, statutory grounds and category of premises, 1980

Marital status	Statutory grounds	NHS hospitals		Non-NHS hospitals		Total	
		Number	Per cent	Number	Per cent	Number	Per cent
Single	1 (with other)	144	71.64	57	28.36	201	100.00
	2	26,398	39.88	39,789	60.12	66,187	100.00
	3 (with other except 1)	1,275	61.74	790	38.26	2,065	100.00
	4 (with 2)	245	81.13	57	18.87	302	100.00
	5 and 6	1	100.00	0	—	1	100.00
Married	1 (with other)	319	83.95	61	16.05	380	100.00
	2	17,084	52.78	15,285	47.22	32,369	100.00
	3 (with other except 1)	5,526	54.98	4,525	45.02	10,051	100.00
	4 (with 2)	1,278	88.32	169	11.68	1,447	100.00
	5 and 6	6	100.00	0	—	6	100.00
Other	1 (with other)	78	78.79	21	21.21	99	100.00
	2	5,984	50.98	5,754	49.02	11,738	100.00
	3 (with other except 1)	2,137	54.38	1,793	45.62	3,930	100.00
	4 (with 2)	119	78.81	32	21.19	151	100.00
	5 and 6	0	—	0	—	0	—
Total	1 (with other)	541	79.56	139	20.44	680	100.00
	2	49,466	44.85	60,828	55.15	110,294	100.00
	3 (with other except 1)	8,938	55.70	7,108	44.30	16,046	100.00
	4 (with 2)	1,642	86.42	258	13.58	1,900	100.00
	5 and 6	7	100.00	0	—	7	100.00

Source: OPCS, *Abortion Statistics, Series AB*

Conditions of the Act and statutory grounds

A legally induced abortion must be:

a) performed by a registered medical practitioner

b) performed, except in an emergency, in a National Health Service hospital or in a place for the time being approved for the purpose of the Act

c) certified by two registered medical practitioners as necessary on any of the grounds:

1 the continuance of the pregnancy would involve risk to the life of the pregnant woman greater than if the pregnancy were terminated

2 the continuance of the pregnancy would involve risk of injury to the physical or mental health of the pregnant woman greater than if the pregnancy were terminated

3 the continuance of the pregnancy would involve risk of injury to the physical or mental health of any existing children in the family greater than if the pregnancy were terminated

4 there is a substantial risk that if the child were born it would suffer from such physical or mental abnormalities as to be seriously handicapped

or in the emergency, certified by the operating practitioner as immediately necessary—

5 to save the life of the pregnant woman, or

6 to prevent grave permanent injury to the physical or mental health of the pregnant woman.

The above numbering of the grounds of termination appears in the notification form itself and is used for brevity in the tables. Combinations of grounds are often recorded and the tabulations distinguish two such: 2 and 4 together and 3 with any others (usually 2 and/or 4). Where ground 1 is stated with any other, the case is treated as ground 1. The Act provides that in relation to grounds numbered above as 2 and 3 the certifying practitioner may take account of the pregnant woman's actual or reasonably forseeable environment.

Table A4.26 Offences recorded by the police and persons tried and found guilty or cautioned for procuring illegal abortion, England and Wales, 1900-81

Year	Offences recorded by the police	Persons sent for trial	Persons found guilty or cautioned
	Average number per year		
1900-04	12	11	..
1905-09	33	20	..
1910-14	40	30	..
1915-19	65	43	..
1920-24	48	32	..
1925-29	82	53	..
1930-34	80	48	..
1935-39	156	72	..
1940-44	347	119	..
1945-49	271	100	..
1950-54	244	60	..
1955-59	164	47	..
1960-64	276	65	..
1965-69	242	65	76
1970-74	82	27	37
1975-79	9	2	3
	Number per year		
1965	184	67	70
1966	208	62	65
1967	314	71	78
1968	247	68	93
1969	257	59	72
1970	212	43	55
1971	80	38	54
1972	62	34	48
1973	36	7	11
1974	21	11	17
1975	14	2	1
1976	9	4	5
1977	11	1	3
1978	7	3	4
1979	3	0	0
1980	2*	4	5
1981	3*	0	3

* *New counting procedure introduced in 1980*

Source: Home Office, *Crime Statistics*

Table A5.1 Live births by social class and legitimacy, England and Wales, 1950, 1964, 1970-80

Year	Percentage of all live births					Number of live births (=100%)
	Legitimate				Illegitimate	
	Social Class I and II	III	IV and V	Other		
1950	15.6	53.3	25.5	0.5	5.1	697,097
1964	15.3	47.1	27.1	3.3	7.2	875,972
1970	18.9	48.1	21.4	3.4	8.3	784,486
1971	19.8	47.7	20.4	3.8	8.4	783,155
1972	20.9	47.3	19.4	3.8	8.6	725,440
1973	21.9	45.9	19.3	4.3	8.6	675,953
1974	22.8	45.6	18.8	3.9	8.8	639,885
1975	23.5	44.9	18.5	4.0	9.1	603,445
1976	24.1	44.5	18.9	3.3	9.2	584,270
1977	25.0	43.3	18.7	3.2	9.7	569,259
1978	25.2	43.0	18.7	2.9	10.2	596,418
1979	24.6	42.9	18.8	2.8	10.9	638,028
1979*	25.1	42.2	19.0	2.8	10.9	638,028
1980*	25.1	41.8	18.3	3.0	11.8	656,234

* *Based on the 1980 Classification of Occupations*

Source: Studies on Medical and Population Subjects Nos. 15 and 19. OPCS *Birth statistics, Series FM1.* Data for 1970-80 are based on a ten per cent sample of all live births.

Table A5.2 Percentage distributions of birthweights in each social class, England and Wales, 1980

Birthweight g	Social class of father (legitimate births only)						Other Legitimate	Illegitimate	Total births
	I Higher professional	II Other professional	IIIN Skilled non manual	IIIM Skilled manual	IV Partly skilled	V Unskilled			
<1500	0.9	0.7	0.9	1.0	1.0	1.0	0.9	1.4	0.9
1500-1999	0.9	1.2	1.1	1.3	1.5	1.4	1.0	1.9	1.4
2000-2499	3.8	3.7	4.1	4.7	5.3	6.3	4.6	6.7	4.8
2500-2999	15.8	15.7	17.3	19.0	20.8	23.1	18.7	23.2	19.2
3000-3499	39.8	39.2	39.0	39.0	39.8	39.8	40.0	39.4	38.9
3500-3999	30.3	29.9	28.7	26.7	24.7	22.6	26.9	22.0	26.7
4000+	8.5	9.6	8.9	8.3	7.0	5.8	7.9	5.3	8.0
Total	100.0	100.0	100.0	100.0	100.0	100.0	100.0	100.0	100.0
Number with birthweight stated	35,643	108,478	52,923	183,195	75,565	28,454	16,860	72,041	573,362
Percent without birthweight stated	13.1	12.8	15.0	14.3	14.5	13.7	16.0	7.7	13.3
Total births (live and still)	41,077	124,331	62,289	213,855	88,407	32,982	20,068	78,068	661,007

Source: Derived from data published in *OPCS Monitor DH3 81/4*. Data for live births are estimated from a ten per cent sample.

Table A5.3   Mortality rates in the first year of life by cause, legitimacy and social class, England and Wales, 1980

Cause	Legitimacy and social class	Stillbirths*	Perinatal deaths*	Neonatal deaths†	Postneonatal deaths†	Infant deaths†
All causes (ICD 000-999)	**Total**	**7.2**	**13.3**	**7.6**	**4.3**	**11.9**
	Legitimate	7.0	12.8	7.3	3.9	11.2
	I	5.0	9.7	5.7	3.2	8.9
	II	6.0	11.1	6.4	3.1	9.5
	III N	6.2	11.8	6.7	3.4	10.2
	III M	7.4	13.0	7.1	3.5	10.7
	IV	8.0	15.0	8.7	4.8	13.5
	V	9.5	17.0	9.8	6.2	16.0
	Others	7.2	14.9	10.1	8.1	18.2
	Illegitimate	8.9	16.9	9.7	6.9	16.7
Congenital anomalies (ICD 740-759)	**Total**	**1.2**	**2.9**	**2.4**	**0.8**	**3.1**
	Legitimate	1.2	3.0	2.4	0.7	3.1
	I	0.8	2.2	2.0	0.7	2.7
	II	1.0	2.5	2.1	0.6	2.7
	III N	1.1	2.8	2.1	0.8	2.9
	III M	1.3	3.0	2.3	0.7	3.0
	IV	1.6	3.5	2.8	0.9	3.7
	V	1.8	4.4	3.5	0.8	4.3
	Others	1.1	3.6	3.5	1.0	4.4
	Illegitimate	1.1	2.6	2.2	1.1	3.2
Other causes	**Total**	**6.0**	**10.4**	**5.2**	**3.5**	**8.8**
	Legitimate	5.8	9.8	4.9	3.0	8.1
	I	4.2	7.5	3.7	2.5	6.2
	II	5.0	8.6	4.3	2.5	6.8
	III N	5.1	9.0	4.6	2.6	7.3
	III M	6.1	10.0	5.8	2.8	7.7
	IV	6.4	11.5	5.9	3.9	9.8
	V	7.7	12.6	6.3	5.4	11.7
	Others	6.1	11.3	6.6	7.1	13.8
	Illegitimate	7.8	14.3	7.5	5.8	13.5

* *Per 1,000 total births.*

† *Per 1,000 live births.*

Source: OPCS, *Mortality statistics: perinatal and infant,* Series DH3 No. 9.

Table A5.4 Mortality in the first year of life by legitimacy, parity, social class and age of mother, England and Wales, 1980
(a) Stillbirths

Legitimacy and parity	Social class of father	Age of mother											
		All ages		Under 20		20-24		25-29		30-34		35 and over	
		Number	Rate*	Number	Rate*	Number	Rate*	Number	Rate*	Number	Rate*	Number	Rate*
Legitimate All parities	Total	**4,077**	**6.99**	**257**	**7.47**	**1,147**	**6.45**	**1,359**	**6.45**	**894**	**7.21**	**420**	**11.61**
	I-V	3,933	6.99	246	7.52	1,089	6.41	1,316	6.45	868	7.19	414	11.70
	I	204	4.97	2	5.84	25	5.07	85	4.96	69	4.71	23	5.82
	II	745	5.99	18	9.42	120	5.72	266	5.18	242	6.13	99	9.38
	IIIN	387	6.21	11	6.31	97	5.80	159	6.19	85	5.83	35	9.88
	IIIM	1,576	7.37	98	6.83	483	6.32	522	6.85	318	8.88	155	13.97
	IV	708	8.01	74	8.13	243	6.72	206	7.92	116	9.31	69	14.85
	V	313	9.49	43	8.14	121	8.26	78	10.19	38	9.99	33	20.81
	Other	144	7.17	11	6.49	58	7.26	43	6.69	26	8.25	6	7.43
0	Total	**1,856**	**7.68**	**216**	**7.78**	**715**	**7.31**	**620**	**7.64**	**225**	**7.74**	**80**	**13.54**
	I-V	1,786	7.69	207	7.88	680	7.28	598	7.61	222	7.86	79	13.72
	I	110	6.36	2	7.08	22	6.42	59	6.91	23	5.62	4	4.23
	II	343	6.56	15	9.05	84	6.19	138	5.69	79	7.38	27	12.73
	IIIN	205	7.20	11	7.27	63	5.81	94	8.09	26	6.82	11	16.12
	IIIM	693	8.04	84	7.35	315	7.61	209	8.34	62	9.14	23	15.28
	IV	315	8.88	60	8.24	138	7.71	80	10.66	24	10.18	13	29.97
	V	120	9.63	35	8.55	58	9.34	18	11.24	8	16.36	1	14.06
	Other	70	7.32	9	6.03	35	7.76	22	8.47	3	3.68	1	6.61
1	Total	**1,130**	**5.41**	**38**	**6.03**	**301**	**4.95**	**411**	**4.88**	**293**	**6.09**	**87**	**9.48**
	I-V	1,093	5.41	36	5.90	285	4.92	401	4.90	287	6.11	84	9.34
	I	47	3.07	0	–	3	2.35	17	2.58	20	3.20	7	6.09
	II	232	4.96	3	11.84	28	4.55	88	4.29	87	5.25	26	8.02
	IIIN	105	4.54	0	–	22	4.32	42	3.93	32	5.30	9	8.10
	IIIM	440	5.78	13	4.65	122	4.65	177	5.63	100	7.54	28	11.51
	IV	190	6.32	12	7.04	72	5.33	57	5.66	37	9.50	12	13.74
	V	79	7.58	8	7.55	38	6.74	20	7.68	11	11.67	2	10.97
	Other	37	5.38	2	9.88	16	5.51	10	4.18	6	5.01	3	16.36

(a) Stillbirths-*continued*

Legitimacy and parity	Social class of father	Age of mother											
		All ages		Under 20		20-24		25-29		30-34		35 and over	
		Number	Rate*	Number	Rate*	Number	Rate*	Number	Rate*	Number	Rate*	Number	Rate*
2	**Total**	**627**	**7.12**	**3**	**8.03**	**100**	**6.28**	**207**	**6.44**	**228**	**7.48**	**89**	**9.70**
	I-V	602	7.03	3	8.03	94	6.11	197	6.33	220	7.38	88	9.82
	I	33	5.08	0	—	0	—	7	4.02	19	5.56	7	6.20
	II	122	6.63	0	—	8	7.27	31	5.71	59	6.56	24	8.36
	IIIN	54	7.07	0	—	8	12.14	20	7.68	19	5.58	7	7.30
	IIIM	231	6.71	1	8.25	37	4.91	79	5.49	90	9.26	24	9.06
	IV	109	8.11	2	17.83	25	6.58	37	7.26	27	7.93	18	17.48
	V	53	10.03	0	—	16	7.73	23	12.32	6	6.76	8	24.35
	Other	25	10.21	0	—	6	11.17	10	9.60	8	12.14	1	4.73
3 and over	**Total**	**464**	**10.47**	**0**	—	**31**	**9.55**	**121**	**9.38**	**148**	**9.11**	**164**	**13.15**
	I-V	452	10.48	0	—	30	9.36	120	9.60	139	8.82	163	13.97
	I	14	7.38	0	—	0	—	2	7.62	7	7.88	5	6.88
	II	48	7.00	0	—	0	—	9	7.69	17	5.31	22	9.46
	IIIN	23	7.57	0	—	4	32.20	3	3.82	8	5.97	8	10.13
	IIIM	212	12.39	0	—	9	7.49	57	10.64	66	10.91	80	17.75
	IV	94	9.98	0	—	8	8.34	32	9.56	28	9.99	26	11.25
	V	61	12.68	0	—	9	12.16	17	10.76	13	8.75	22	21.92
	Other	12	10.22	0	—	1	24.35	1	24.35	9	18.76	1	3.82
Illegitimate		**696**	**8.92**	**251**	**9.74**	**240**	**8.83**	**101**	**7.70**	**59**	**7.22**	**145**	**11.74**
Total		**4,773**	**7.27**	**508**	**8.51**	**1,387**	**6.81**	**1,460**	**6.57**	**953**	**7.27**	**465**	**11.76**

* *Per 1,000 total births*

125

Table A5.4 Mortality in the first year of life by legitimacy, parity, social class and age of mother, England and Wales, 1980 - *continued*

(b) Perinatal deaths

Legitimacy and parity	Social class	Age of mother											
		All ages		Under 20		20-24		25-29		30-34		35 and over	
		Number	Rate*	Number	Rate*	Number	Rate*	Number	Rate*	Number	Rate*	Number	Rate*
Legitimate													
All parities	**Total**	**7,480**	**12.83**	**532**	**15.46**	**2,254**	**12.67**	**2,495**	**11.85**	**1,541**	**12.43**	**658**	**18.18**
	I-V	7,180	12.76	501	15.31	2,134	12.56	2,407	11.79	1,496	12.39	642	18.15
	I	398	9.71	3	8.76	60	12.16	163	9.51	121	8.27	51	12.91
	II	1,377	11.08	34	17.79	248	11.82	505	9.83	425	10.76	165	15.63
	IIIN	732	11.75	28	16.05	180	10.76	301	11.72	172	11.79	51	14.40
	IIIM	2,789	13.04	196	13.66	927	12.14	929	12.19	519	14.50	218	19.65
	IV	1,324	14.98	156	17.14	494	13.65	373	14.33	190	15.25	111	23.88
	V	560	16.98	84	15.90	225	15.35	136	17.77	69	18.13	46	29.01
	Other	300	14.95	31	18.30	120	15.01	88	13.70	45	14.28	16	19.82
0	**Total**	**3,384**	**14.00**	**436**	**15.71**	**1,312**	**13.41**	**1,090**	**13.42**	**419**	**14.42**	**127**	**21.49**
	I-V	3,229	13.91	411	15.65	1,235	13.23	1,050	13.36	411	14.55	122	21.18
	I	210	12.14	3	10.62	46	13.42	102	11.94	46	11.25	13	13.75
	II	625	11.95	24	14.48	165	12.16	256	10.55	141	13.17	39	18.39
	IIIN	382	13.41	23	15.19	121	11.15	162	13.95	59	15.47	17	24.92
	IIIM	1,223	14.19	162	14.18	556	13.43	368	14.68	105	15.48	32	21.25
	IV	579	16.32	133	18.26	250	13.97	131	17.46	47	19.93	18	41.50
	V	210	16.85	66	16.13	97	15.62	31	19.36	13	26.59	3	42.18
	Other	155	16.20	25	16.76	77	17.06	40	15.40	8	9.82	5	33.05
1	**Total**	**2,168**	**10.39**	**86**	**13.65**	**660**	**10.85**	**813**	**9.65**	**484**	**10.05**	**125**	**13.63**
	I-V	2,094	10.37	80	13.12	632	10.91	788	9.62	473	10.07	121	13.46
	I	102	6.66	0	–	11	8.63	42	6.36	35	5.61	14	12.18
	II	440	9.41	9	35.51	66	10.72	175	8.53	154	9.28	36	11.10
	IIIN	212	9.16	5	22.69	45	8.84	92	8.61	56	9.28	14	12.60
	IIIM	820	10.77	31	11.08	263	10.02	325	10.35	163	12.30	381	15.62
	IV	373	12.41	19	11.14	169	12.50	119	11.81	49	12.58	17	19.46
	V	147	14.10	16	15.10	78	13.83	35	13.44	16	16.97	2	10.97
	Other	74	10.76	6	29.65	28	9.65	25	10.44	11	9.18	4	21.82

(b) Perinatal deaths-*continued*

Legitimacy and parity	Social class of father	Age of mother											
		All ages		Under 20		20-24		25-29		30-34		35 and over	
		Number	Rate*	Number	Rate*	Number	Rate*	Number	Rate*	Number	Rate*	Number	Rate*
2	**Total**	**1,155**	**13.11**	**10**	**26.76**	**222**	**13.95**	**384**	**11.94**	**388**	**12.73**	**151**	**16.46**
	I-V	1,113	12.99	10	26.76	211	13.72	368	11.82	374	12.54	150	16.73
	I	59	9.08	0	—	2	9.51	17	9.77	30	8.78	10	8.86
	II	228	12.39	1	—	17	15.45	59	10.86	101	11.23	50	17.43
	IIIN	99	12.96	0	—	9	13.65	39	14.97	42	12.33	9	9.39
	IIIM	426	12.38	3	24.75	89	11.80	149	10.36	141	14.51	44	16.61
	IV	198	14.73	4	35.65	59	15.52	62	12.17	48	14.10	25	24.28
	V	103	19.50	2	15.36	35	16.91	42	22.50	12	13.52	12	36.52
	Other	42	17.15	0	—	11	20.49	16	15.36	14	21.24	1	4.73
3 and over	**Total**	**773**	**17.44**	**0**	**—**	**60**	**18.48**	**208**	**16.13**	**250**	**15.39**	**255**	**21.38**
	I-V	744	17.25	0	—	56	17.47	201	16.08	238	15.09	249	21.35
	I	27	14.23	0	—	1	49.91	2	7.62	10	11.25	14	19.28
	II	84	12.24	0	—	0	—	15	12.81	29	9.05	40	17.20
	IIIN	39	12.84	0	—	5	40.25	8	10.20	15	11.19	11	13.93
	IIIM	320	18.70	0	—	19	15.82	87	16.24	110	18.19	104	23.07
	IV	174	18.47	0	—	16	16.67	61	18.22	46	16.41	51	22.08
	V	100	20.79	0	—	15	20.26	28	17.72	28	18.85	29	28.89
	Other	29	24.70	0	—	4	97.39	7	17.87	12	25.01	6	22.95
Illegitimate		**1,316**	**16.86**	**483**	**18.74**	**444**	**16.34**	**205**	**15.63**	**114**	**13.96**	**70**	**18.26**
Total		**8,796**	**13.40**	**1,015**	**17.01**	**2,698**	**13.25**	**2,700**	**12.15**	**1,655**	**12.62**	**728**	**18.41**

* *Per 1,000 total births*

127

Table A5.4 Mortality in the first year of life by legitimacy, parity, social class and age of mother, England and Wales, 1980 - *continued*

(c) Neonatal deaths

Legitimacy and parity	Social class	Age of mother											
		All ages		Under 20		20-24		25-29		30-34		35 and over	
		Number	Rate*	Number	Rate*	Number	Rate*	Number	Rate*	Number	Rate*	Number	Rate*
Legitimate All parities	**Total**	**4,233**	**7.31**	**340**	**9.95**	**1,369**	**7.75**	**1,428**	**6.83**	**803**	**6.53**	**293**	**8.19**
	I-V	4,032	7.21	317	9.76	1,293	7.66	1,366	6.74	775	6.46	281	8.04
	I	232	5.69	1	2.94	36	7.33	92	5.39	67	4.60	36	9.17
	II	787	6.37	18	9.51	153	7.33	315	6.16	226	5.76	75	7.17
	IIIN	417	6.74	19	10.96	104	6.25	170	6.66	104	7.17	20	5.70
	IIIM	1,516	7.14	124	8.70	564	7.43	509	6.72	241	6.79	78	7.13
	IV	761	8.68	101	11.19	307	8.54	206	7.98	94	7.62	53	11.58
	V	319	9.76	54	10.31	129	8.87	74	9.77	43	11.42	19	12.24
	Other	201	10.09	23	13.67	76	9.58	62	9.72	28	8.96	12	14.97
0	**Total**	**1,889**	**7.87**	**270**	**9.81**	**739**	**7.61**	**592**	**7.35**	**232**	**8.05**	**56**	**9.60**
	I-V	1,782	7.73	252	9.67	690	7.45	563	7.22	225	8.03	52	9.15
	I	117	6.81	1	3.56	24	7.05	54	6.36	27	6.64	11	11.68
	II	353	6.79	11	6.70	96	7.12	157	6.51	76	7.15	13	6.21
	IIIN	215	7.60	14	9.32	71	6.58	81	7.03	41	10.83	8	11.92
	IIIM	659	7.71	99	8.73	307	7.47	192	7.72	51	7.59	10	6.74
	IV	321	9.13	89	12.32	141	7.94	62	8.35	23	9.85	6	14.26
	V	117	9.48	38	9.37	51	8.29	17	10.74	7	14.56	4	57.04
	Other	107	11.27	18	12.14	49	10.94	29	11.26	7	8.63	4	26.62
1	**Total**	**1,313**	**6.32**	**62**	**9.90**	**455**	**7.52**	**502**	**5.99**	**241**	**5.04**	**53**	**5.83**
	I-V	1,261	6.28	57	9.40	436	7.56	482	5.91	235	5.04	51	5.73
	I	69	4.52	0	—	9	7.07	28	4.25	23	3.70	9	7.88
	II	254	5.46	6	23.96	45	7.34	108	5.29	81	4.91	14	4.35
	IIIN	135	5.86	5	22.69	31	6.12	63	5.92	30	5.00	6	5.44
	IIIM	483	6.38	22	7.90	183	7.00	189	6.05	75	5.70	14	5.82
	IV	230	7.70	10	5.91	119	8.85	74	7.39	20	5.19	7	8.12
	V	90	8.70	14	13.31	49	8.75	20	7.74	6	6.44	1	5.55
	Other	52	7.60	5	24.95	19	6.59	20	8.39	6	5.03	2	11.09

(c) **Neonatal deaths**-*continued*

Legitimacy and parity	Social class of father	Age of mother											
		All ages		Under 20		20-24		25-29		30-34		35 and over	
		Number	Rate*	Number	Rate*	Number	Rate*	Number	Rate*	Number	Rate*	Number	Rate*
2	**Total**	**642**	**7.34**	**8**	**21.58**	**142**	**8.98**	**229**	**7.17**	**190**	**6.28**	**73**	**8.03**
	I-V	619	7.28	8	21.58	137	8.96	222	7.18	179	6.05	73	8.22
	I	29	4.49	0	—	2	9.51	10	5.77	12	3.53	5	4.46
	II	152	7.22	1	—	12	10.99	41	7.59	50	5.60	28	9.84
	IIIN	51	6.72	0	—	1	1.54	21	8.12	26	7.68	3	3.15
	IIIM	239	6.99	3	24.95	62	8.26	90	6.29	60	6.23	24	9.14
	IV	111	8.32	2	:8.15	38	10.06	38	7.51	24	7.11	9	8.89
	V	57	10.90	2	15.36	22	10.71	22	11.93	7	7.94	4	12.48
	Other	23	9.49	0	—	5	9.42	7	6.78	11	16.89	0	—
3 and over	**Total**	**389**	**8.87**	**0**	**—**	**33**	**10.26**	**105**	**8.22**	**140**	**8.70**	**111**	**9.44**
	I-V	370	8.67	0	—	30	9.45	99	8.00	136	8.70	105	9.13
	I	17	9.03	0	—	1	49.91	0	—	5	5.67	11	15.25
	II	48	7.05	0	—	0	—	9	7.74	19	5.96	20	8.68
	IIIN	16	5.31	0	—	1	8.32	5	6.40	7	5.25	3	3.84
	IIIM	135	7.99	0	—	12	10.07	38	7.17	55	9.20	30	6.77
	IV	99	10.61	0	—	9	9.46	32	9.65	27	9.73	31	13.57
	V	55	11.58	0	—	7	9.57	15	9.60	23	15.62	10	10.19
	Other	19	16.35	0	—	3	74.86	6	15.36	4	8.50	6	23.03
Illegitimate		**754**	**9.75**	**278**	**10.89**	**256**	**9.50**	**118**	**9.07**	**71**	**8.76**	**31**	**8.18**
Total		**4,387**	**7.60**	**613**	**10.35**	**1,625**	**7.98**	**1,546**	**6.96**	**874**	**6.66**	**324**	**8.19**

* Per 1,000 live births

Table A5.4 Mortality in the first year of life by legitimacy, parity, social class and age of mother, England and Wales, 1980 - *continued*
(d) Postneonatal deaths

Legitimacy and parity	Social class	Age of mother											
		All ages		Under 20		20-24		25-29		30-34		35 and over	
		Number	Rate*	Number	Rate*	Number	Rate*	Number	Rate*	Number	Rate*	Number	Rate*
Legitimate													
All parities	**Total**	**2,266**	**3.91**	**246**	**7.20**	**788**	**4.46**	**733**	**3.50**	**375**	**3.05**	**124**	**3.47**
	I-V	2,104	3.76	219	6.74	710	4.21	691	3.41	362	3.02	122	3.49
	I	132	3.23	0	—	18	3.67	52	3.05	46	3.16	16	4.07
	II	384	3.11	9	4.75	58	2.78	177	3.46	112	2.85	28	2.68
	IIIN	212	3.42	8	4.62	52	3.13	92	3.60	47	3.24	13	3.71
	IIIM	748	3.52	77	5.41	301	3.97	237	3.13	98	2.76	35	3.20
	IV	424	4.83	76	8.42	185	5.15	93	3.60	46	3.73	24	5.24
	V	204	6.24	49	9.35	96	6.60	40	5.28	13	3.45	6	3.86
	Other	162	8.13	27	16.04	78	9.83	42	6.58	13	4.16	2	2.50
0	**Total**	**675**	**2.81**	**151**	**5.48**	**261**	**2.69**	**188**	**2.33**	**63**	**2.19**	**12**	**2.06**
	I-V	606	2.63	127	4.88	228	2.46	177	2.27	62	2.21	12	2.11
	I	42	2.44	0	—	11	3.23	19	2.24	11	2.70	1	1.06
	II	108	2.08	5	3.04	28	2.08	52	2.16	17	1.60	6	2.87
	IIIN	70	2.48	6	3.99	24	2.22	27	2.34	11	2.90	2	2.98
	IIIM	203	2.37	42	3.70	91	2.22	56	2.25	13	1.93	1	0.67
	IV	125	3.55	48	6.65	51	2.87	16	2.16	8	3.43	2	4.75
	V	58	4.70	26	6.41	23	3.74	7	4.42	2	4.16	2	—
	Other	69	7.27	24	16.19	33	7.37	11	4.27	1	1.23	0	—
1	**Total**	**928**	**4.47**	**84**	**13.42**	**368**	**6.08**	**309**	**3.68**	**137**	**2.86**	**30**	**3.30**
	I-V	876	4.36	82	13.53	336	5.83	296	3.63	132	2.83	30	3.37
	I	56	3.67	0	—	6	4.72	30	4.56	18	2.89	2	1.75
	II	178	3.83	3	11.98	24	3.91	94	4.60	46	2.79	11	3.42
	IIIN	96	4.17	2	9.07	24	4.73	48	4.51	20	3.33	2	1.81
	IIIM	312	4.12	32	11.49	149	5.70	83	2.66	38	2.89	10	4.16
	IV	155	5.19	24	14.18	89	6.62	31	3.09	6	1.56	5	5.80
	V	79	7.63	21	19.96	44	7.86	10	3.87	4	4.29	0	—
	Other	52	7.60	2	9.98	32	11.09	13	5.45	5	4.19	0	—

(d) Postneonatal deaths-*continued*

Legitimacy and parity	Social class of father	Age of mother											
		All ages		Under 20		20-24		25-29		30-34		35 and over	
		Number	Rate*	Number	Rate*	Number	Rate*	Number	Rate*	Number	Rate*	Number	Rate*
2	**Total**	**422**	**4.82**	**11**	**29.68**	**128**	**8.09**	**149**	**4.66**	**102**	**3.37**	**32**	**3.52**
	I-V	393	4.62	10	26.98	116	7.59	135	4.37	100	3.38	32	3.61
	I	27	4.18	0	—	1	4.75	3	1.73	15	4.42	8	7.13
	II	59	3.78	1	—	5	4.58	24	4.44	32	3.58	7	2.46
	IIIN	31	4.09	0	—	3	4.61	13	5.03	12	3.54	3	3.15
	IIIM	151	4.42	3	24.95	51	6.80	62	4.33	26	2.70	9	3.43
	IV	77	5.77	4	36.30	35	9.27	21	4.15	13	3.85	4	3.95
	V	38	7.27	2	15.36	21	10.23	12	6.51	2	2.27	1	3.12
	Other	29	11.96	1	—	12	22.60	14	13.57	2	3.07	0	—
3 and over	**Total**	**241**	**5.50**	**0**	**—**	**31**	**9.64**	**87**	**6.81**	**73**	**4.53**	**50**	**4.25**
	I-V	229	5.36	0	—	30	9.45	83	6.70	68	4.35	48	4.17
	I	7	3.72	0	—	0	—	0	—	2	2.27	5	6.93
	II	29	4.26	0	—	1	6.24	7	6.02	17	5.34	4	1.74
	IIIN	15	4.97	0	—	1	8.32	4	5.12	4	3.00	6	7.68
	IIIM	82	4.85	0	—	10	8.39	36	6.79	21	3.51	15	3.39
	IV	67	7.18	0	—	10	10.51	25	7.54	19	6.85	13	5.69
	V	29	6.11	0	—	8	10.94	11	7.04	5	3.40	5	5.09
	Other	12	10.33	0	—	1	24.95	4	10.24	5	10.62	2	7.68
Illegitimate		**537**	**6.94**	**202**	**7.91**	**199**	**7.39**	**82**	**6.30**	**34**	**4.19**	**20**	**5.28**
Total		**2,303**	**4.27**	**448**	**7.51**	**987**	**4.85**	**815**	**3.67**	**409**	**3.12**	**144**	**3.64**

* Per 1,000 live births
Source: OPCS, *Mortality statistics; perinatal and infant, Series DH3 No 9*

Table A5.5 Live births by parity, social class and age of mother, England and Wales, 1980

Parity	Social-class	Age of mother					
		All ages	Under 20	20-24	25-29	30-34	35 and over
All live births		**656,234**	**59,686**	**203,649**	**222,194**	**131,153**	**39,553**
All Legitimate	**Total**	**578,862**	**34,162**	**176,711**	**209,180**	**123,044**	**35,765**
	I-V	558,936	32,479	168,777	202,799	119,918	34,964
	I	40,804	341	4,909	17,061	14,566	3,927
	II	123,585	1,893	20,868	51,113	39,251	10,459
	IIIN	61,902	1,733	16,630	25,526	14,506	3,506
	IIIM	212,276	14,246	75,898	75,708	35,484	10,940
	IV	87,699	9,026	35,935	25,817	12,342	4,578
	V	32,669	5,240	14,536	7,574	3,767	1,553
	Other	19,926	1,683	7,934	6,382	3,126	801
0	**Total**	**239,916**	**27,530**	**97,147**	**80,576**	**28,832**	**5,831**
	I-V	230,419	26,047	92,668	78,002	28,021	5,680
	I	17,181	281	3,406	8,485	4,067	942
	II	51,974	1,643	13,485	24,124	10,629	2,094
	IIIN	28,271	1,503	10,790	11,521	3,787	671
	IIIM	85,485	11,341	41,075	24,865	6,722	1,483
	IV	35,164	7,223	17,762	7,423	2,334	421
	V	12,342	4,057	6,151	1,583	481	70
	Other	9,497	1,483	4,478	2,575	811	150
1	**Total**	**207,607**	**6,261**	**60,530**	**83,872**	**47,857**	**9,087**
	I-V	200,765	5,061	57,645	81,488	46,665	8,906
	I	15,278	60	1,272	6,582	6,221	1,142
	II	46,525	250	6,131	20,427	16,500	3,216
	IIIN	23,032	220	5,069	10,639	6,001	1,102
	IIIM	75,708	2,785	26,127	31,237	13,154	2,404
	IV	29,874	1,693	13,444	10,018	3,857	862
	V	10,349	1,052	5,600	2,585	932	180
	Other	6,842	200	2,885	2,384	1,192	180
2	**Total**	**87,489**	**371**	**15,819**	**31,958**	**30,255**	**9,087**
	I-V	85,065	371	15,288	30,926	29,604	8,876
	I	6,462	-	210	1,733	3,396	1,122
	II	18,273	-	1,091	5,400	8,936	2,845
	IIIN	7,584	10	651	2,585	3,386	952
	IIIM	34,182	120	7,504	14,306	9,627	2,625
	IV	13,334	110	3,777	5,059	3,376	1,012
	V	5,230	130	2,054	1,843	882	321
	Other	2,424	-	531	1,032	651	210
3 and over	**Total**	**43,850**	**-**	**3,216**	**12,773**	**16,099**	**11,761**
	I-V	42,688	-	3,176	12,383	15,628	11,501
	I	1,883	-	20	260	882	721
	II	6,812	-	160	1,162	3,186	2,304
	IIIN	3,015	-	120	781	1,332	781
	IIIM	16,901	-	1,192	5,300	5,981	4,428
	IV	9,327	-	952	3,316	2,775	2,284
	V	4,749	-	731	1,563	1,473	982
	Other	1,162	-	40	391	471	260
Illegitimate		**77,372**	**25,524**	**26,938**	**13,014**	**8,109**	**3,788**

Source: OPCS, *Mortality statistics: perinatal and infant. Series DH3 No. 9*

132

Table A5.6   Singleton and multiple births by birthweight and social class, Scotland, 1979

Birthweight g	Social Class						Total
	I	II	III	IV	V	Not known	
Singleton births							
	Numbers						
1- 499	2	0	2	1	0	2	7
500- 999	7	11	51	25	9	31	134
1,000-1,499	14	30	145	49	40	117	395
1,500-1,999	23	64	265	101	72	182	707
2,000-2,499	88	206	964	415	288	760	2,721
2,500-2,999	608	1,047	4,548	1,621	1,133	2,721	11,678
3,000-3,499	1,708	2,998	10,373	3,611	2,043	5,123	25,856
3,500-3,999	1,525	2,399	7,572	2,556	1,214	3,184	18,450
4,000-4,499	411	768	2,163	708	311	816	5,177
4,500 and over	78	109	338	121	39	119	804
Total known	4,464	7,632	26,421	9,208	5,149	13,055	65,929
Not known	9	25	118	47	33	82	314
Total	**4,473**	**7,657**	**26,539**	**9,255**	**5,182**	**13,137**	**66,243**
	Percentage distribution of birthweights in each social class						
1- 499	0.00	0.00	0.00	0.00	0.00	0.00	0.00
500- 999	0.16	0.14	0.19	0.27	0.17	0.24	0.20
1,000-1,499	0.31	0.39	0.55	0.53	0.78	0.90	0.60
1,500-1,999	0.52	0.84	1.00	1.10	1.40	1.39	1.07
2,000-2,499	1.97	2.70	3.65	4.51	5.59	5.82	4.13
2,500-2,999	13.62	13.72	17.21	17.60	22.00	20.84	17.71
3,000-3,499	38.26	39.28	39.26	39.22	39.68	39.24	39.22
3,500-3,999	34.16	31.43	28.66	27.76	23.58	24.39	27.98
4,000-4,499	9.21	10.06	8.19	7.69	6.04	6.25	7.85
4,500 and over	1.75	1.43	1.28	1.31	0.76	0.91	1.22
Total known	100	100	100	100	100	100	100
Not known as a percentage of total	0.20	0.33	0.44	0.51	0.64	0.62	0.47

Birthweight g	Social Class						Total
	I	II	III	IV	V	Not known	
Multiple births							
Numbers							
1- 499	0	0	2	0	0	2	4
500- 999	0	0	12	2	4	8	26
1,000-1,499	6	4	30	10	4	10	64
1,500-1,999	6	24	66	18	12	28	154
2,000-2,499	28	32	118	48	36	72	334
2,500-2,999	50	56	176	62	34	62	440
3,000-3,499	10	26	80	20	8	32	176
3,500-3,999	0	8	10	6	0	2	26
4,000-4,499	0	2	2	0	0	0	4
4,500 and over	0	0	0	0	0	0	0
Total known	100	152	496	166	98	216	1,228
Not known	0	4	6	2	4	2	18
Total	**100**	**156**	**502**	**168**	**102**	**218**	**1,246**
Percentage distribution of birthweights in each social class							
1- 499	—	—	0.40	—	—	0.93	0.33
500- 999	—	—	2.42	1.20	4.08	3.70	2.12
1,000-1,499	6.00	2.63	6.05	6.02	4.08	4.63	5.21
1,500-1,999	6.00	15.79	13.31	10.84	12.24	12.96	12.54
2,000-2,499	28.00	21.05	23.79	28.92	36.73	33.33	27.20
3,500-2,999	50.00	36.84	35.48	37.35	34.69	28.70	35.83
3,000-3,499	10.00	17.11	16.13	12.05	8.16	14.81	14.33
3,500-3,999	—	5.26	2.02	3.61	—	0.93	2.12
4,000-4,499	—	1.32	0.40	—	—	—	0.33
4,500 and over	—	—	—	—	—	—	—
Total known	100	100	100	100	100	100	100
Not known as a percentage of total	—	2.56	1.20	1.19	3.92	0.92	1.44

Source: SHHD Information Services Division unpublished SMR2 data

Table A5.7   Perinatal and postneonatal mortality by social class, England and Wales 1970-80

Year	Legitimate							Illegitimate	Total
	Social Class								
	I	II	III N	III M	IV	V	Other		
Perinatal deaths (per 1,000 total births)									
1970-72	16.3	18.6	20.6	22.1	23.9	32.1	31.7	29.6	23.0
1975	13.8	15.6	16.0	18.9	21.4	27.0	20.9	26.4	19.2
1976	12.7	14.3	15.6	17.1	19.2	24.9	21.9	24.3	17.7
1977	11.6	13.0	14.1	17.1	18.8	22.0	21.8	23.3	16.9
1978	11.9	12.3	13.9	15.1	16.7	20.3	20.4	21.1	15.5
1979*	10.3	11.8	12.7	14.3	16.5	18.7	16.8	19.5	14.6
1980*	9.7	11.1	11.8	13.0	15.0	17.0	14.9	16.9	13.3
Postneonatal deaths (per 1,000 live births)									
1970-72	2.9	3.7	3.9	5.6	6.7	13.1	9.7	8.5	6.0
1975	3.0	3.3	3.5	4.4	5.7	8.7	7.5	7.6	4.8
1976	2.6	2.8	3.1	4.0	5.1	8.4	8.8	7.1	4.4
1977	2.9	3.0	3.2	3.7	5.0	8.0	8.7	7.2	4.4
1978	3.0	3.1	3.2	4.2	4.3	7.1	8.9	6.4	4.3
1979*	3.3	2.8	2.6	3.9	5.2	8.1	9.0	7.5	4.5
1980*	3.2	3.1	3.4	3.5	4.8	6.2	8.1	6.9	4.3

* Classified using the *1980 Classification of Occupations*

Source: OPCS, unpublished data from the *Decennial Supplement on Occupational Mortality 1970-72* and *Mortality statistics: perinatal and infant, Series DH3*

Table A5.8 Total births by social class, legitimacy and area of residence, England and Wales, 1979-80

Area of residence	Percentage of total births							Total number of births 1979-80 (=100%)
	Legitimate by social class						Illegitimate	
	I	II	III	IV	V	Other		
ENGLAND AND WALES	**6.1**	**18.9**	**42.0**	**13.6**	**5.1**	**2.9**	**11.4**	**1,304,160**
ENGLAND	**6.2**	**19.0**	**41.9**	**13.6**	**4.8**	**2.9**	**11.5**	**1,229,021**
Northern RHA	**4.5**	**14.9**	**43.9**	**15.4**	**7.8**	**1.8**	**11.7**	**83,538**
Cleveland AHA	5.0	11.8	42.3	15.2	9.6	0.9	15.2	17,484
Cumbria AHA	4.4	19.1	46.2	12.7	7.5	1.3	8.7	11,359
Durham AHA	3.9	16.0	44.0	17.5	7.5	1.8	9.3	16,161
Northumberland AHA	5.3	20.2	42.6	18.2	3.6	3.0	7.0	7,743
Gateshead AHA	3.7	12.3	44.7	14.9	8.6	3.5	12.4	5,596
Newcastle upon Tyne AHA	7.8	16.1	36.9	14.3	7.1	2.3	15.4	7,238
North Tyneside AHA	4.0	15.1	48.7	13.5	5.1	1.0	12.5	5,083
South Tyneside AHA	3.0	12.3	47.9	12.9	9.2	1.4	13.3	4,126
Sunderland AHA	2.2	11.4	45.9	16.3	9.4	2.1	12.8	8,748
Yorkshire RHA	**4.7**	**16.7**	**41.3**	**16.3**	**6.3**	**2.4**	**12.3**	**94,867**
Humberside AHA	4.5	15.3	42.8	13.2	7.9	2.4	13.9	22,313
North Yorkshire AHA	5.4	23.3	38.5	14.1	4.1	6.6	8.0	15,302
Bradford AHA	3.2	15.0	38.0	20.9	7.8	1.5	13.6	15,125
Calderdale AHA	3.9	12.9	44.6	18.3	4.9	0.8	14.5	5,142
Kirklees AHA	4.7	15.5	39.1	22.4	6.2	1.1	11.0	10,697
Leeds AHA	6.3	17.5	42.2	12.9	4.9	1.5	14.7	17,973
Wakefield AHA	3.4	13.7	47.5	18.2	6.9	1.0	9.2	8,315
Trent RHA	**5.2**	**16.7**	**44.9**	**15.3**	**4.8**	**1.9**	**11.2**	**119,270**
Derbyshire AHA	5.7	18.2	45.7	15.8	4.4	0.7	9.4	23,256
Leicestershire AHA	6.3	19.6	44.6	14.0	2.6	2.1	10.8	23,933
Lincolnshire AHA	5.4	20.0	40.6	13.3	4.1	6.7	9.8	13,575
Nottinghamshire AHA	5.0	16.4	41.0	17.5	4.8	1.1	14.2	25,505
Barnsley AHA	2.7	8.1	60.5	13.0	4.6	0.7	10.4	5,814
Doncaster AHA	2.8	10.7	49.6	16.4	7.9	2.2	10.5	7,930
Rotherham AHA	3.5	12.5	46.4	16.1	9.4	1.0	11.1	7,014
Sheffield AHA	6.1	15.2	45.5	14.9	5.9	0.9	11.4	12,243
East Anglian RHA	**6.7**	**18.6**	**41.7**	**12.9**	**3.9**	**7.7**	**8.4**	**48,902**
Cambridgeshire AHA	9.1	18.7	39.1	14.1	3.9	7.3	7.8	16,105
Norfolk AHA	5.4	18.5	44.6	12.9	3.9	5.7	8.9	16,938
Suffolk AHA	5.7	18.7	41.3	11.7	3.9	10.2	8.6	15,859
North West Thames RHA	**9.2**	**23.4**	**38.7**	**11.5**	**3.1**	**2.6**	**11.4**	**94,980**
Bedfordshire AHA	7.3	19.0	41.8	16.6	2.7	3.4	9.2	16,406
Hertfordshire AHA	9.3	26.5	42.3	10.9	2.5	1.2	7.3	24,652
Barnet AHA	13.2	31.8	31.3	7.7	2.6	5.3	8.0	7,527
Brent and Harrow AHA	10.8	23.1	37.8	8.9	3.4	1.6	14.4	13,178

Table A5.8   Total births by social class, legitimacy and area of residence, England and Wales, 1979-80
  —continued

Area of residence	Percentage of total births							Total number of births 1979-80 (=100%)
	Legitimate by social class						Illegitimate	
	I	II	III	IV	V	Other		
North West Thames RHA *—continued*								
Ealing, Hammersmith and Hounslow AHA	7.8	20.3	38.4	12.7	4.1	1.7	14.8	19,023
Hillingdon AHA	7.5	19.6	47.5	9.4	3.2	3.6	9.3	6,186
Kensington, Chelsea and Westminster AHA	10.4	26.6	23.6	9.3	3.4	6.4	20.2	8,008
North East Thames RHA	**5.8**	**19.6**	**42.3**	**13.5**	**3.8**	**2.3**	**12.9**	**101,965**
Essex AHA	6.4	23.8	45.4	11.4	3.3	1.9	7.7	39,063
Barking and Havering AHA	4.1	16.8	52.1	14.2	3.7	0.0	9.0	9,893
Camden and Islington AHA	8.9	18.0	31.4	9.8	4.3	4.0	23.6	8,805
City and East London AHA	2.4	11.0	34.8	20.2	6.0	4.3	21.3	19,053
Enfield and Haringey AHA	7.8	19.9	41.8	11.8	2.7	2.1	13.9	13,028
Redbridge and Waltham Forest AHA	5.9	22.5	44.1	13.1	2.3	1.4	10.6	12,123
South East Thames RHA	**6.1**	**20.7**	**40.8**	**11.0**	**4.6**	**2.6**	**14.3**	**90,769**
East Sussex AHA	7.7	25.2	38.7	10.9	3.6	1.9	11.9	13,627
Kent AHA	5.6	21.8	44.5	11.0	4.9	2.6	9.6	38,975
Greenwich and Bexley AHA	4.2	17.9	45.8	11.7	5.9	2.4	12.0	11,664
Bromley AHA	11.7	31.3	36.7	7.6	2.6	0.9	9.1	6,622
Lambeth, Southwark and Lewisham AHA	5.2	13.6	33.3	11.4	4.4	3.7	28.4	19,881
South West Thames RHA	**11.3**	**27.6**	**37.7**	**9.4**	**2.5**	**1.8**	**9.7**	**70,522**
Surrey AHA	13.8	30.0	35.3	9.4	2.6	2.3	6.6	23,349
West Sussex AHA	8.3	26.6	43.6	10.1	3.3	1.3	6.7	15,529
Croydon AHA	9.4	26.7	36.2	11.2	1.8	1.4	13.4	8,844
Kingston and Richmond AHA	15.2	34.8	33.5	5.6	1.3	1.7	7.9	7,105
Merton, Sutton and Wandsworth AHA	9.7	22.4	38.3	9.4	2.6	1.6	15.9	15.695
Wessex RHA	**7.3**	**19.9**	**39.8**	**10.4**	**3.1**	**10.5**	**9.0**	**67,577**
Dorset AHA	6.8	21.2	43.0	9.4	3.2	6.9	9.5	12,554
Hampshire AHA	7.6	19.7	39.1	10.2	2.9	11.7	8.8	39,113
Wiltshire AHA	7.4	19.3	38.5	11.3	3.2	11.9	8.4	13,451
Isle of Wight AHA	5.9	20.3	41.7	14.4	4.8	1.3	11.7	2,459
Oxford RHA	**8.8**	**22.8**	**40.5**	**12.1**	**3.4**	**3.7**	**8.7**	**65,214**
Berkshire AHA	9.8	25.1	39.8	12.1	2.0	2.7	8.4	19,521
Buckinghamshire AHA	10.3	25.5	39.9	11.6	2.3	2.4	8.0	16,444

Table A5.8 **Total births by social class, legitimacy and area of residence, England and Wales, 1979-80**
 −continued

Area of residence	Percentage of total births							Total number of births 1979-80 (=100%)
	Legitimate by social class						Illegitimate	
	I	II	III	IV	V	Other		
Oxford RHA − continued								
Northamptonshire AHA	5.1	17.5	45.9	13.0	5.5	2.0	11.0	15,030
Oxfordshire AHA	9.6	22.3	36.5	11.5	4.4	8.1	7.6	14,219
South Western RHA	**5.8**	**20.9**	**42.4**	**12.1**	**4.5**	**4.9**	**9.4**	**77,442**
Avon AHA	7.0	20.4	44.8	11.7	4.1	1.8	10.2	22,868
Cornwall (and Scilly) AHA	4.7	21.5	40.2	14.5	4.2	5.6	9.3	10,252
Devon AHA	4.7	20.7	40.7	10.0	5.5	9.0	9.4	21,792
Gloucestershire AHA	6.7	21.9	42.0	12.9	4.5	2.8	9.3	12,566
Somerset AHA	5.2	20.5	43.6	14.2	3.9	5.0	7.6	9,964
West Midlands RHA	**4.8**	**16.6**	**44.4**	**16.3**	**5.1**	**1.5**	**11.3**	**140,602**
Hereford and Worcester AHA	5.6	24.6	44.6	12.0	3.7	1.7	7.8	16,686
Salop AHA	5.3	20.9	38.2	16.6	5.9	4.3	8.9	9,642
Staffordshire AHA	4.1	18.1	49.1	14.2	5.2	1.2	8.1	27,447
Warwickshire AHA	7.8	20.0	41.6	16.9	3.4	1.7	8.5	11,983
Birmingham AHA	4.1	12.2	39.6	18.5	6.3	1.5	17.8	30,235
Coventry AHA	5.0	12.1	44.0	19.9	4.0	0.9	14.1	9,019
Dudley AHA	5.7	19.5	51.6	12.8	2.8	0.5	7.2	7,891
Sandwell AHA	3.0	7.8	50.0	19.2	7.7	0.5	11.8	8,324
Solihull AHA	7.9	22.9	42.3	12.6	2.1	0.9	11.2	4,847
Walsall AHA	2.5	13.4	48.5	19.1	5.9	0.8	9.8	7,181
Wolverhampton AHA	4.0	10.7	43.5	19.3	6.1	1.6	14.7	7,347
Mersey RHA	**4.6**	**16.4**	**41.5**	**15.8**	**7.6**	**1.4**	**12.6**	**64,972**
Cheshire AHA	6.3	20.7	43.7	14.7	4.5	1.4	8.7	24,145
Liverpool AHA	2.9	9.9	37.9	17.1	11.3	1.2	19.6	13,896
St Helens and Knowsley AHA	2.7	11.3	42.2	18.2	10.5	1.7	13.4	10,844
Sefton AHA	4.7	19.6	42.9	13.1	8.0	0.9	10.9	7,118
Wirral AHA	4.9	18.9	39.1	16.1	6.5	1.8	12.7	8,969
North Western RHA	**5.0**	**16.2**	**42.9**	**14.9**	**6.0**	**1.4**	**13.7**	**108,401**
Lancashire AHA	4.5	18.3	43.8	15.4	5.5	1.2	11.2	36,059
Bolton AHA	4.8	15.1	41.9	18.2	7.3	1.1	11.5	7,481
Bury AHA	6.5	21.1	44.2	11.2	4.0	1.9	11.0	4,825
Manchester AHA	3.7	10.1	35.3	14.1	7.5	3.0	26.2	12,688
Oldham AHA	2.9	14.3	40.7	17.2	7.9	1.6	15.4	6,542
Rochdale AHA	3.6	14.4	40.8	18.6	6.0	0.9	15.7	6,706
Salford AHA	5.0	10.5	40.1	15.9	8.2	1.3	19.0	6,323
Stockport AHA	10.7	20.8	45.3	8.3	3.0	1.1	10.8	7,511
Tameside AHA	4.2	12.7	48.0	14.5	7.0	0.8	12.9	5,943
Trafford AHA	8.1	20.0	43.3	12.3	3.0	1.1	12.1	5,608
Wigan AHA	3.9	17.0	49.2	15.3	7.2	0.6	6.9	8,715

Table A5.8 Total births by social class, legitimacy and area of residence, England and Wales, 1979-80
−continued

Area of residence	Percentage of total births							Total number of births 1979-80 (=100%)
	Legitimate by social class						Illegitimate	
	I	II	III	IV	V	Other		
WALES	**4.8**	**16.9**	**43.4**	**13.6**	**9.0**	**2.5**	**9.9**	**74,083**
Clwyd AHA	4.6	19.1	44.6	12.4	9.1	2.0	8.2	10,092
Dyfed AHA	5.0	21.6	41.2	13.0	6.1	5.5	7.6	8,125
Gwent AHA	4.4	14.6	41.5	13.4	13.8	1.7	10.6	11,856
Gwynedd AHA	4.7	18.4	42.4	12.3	8.0	3.7	10.5	5,687
Mid Glamorgan AHA	3.7	13.2	46.0	15.4	10.1	1.5	10.0	15,533
Powys AHA	4.7	29.3	38.5	12.2	6.4	1.2	7.7	2,562
South Glamorgan AHA	7.7	18.5	40.9	10.1	5.8	3.3	13.7	10,517
West Glamorgan AHA	4.3	13.1	46.7	17.5	8.4	1.4	8.7	9,711

Source: Data derived from unpublished reference tables for each RHA and AHA. As explained in OPCS *Monitor DH3 82/3*, which contains data for 1980 for RHA's only, the reference tables can be obtained from Medical Statistics Division, OPCS.

Table A5.9 Legitimate stillbirths and infant deaths by 1970 and 1980 social class classifications, England and Wales, 1979

		Total		I		II		III		IV		V	
		Number	Rate	Number	Rate	Number	Rate	Number	Rate	Number	Rate	Number	Rate
Stillbirths*	1970	4,410	7.7	252	5.6	704	6.3	2,161	7.8	850	9.2	282	9.7
	1980	4,410	7.7	200	5.2	771	6.3	2,128	7.8	835	9.2	316	9.6
Perinatal deaths*	1970	8,034	14.0	487	10.7	1,324	11.8	3,858	14.0	1,511	16.4	551	19.0
	1980	8,034	14.0	400	10.3	1,442	11.8	3,798	14.0	1,479	16.5	615	18.7
Neonatal deaths†	1970	4,411	7.8	293	6.5	768	6.9	2,035	7.4	826	9.1	313	10.9
	1980	4,411	7.8	251	6.5	835	6.9	2,000	7.4	806	9.1	348	10.7
Postneonatal deaths†	1970	2,326	4.1	144	3.2	219	2.8	991	3.6	454	5.0	261	9.1
	1980	2,326	4.1	129	3.3	341	2.8	970	3.6	464	5.2	263	8.1
Infant deaths†	1970	6,737	11.8	437	9.7	1,087	9.7	3,026	11.1	1,280	14.1	574	19.9
	1980	6,737	11.8	380	9.8	1,176	9.7	2,970	11.0	1,270	14.3	611	18.7
Live births	1970	568,561		45,094		111,935		273,834		91,101		28,790	
	1980	568,561		38,579		121,560		269,515		88,562		32,637	

* Rates are per 1,000 total births
† Rates are per 1,000 live births
Source: OPCS Monitor DH3 82/5.

Table A5.10 Illegitimate births and pre-marital conceptions, England and Wales, 1938-80

Year	Numbers				Percentages			
	Illegitimate births		Total	Conceived before marriage*	Illegitimate births as percentage of total births	Joint registrations as percentages of total births	Sole registrations as percentages of total births	Conceived before marriage as percentage of total births*
	Joint registration	Sole registration						
1938	-	-	27,755	64,530	4.30	-	-	-
1939	-	-	26,842	60,346	4.20	-	-	-
1940	-	-	26,915		4.39	-	-	-
1941	-	-	32,550	43,146†	5.43	-	-	-
1942	-	-	38,016		5.64	-	-	-
1943	-	-	45,411		6.44	-	-	-
1944	-	-	57,130		7.39	-	-	-
1945	-	-	65,483		9.36	-	-	-
1946	-	-	55,768	52,557†	6.61	-	-	-
1947	-	-	48,075		5.32	-	-	-
1948	-	-	42,932		5.41	-	-	-
1949	-	-	38,030		5.09	-	-	-
1950	-	-	36,306	54,188	5.09	-	-	-
1951	-	-	33,839	50,477	4.88	-	-	6.4
1952	-	-	33,545	44,239	4.87	-	-	6.3
1953	-	-	33,503	43,988	4.79	-	-	6.4
1954	-	-	32,560	44,319	4.72	-	-	6.4
1955	-	-	32,067	43,601	4.69	-	-	
1956	-	-	34,536	47,377	4.82	-	-	6.6
1957	-	-	35,585	48,611	4.81	-	-	6.6
1958	-	-	37,232	49,775	4.92	-	-	6.6
1959	-	-	39,235	50,871	5.13	-	-	6.7
1960	-	-	43,799	54,576	5.47	-	-	6.8
1961	18,456	31,235	49,691	59,115	6.01	2.23	3.78	7.1
1962	21,748	34,917	56,665	62,455	6.63	2.55	4.09	7.3
1963	23,944	36,395	60,340	64,427	6.94	2.76	4.19	7.4
1964	25,746	38,903	64,649	67,933	7.26	2.89	4.37	7.6
1965	25,884	41,649	67,533	70,457	7.70	2.95	4.75	8.0

141

Table A5.10 Illegitimate births and pre-marital conceptions, England and Wales, 1938-80 - *continued*

Year	Numbers				Percentages			
	Illegitimate births			Conceived before marriage*	Illegitimate births as percentage of total births	Joint registrations as percentages of total births	Sole registrations as percentages of total births	Conceived before marriage as percentage of total births
	Joint registration	Sole registration	Total					
1966	25,842	43,382	69,224	71,648	8.02	2.99	5.03	8.3
1967	26,562	44,698	71,260	73,667	8.44	3.14	5.29	8.7
1968	27,432	43,606	71,038	74,531	8.55	3.30	5.25	9.0
1969	27,601	40,547	68,148	72,595	8.43	3.42	5.02	9.0
1970	28,425	37,364	65,789	70,623	8.28	3.58	4.70	8.9
1971	30,093	36,657	66,750	67,294	8.42	3.79	4.62	8.5
1972	29,028	34,434	63,462	59,836	8.64	3.95	4.69	8.1
1973	27,113	31,863	58,976	52,293	8.62	3.96	4.66	7.6
1974	27,257	30,063	57,320	45,981	8.86	4.21	4.65	7.1
1975	27,066	28,541	55,607	40,293	9.12	4.44	4.68	6.6
1976	27,568	26,885	54,453	35,383	9.23	4.67	4.56	6.0
1977	29,483	26,595	56,078	32,913	9.76	5.13	4.63	5.7
1978	32,986	28,350	61,336	34,533	10.20	5.48	4.71	5.7
1979	38,553	31,629	70,182	37,448	10.91	5.99	4.92	5.8
1980	44,410	33,658	78,068	39,798	11.81	6.72	5.09	6.0

* From 1952 onwards the figures relate to women married only once. Until 1951 the figures are for births occurring with 8½ months of marriage, thereafter within 8 months
† Annual average

Source: OPCS, *Birth Statistics, Series FM1*

Table A5.11 Adoptions, England and Wales, 1980

Age of children at adoption	Sex	All children	Legitimate children				Illegitimate children			
			Total	Joint adopters		Sole adopter	Total	Joint adopters		Sole adopter
				One or both a parent	Neither a parent			One or both a parent	Neither a parent	
Total	**All**	**10,609**	**4,535**	**3,668**	**835**	**32**	**6,074**	**2,482**	**3,529**	**63**
	Males	**5,428**	**2,283**	**1,839**	**428**	**16**	**3,145**	**1,244**	**1,876**	**25**
	Females	**5,181**	**2,252**	**1,829**	**407**	**16**	**2,929**	**1,238**	**1,653**	**38**
Under 6 months	Males	514	17	-	17	-	497	7	490	-
	Females	480	11	2	9	-	469	5	463	1
6-8 months	Males	715	34	-	34	-	681	6	675	-
	Females	603	34	-	34	-	569	8	561	-
9-11 months	Males	154	19	2	17	-	135	6	127	2
	Females	135	11	-	11	-	122	6	115	1
1 year	Males	205	33	8	23	2	172	26	146	-
	Females	212	39	4	35	-	173	27	146	-
2 years	Males	199	57	27	30	-	142	75	67	-
	Females	180	63	22	40	1	117	57	58	2
3-4 years	Males	665	248	182	65	1	418	305	110	3
	Females	623	234	176	57	1	394	291	95	8
5-9 years	Males	1,723	1,042	876	163	3	681	521	153	7
	Females	1,691	978	836	137	5	713	566	130	17
10-14 years	Males	1,016	697	627	64	6	319	242	69	8
	Females	1,025	722	650	66	6	303	234	62	7
15-17 years	Males	236	136	117	15	4	100	56	39	5
	Females	229	160	139	18	3	69	44	23	2

Source: *OPCS Monitor FM3 81/1*

143

Table A5.12 Divorce decrees made absolute by duration of marriage and number of children aged under 16, England and Wales, 1980

Duration of marriage (completed years)	Couples with no children under 16*	Couples with one or more child(ren) under 16*	Total number of divorcing couples	Percentage of divorcing couples with:	
				no children under 16*	no children
Total all durations	**60,099**	**88,202**	**148,301**	**41**	**31**
0-2	1,136	440	1,576	72	71
3	9,062	4,583	13,645	66	66
4	7,434	5,862	13,296	56	55
5	5,448	5,470	10,918	50	49
6	4,168	5,577	9,745	43	42
7	3,418	5,596	9,014	38	37
8	2,498	5,571	8,069	31	30
9	1,930	5,476	7,406	26	25
10-14	4,721	23,899	28,620	16	15
15-19	2,789	15,752	18,541	15	9
20-24	5,505	7,179	12,684	43	12
25-29	5,187	2,232	7,419	70	19
30 or more	6,803	565	7,368	92	26
Median duration (yrs)	7.8	11.2†	10.1		

* *Age at date petition filed*
† *Estimated*
Source: *OPCS Monitor FM2 82/1*

Table A5.13 Family type by number of dependent children and age of youngest child, Great Britain, 1979-80

Family type	Number of dependent children				Base =100%	Average (mean) number of children	Age of youngest child				Base =100%	Total
	1	2	3	4 or more			0-4	5-9	10-15	16 or over		
Married couple*	% 38	43	14	5	7,505	1.9	37	28	31	4	7,505	88
Lone mother	% 57	29	9	5	856	1.6	29	29	37	6	856	10
Lone father	% 50	35	13	1	127	1.6	5	27	61	8	127	1
Total	% 40	41	14	5	8,488	1.9	36	28	32	4	8,488	100

* Including married women whose husbands were not defined as resident in the household
Source: OPCS *General Household Survey* 1980

145

Table A5.14 Live births by mother's country of birth, England and Wales, 1973-80

Birthplace of mother		1973	1974	1975	1976	1977	1978	1979	1980
All countries	percentage	100.0	100.0	100.0	100.0	100.0	100.0	100.0	100.0
	number	675,953	639,885	603,445	584,270	569,259	596,418	638,028	656,234
United Kingdom*		88.3	88.2	87.9	87.5	86.9	86.8	86.9	86.7
Total outside United Kingdom		11.5	11.6	11.9	12.4	13.0	13.1	13.1	13.2
Irish Republic†		2.4	2.3	2.1	1.9	1.8	1.6	1.5	1.4
Australia, Canada, New Zealand		0.4	0.4	0.4	0.4	0.4	0.4	0.4	0.4
New Commonwealth and Pakistan		6.1	6.2	6.6	7.2	7.8	8.0	8.2	8.5
Bangladesh		0.1	0.1	0.2	0.2	0.3	0.3	0.3	0.4
India		1.9	1.9	2.0	2.1	2.2	2.1	2.1	2.0
Sri Lanka ø		0.1	0.1	0.1	0.1	0.1	0.1	0.1	0.1
Hong Kong		0.2	0.2	0.2	0.2	0.2	0.2	0.2	0.2
South East Asia‡		0.1	0.1	0.1	0.2	0.2	0.2	0.3	0.3
East African Commonwealth§		0.4	0.5	0.6	0.7	0.9	0.9	1.0	1.0
Other African Commonwealth**		0.4	0.4	0.4	0.4	0.5	0.5	0.5	0.5
Caribbean††		1.3	1.3	1.3	1.2	1.2	1.2	1.1	1.1
Malta, Gibralta, Cyprus		0.4	0.4	0.5	0.5	0.5	0.5	0.5	0.5
Remainder of New Commonwealth		0.1	0.1	0.1	0.1	0.1	0.1	0.2	0.2
Pakistan		1.0	1.1	1.2	1.4	1.7	1.9	2.0	2.1
European Community‡‡		0.9	1.0	0.9	0.9	0.9	0.9	0.9	0.9
Other Europe		0.7	0.7	0.7	0.6	0.6	0.6	0.6	0.6
United States of America		0.3	0.4	0.4	0.4	0.4	0.4	0.4	0.4
South Africa		0.1	0.1	0.1	0.1	0.1	0.1	0.1	0.1
South East Asia (excluding Commonwealth)øø		0.0	0.1	0.1	0.1	0.1	0.1	0.1	0.2
Other foreign (including USSR)		0.5	0.6	0.7	0.7	0.8	0.9	0.9	0.8
Not stated		0.2	0.2	0.2	0.1	0.1	0.1	0.1	0.0

* Including Isle of Man and Channel Islands
† Including Ireland, part not stated
ø Including Laccadive and Maldive Islands
‡ Including Malaysia, Brunei, Singapore and other Asian Commonwealth not listed
§ Including Kenya, Malawi, Tanzania, Uganda, Zambia and other East African Commonwealth not listed

** Including Botswana, Ghana, Gambia, Lesotho, Nigeria, Sierra Leone, Swaziland and Zimbabwe
†† Including Guyana and Belize
‡‡ Excluding UK and Irish Republic
øø Including Vietnam, Indonesia, Phillipines and Thailand

Source: OPCS Birth statistics, Series FM1

Table A5.15 Live births by mother's country of birth by area of residence, England and Wales, 1980

Percentages of all live births in area

Area of residence	Mother's country of birth							
	United Kingdom	Irish Republic	India	Bangladesh	African Commonwealth	Rest of New Commonwealth	Pakistan	Elsewhere
ENGLAND AND WALES	**86.7**	**1.4**	**2.1**	**0.4**	**1.5**	**2.3**	**2.1**	**3.4**
ENGLAND	**86.2**	**1.4**	**2.2**	**0.4**	**1.6**	**2.4**	**2.2**	**3.5**
Northern RHA	**96.5**	**0.3**	**0.4**	**0.1**	**0.2**	**0.5**	**0.7**	**1.2**
Cleveland AHA	95.0	0.5	0.5	0.0	0.3	0.5	2.2	0.9
Hartlepool HD	98.5	0.2	0.2	–	0.2	0.3	0.5	0.2
North Tees HD	95.3	0.7	0.4	0.0	0.1	0.7	1.9	0.8
South Tees HD	94.0	0.4	0.7	0.1	0.3	0.4	2.8	1.3
Cumbria AHA	97.6	0.4	0.1	0.0	0.2	0.5	0.0	1.0
East Cumbria HD	97.2	0.4	0.1	0.0	0.3	0.6	0.1	1.3
South West Cumbria HD	96.8	0.6	0.2	–	–	0.8	–	1.5
West Cumbria HD	98.6	0.3	0.1	–	0.1	0.2	–	0.7
Durham AHA	97.7	0.1	0.3	0.1	0.1	0.5	0.0	1.2
Darlington HD	95.5	0.3	0.9	0.3	0.2	0.7	0.1	2.0
Durham HD	97.9	0.2	0.1	0.0	0.1	0.4	–	1.2
North West Durham HD	98.7	0.1	0.4	–	–	0.3	0.1	0.5
South West Durham HD	98.2	0.0	0.1	0.0	–	0.6	–	1.0
Northumberland AHA	97.4	0.2	0.2	0.0	0.1	0.6	0.0	1.5
Gateshead AHA	97.2	0.3	0.2	0.0	0.1	0.3	0.3	1.5
Newcastle upon Tyne AHA	97.4	0.5	1.4	0.5	0.4	1.0	2.2	2.6
North Tyneside AHA	97.5	0.3	–	0.2	0.1	0.7	0.1	1.1
South Tyneside AHA	97.8	0.1	0.2	0.3	0.2	0.3	0.2	0.8
Sunderland AHA	98.2	0.1	0.3	0.1	0.1	0.4	0.0	0.8

Table A5.15 Live births by mother's country of birth by area of residence, England and Wales, 1980 - *continued*

Area of residence	Mother's country of birth							
	United Kingdom	Irish Republic	India	Bangladesh	African Common-wealth	Rest of New Common-wealth	Pakistan	Elsewhere
Yorkshire RHA	**87.6**	**0.8**	**1.9**	**0.3**	**0.6**	**1.0**	**5.9**	**1.7**
Humberside AHA	96.4	0.4	0.3	0.3	0.3	0.6	0.1	1.6
Hull HD	96.9	0.2	0.2	0.1	0.5	0.6	0.1	1.6
Beverley HD	96.3	0.6	0.1	-	0.3	0.5	0.2	2.0
Grimsby HD	97.0	0.3	0.1	0.1	0.3	0.7	0.1	1.4
Scunthorpe HD	95.2	0.6	0.9	1.0	0.1	0.5	0.1	1.5
North Yorkshire AHA	94.8	0.5	0.2	0.1	0.3	0.9	0.2	2.9
Northallerton HD	94.9	0.3	0.2	-	0.2	1.3	-	3.2
York HD	95.5	0.5	0.3	0.1	0.4	0.9	0.0	2.3
Scarborough HD	96.0	0.4	0.2	-	0.1	0.8	0.1	2.3
Harrogate HD	92.2	0.6	0.1	-	0.4	1.2	0.1	5.3
Bradford AHA	69.9	0.6	4.4	1.0	1.1	1.0	20.5	1.5
Bradford HD	65.8	0.7	5.5	0.8	1.4	1.1	23.1	1.6
Airedale HD	86.4	0.4	0.4	1.2	0.1	0.6	9.4	1.5
Calderdale AHA	85.9	1.6	0.5	0.4	0.2	0.8	9.6	1.0
Kirklees AHA	77.0	1.1	6.3	0.1	0.8	1.5	12.1	1.2
Huddersfield HD	78.5	1.7	3.7	0.0	0.7	2.6	11.5	1.3
Dewsbury HD	75.2	0.4	9.4	0.1	1.0	0.2	12.8	1.0
Leeds AHA	88.8	1.4	2.0	0.4	1.1	1.6	2.8	1.7
Western HD	90.1	1.1	1.5	0.3	1.2	1.2	2.8	1.7
Eastern HD	87.6	1.7	2.4	0.6	1.0	2.0	2.8	1.9
Wakefield AHA	96.0	0.4	0.3	0.0	0.2	0.4	1.8	0.9
Western (Wakefield) HD	93.3	0.7	0.5	0.1	0.3	0.6	3.8	0.8
Eastern (Pontefract) HD	98.3	0.2	0.1	-	0.0	0.4	0.0	1.0
Trent RHA	**91.4**	**0.6**	**2.0**	**0.1**	**1.5**	**1.2**	**1.5**	**1.7**
Derbyshire AHA	92.8	0.7	2.1	0.0	0.3	0.9	1.8	1.4
Central Derbyshire HD	97.0	0.5	0.4	-	0.2	0.5	0.1	1.3
North Derbyshire HD	97.3	0.5	0.1	0.0	0.1	0.5	0.2	1.3
South Derbyshire HD	84.4	1.0	5.8	0.1	0.5	1.7	5.0	1.6

Table A5.15 Live births by mother's country of birth by area of residence, England and Wales, 1980 - *continued*

Area of residence	Mother's country of birth							
	United Kingdom	Irish Republic	India	Bangladesh	African Commonwealth	Rest of New Commonwealth	Pakistan	Elsewhere
Trent RHA - continued								
Leicestershire AHA	82.2	0.8	6.0	0.3	6.5	1.5	0.4	2.3
East Leicestershire HD	67.3	0.8	12.2	0.4	14.0	1.8	1.2	2.2
North West Leicestershire HD	88.8	0.6	3.3	0.4	3.0	1.2	0.1	2.4
South West Leicestershire HD	90.0	1.0	2.5	0.1	2.5	1.5	0.1	2.3
Lincolnshire AHA	95.1	0.8	0.2	0.1	0.3	1.2	0.0	2.0
Lincolnshire South HD	95.3	0.4	0.3	-	0.4	1.1	0.0	2.0
Lincolnshire North HD	94.4	1.2	0.2	0.1	0.3	1.3	0.1	2.5
Nottinghamshire AHA	93.0	0.7	0.9	0.0	0.5	1.5	1.5	1.8
Central Nottinghamshire HD	97.4	0.3	0.1	0.0	0.1	1.0	0.1	0.9
Worksop and Retford HD	98.2	0.2	-	-	-	0.8	-	0.9
North Nottingham HD	91.1	0.9	1.8	-	0.8	1.6	1.9	1.9
South Nottingham HD	89.4	0.9	1.2	0.1	0.7	2.1	2.9	2.6
Barnsley AHA	98.2	0.3	0.3	0.0	0.1	0.4	0.0	0.7
Doncaster AHA	96.2	0.5	0.6	-	0.2	0.6	0.8	1.2
Rotherham AHA	94.8	0.5	0.3	-	0.1	0.4	3.2	0.7
Sheffield AHA	90.8	0.4	0.3	0.3	0.2	1.3	4.7	1.9
Northern HD	90.2	0.3	0.3	0.4	0.1	0.8	6.8	1.1
Southern HD	91.3	0.5	0.4	0.2	0.4	1.8	3.1	2.5
East Anglian RHA	**90.5**	**0.6**	**0.4**	**0.1**	**0.5**	**1.3**	**0.7**	**5.9**
Cambridgeshire AHA	88.6	0.8	0.6	0.1	0.9	1.4	1.9	5.7
Cambridge HD	88.7	0.8	0.4	0.2	0.7	1.4	0.4	7.4
Peterborough HD	87.2	1.0	1.0	0.0	1.4	1.2	4.7	3.6

Table A5.15 Live births by mother's country of birth by area of residence, England and Wales, 1980 - *continued*

Area of residence	Mother's country of birth							
	United Kingdom	Irish Republic	India	Bangladesh	African Common-wealth	Rest of New Common-wealth	Pakistan	Elsewhere
East Anglian RHA - continued								
Norfolk AHA	93.9	0.4	0.2	0.1	0.4	1.3	0.0	3.6
Norwich HD	94.6	0.2	0.2	0.1	0.4	1.2	0.0	3.3
Great Yarmouth and Waveney HD	95.5	0.6	-	0.1	0.3	1.2	0.0	2.3
King's Lynn HD	93.0	0.4	0.1	0.0	0.4	1.2	0.0	4.7
Suffolk AHA	88.8	0.6	0.3	0.2	0.3	1.2	0.0	8.6
Bury St Edmunds HD	84.4	0.8	0.2	-	0.4	1.4	0.0	12.7
Ipswich HD	89.8	0.4	0.4	0.5	0.1	1.3	0.0	7.4
North West Thames RHA	**67.9**	**3.7**	**5.7**	**0.7**	**5.2**	**5.1**	**2.3**	**9.3**
Bedfordshire AHA	80.2	2.1	3.0	1.6	1.6	2.8	4.5	4.2
Northern HD	82.4	1.4	4.0	0.8	1.2	2.6	1.3	6.4
Southern HD	78.5	2.6	2.3	2.2	1.9	2.9	7.0	2.5
Hertfordshire AHA	87.6	1.8	1.4	0.3	1.0	2.1	1.1	4.8
North Hertfordshire HD	88.5	1.2	4.2	0.6	0.7	1.7	0.6	2.5
East Hertfordshire HD	90.8	1.5	0.2	0.1	0.7	1.8	0.1	4.7
North West Hertfordshire HD	88.2	1.7	0.4	0.5	1.0	2.1	1.1	5.0
South West Hertfordshire HD	80.2	2.9	1.6	-	1.8	3.1	3.5	6.9
Barnet AHA	61.2	4.4	4.7	0.3	8.4	6.0	0.9	14.1
Barnet and Finchley HD	70.6	3.3	3.2	0.2	5.7	5.9	0.2	11.0
Edgware and Hendon HD	55.3	5.6	6.3	0.5	11.4	5.1	1.9	13.8
Brent and Harrow AHA	46.9	7.5	9.3	0.4	14.4	10.0	3.0	8.5
Brent HD	34.8	9.5	12.0	0.4	15.6	13.3	4.5	9.8
Harrow HD	62.5	4.4	6.3	0.4	12.1	5.5	1.5	7.2

Table A5.15 Live births by mother's country of birth by area of residence, England and Wales, 1980 - *continued*

Area of residence	Mother's country of birth							
	United Kingdom	Irish Republic	India	Bangladesh	African Common-wealth	Rest of New Common-wealth	Pakistan	Elsewhere
North West Thames RHA - continued								
Ealing, Hammersmith and Hounslow AHA	54.3	5.0	13.3	0.5	7.2	7.2	3.0	9.3
Hounslow HD	63.2	3.3	12.3	0.3	7.4	3.5	2.6	7.5
South Hammersmith HD	60.5	5.1	1.2	0.7	3.5	8.6	1.4	19.0
North Hammersmith HD	53.2	9.9	4.0	0.7	4.9	11.9	3.1	12.4
Ealing HD	45.2	4.3	23.6	0.5	9.6	7.5	3.6	5.9
Hillingdon AHA	80.1	3.2	5.7	0.2	3.1	2.9	0.8	4.0
Kensington, Chelsea and Westminster AHA	44.7	4.0	1.6	1.5	4.5	7.3	0.9	35.2
North West HD	45.0	6.6	2.1	1.1	6.5	11.4	1.3	26.1
North East HD	41.7	2.7	2.5	3.7	4.3	8.2	0.9	36.1
South HD	43.8	2.9	1.4	0.9	3.3	3.6	0.6	43.5
North East Thames RHA	**74.7**	**2.7**	**2.8**	**1.9**	**3.4**	**7.2**	**2.3**	**5.1**
Essex AHA	93.2	1.0	0.5	0.1	0.5	1.5	0.2	2.9
Basildon and Thurrock HD	94.0	1.2	1.0	-	0.4	1.3	0.2	1.9
Chelmsford HD	93.4	1.1	0.3	0.0	0.4	1.3	0.2	3.2
Colchester HD	93.0	0.7	0.3	0.1	0.5	1.6	0.1	3.8
Harlow HD	92.0	1.1	0.7	0.1	0.8	2.0	0.5	3.0
Southend HD	93.5	1.0	0.4	0.1	0.5	1.3	0.3	2.9
Barking and Havering AHA	91.3	1.6	1.7	0.0	0.7	1.7	1.1	1.7
Barking HD	89.4	1.6	2.3	0.0	0.7	2.0	2.4	1.5
Havering HD	92.7	1.7	1.2	0.0	0.7	1.5	0.2	1.9
Camden and Islington AHA	56.2	7.4	1.8	2.1	4.8	10.5	0.8	16.3
North Camden HD	52.4	7.2	2.0	0.7	4.5	8.0	1.0	24.1
South Camden HD	54.6	5.0	2.3	6.4	3.5	7.0	1.2	20.0
Islington HD	59.0	8.4	1.4	1.4	5.5	13.2	0.6	10.5

Table A5.15 Live births by mother's country of birth by area of residence, England and Wales, 1980 - *continued*

Area of residence	Mother's country of birth							
	United Kingdom	Irish Republic	India	Bangladesh	African Common- wealth	Rest of New Common- wealth	Pakistan	Elsewhere
North East Thames RHA - continued								
City and East London AHA	53.6	2.5	7.1	7.6	7.7	11.5	4.7	5.3
City and Hackney HD	49.9	3.9	4.6	2.0	8.6	18.2	2.0	10.8
Newham HD	55.5	1.7	12.4	0.5	10.1	8.9	8.7	2.1
Tower Hamlets HD	55.7	1.7	2.1	25.9	3.0	6.7	2.0	3.0
Enfield and Haringey AHA	59.3	4.8	2.0	1.2	5.3	18.6	1.0	7.7
Enfield HD	71.1	3.7	1.6	1.1	2.8	13.6	0.5	5.5
Haringey HD	46.8	6.0	2.4	1.3	7.9	24.0	1.5	10.1
Redbridge and Waltham Forest AHA	65.7	3.5	5.3	0.7	4.9	8.3	8.1	3.5
East Roding HD	70.3	3.4	7.3	0.5	5.0	5.5	3.4	4.5
West Roding HD	61.6	3.5	3.5	0.8	4.8	10.9	12.2	2.7
South East Thames RHA	**85.0**	**1.7**	**1.5**	**0.3**	**2.3**	**4.6**	**0.4**	**4.3**
East Sussex AHA	90.9	0.8	0.5	0.2	0.7	1.5	0.1	5.2
Brighton HD	89.9	0.8	0.6	0.2	0.8	1.6	0.2	6.0
Eastbourne HD	91.0	1.2	0.3	0.1	0.6	1.4	0.1	5.2
Hastings HD	92.7	0.4	0.4	0.4	0.6	1.6	0.1	3.8
Kent AHA	92.1	1.0	1.6	0.1	0.7	1.4	0.2	3.0
South East Kent HD	93.5	0.8	0.2	0.1	0.3	1.2	0.0	3.8
Canterbury and Thanet HD	93.5	0.7	0.2	0.1	0.5	1.1	0.1	3.7
Dartford and Gravesham HD	88.9	1.1	5.3	0.2	0.8	1.7	0.2	1.9
Maidstone HD	93.6	0.9	0.4	0.1	0.6	1.6	0.2	2.7
Medway HD	91.2	1.2	2.2	0.1	1.0	1.6	0.3	2.5
Tunbridge Wells HD	93.0	0.9	0.3	0.0	0.8	1.0	-	4.0
Greenwich and Bexley AHA	85.0	1.8	3.5	0.2	2.3	3.3	0.7	3.2
Bexley HD	89.1	1.4	3.2	0.2	1.3	2.1	0.1	2.7
Greenwich HD	81.3	2.2	3.8	0.2	3.3	4.4	1.3	3.6
Bromley AHA	88.7	1.5	0.7	0.2	1.2	2.0	0.2	5.5

Table A5.15 Live births by mother's country of birth by area of residence, England and Wales, 1980 - *continued*

Area of residence	Mother's country of birth							
	United Kingdom	Irish Republic	India	Bangladesh	African Common-wealth	Rest of New Common-wealth	Pakistan	Elsewhere
South East Thames RHA - continued								
Lambeth, Southwark and Lewisham AHA	66.-	3.6	1.0	0.8	6.8	14.4	0.8	6.5
St Thomas' HD	58.0	3.5	1.3	1.0	10.4	14.9	1.3	9.7
Kings' HD	63.6	4.2	1.1	0.6	6.9	16.7	0.8	6.3
Guy's HD	69.3	3.5	0.6	1.3	5.9	14.4	0.5	4.5
Lewisham HD	75.8	3.1	1.0	0.4	3.5	10.4	0.5	5.4
South West Thames RHA	**82.0**	**1.8**	**1.5**	**0.3**	**2.6**	**3.8**	**1.1**	**6.7**
Surrey AHA	87.3	1.3	0.7	0.1	0.8	1.4	1.0	6.9
North Surrey HD	87.0	1.9	2.0	-	1.4	2.0	0.9	4.7
North West Surrey HD	82.9	1.5	0.9	0.2	0.5	1.6	3.2	9.2
West Surrey and North East Hampshire HD	90.5	0.9	0.4	0.1	0.7	1.7	0.3	5.5
South West Surrey HD	90.7	0.8	0.5	0.1	1.0	1.0	0.1	5.9
Mid Surrey HD	85.9	1.5	0.5	0.3	0.8	3.1	0.2	7.7
East Surrey HD	89.7	1.3	0.7	0.1	0.7	1.6	0.8	5.0
West Sussex AHA	90.5	0.8	0.7	0.1	1.2	1.2	0.5	4.6
Chichester HD	92.4	0.2	0.2	0.1	0.6	0.8	0.1	5.6
Cuckfield and Crawley HD	88.9	1.0	1.2	0.1	1.7	1.3	1.0	4.9
Worthing HD	92.1	0.8	0.4	0.3	1.0	1.3	0.1	4.1
Croydon AHA	75.8	2.7	3.1	0.1	4.0	7.5	1.5	5.2
Kingston and Richmond AHA	80.5	2.1	1.6	0.1	1.5	3.4	0.5	10.3
Merton, Sutton and Wandsworth AHA	70.1	2.9	2.4	0.8	6.2	7.7	2.1	7.8
Roehampton HD	70.5	3.7	1.6	0.1	2.7	4.0	1.0	16.3
Wandsworth and East Merton HD	60.1	3.0	3.2	1.0	10.4	12.5	2.9	7.0
Sutton and West Merton HD	80.8	2.6	1.6	0.6	2.4	3.3	1.5	7.2

Table A5.15 Live births by mother's country of birth by area of residence, England and Wales, 1980 - *continued*

Area of residence	Mother's country of birth							
	United Kingdom	Irish Republic	India	Bangladesh	African Common-wealth	Rest of New Common-wealth	Pakistan	Elsewhere
Wessex RHA	**92.5**	**0.7**	**0.5**	**0.2**	**0.6**	**1.7**	**0.1**	**3.7**
Dorset AHA	94.0	0.5	0.1	0.1	0.5	1.0	-	3.7
East Dorset HD	93.9	0.5	0.2	0.1	0.5	0.8	-	4.0
West Dorset HD	94.3	0.6	0.1	0.0	0.4	1.3	-	3.3
Hampshire AHA	91.8	0.7	0.6	0.3	0.7	2.0	0.2	3.7
Portsmouth and South East Hampshire HD	92.3	0.7	0.2	0.4	0.6	2.6	0.0	3.2
Southampton and South West Hampshire HD	90.5	0.7	1.5	0.3	0.9	1.8	0.6	3.8
Winchester and Central Hampshire HD	92.6	0.7	0.6	0.2	0.5	1.3	0.2	4.0
Basingstoke and North Hampshire HD	92.3	1.1	0.5	0.0	1.0	1.7	0.1	3.4
Wiltshire AHA	92.3	0.9	0.7	0.1	0.4	1.6	0.1	3.8
Salisbury HD	92.0	0.6	0.4	0.2	0.2	2.4	0.1	4.2
Swindon HD	91.4	1.1	1.2	0.2	0.4	1.5	0.2	4.0
Bath HD	93.8	0.6	0.4	0.0	0.4	1.3	0.0	3.5
Isle of Wight AHA	95.9	0.5	0.2	0.1	0.3	0.7	-	2.3
Oxford RHA	**86.1**	**1.4**	**1.7**	**0.2**	**1.2**	**2.0**	**2.6**	**4.8**
Berkshire AHA	82.6	1.3	3.4	0.1	1.7	2.4	4.1	4.4
East Berkshire HD	76.3	1.5	5.8	0.1	2.4	2.3	6.3	5.3
West Berkshire HD	89.1	1.1	0.9	0.1	1.0	2.3	1.5	4.0
Buckinghamshire AHA	85.6	1.4	0.7	0.1	1.1	2.4	4.0	4.5
Aylesbury HD	88.8	1.6	0.6	0.1	1.3	2.3	1.7	3.6
High Wycombe HD	81.6	1.1	0.6	0.0	0.9	2.7	7.4	5.7
Northamptonshire AHA	90.6	1.5	1.2	0.6	1.2	1.6	0.2	3.1
Kettering HD	91.0	1.1	1.7	0.3	1.6	1.3	0.1	2.8
Northampton HD	90.2	1.9	0.7	0.8	0.9	1.8	0.4	3.5
Oxfordshire AHA	86.5	1.2	0.8	0.1	0.7	1.8	1.4	7.5

Table A5.15 Live births by mother's country of birth by area of residence, England and Wales, 1980 - *continued*

Area of residence	Mother's country of birth							
	United Kingdom	Irish Republic	India	Bangladesh	African Commonwealth	Rest of New Commonwealth	Pakistan	Elsewhere
South Western RHA	**94.3**	**0.6**	**0.4**	**0.1**	**0.4**	**1.3**	**0.3**	**2.6**
Avon AHA	92.5	1.0	0.5	0.1	0.6	1.7	0.8	2.9
Bristol and Weston HD	92.0	0.9	0.6	0.1	0.7	1.7	1.4	2.7
Frenchay HD	94.1	0.9	0.6	-	0.4	1.2	0.4	2.3
Southmead HD	91.9	1.4	0.3	0.1	0.5	1.9	0.5	3.3
Cornwall (and Scilly) AHA	95.9	0.4	0.1	0.0	0.2	0.9	0.0	2.4
Devon AHA	95.1	0.4	0.2	0.0	0.5	1.2	0.1	2.4
Exeter HD	94.9	0.3	0.2	0.1	0.4	1.0	0.1	3.0
North Devon HD	96.1	0.4	0.4	-	0.2	0.6	0.1	2.2
Plymouth HD	94.3	0.5	0.2	-	0.8	1.8	0.0	2.0
Torbay HD	95.5	0.5	0.3	-	0.1	0.9	0.0	2.6
Gloucester AHA	93.7	0.9	0.8	-	0.5	1.3	0.1	2.8
Cheltenham HD } Gloucester HD }	93.7	0.9	0.8	-	0.5	1.3	0.1	2.8
Somerset AHA	96.1	0.2	0.2	0.0	0.4	0.9	0.1	2.0
West Somerset HD } East Somerset HD }	95.9	0.2	0.2	0.0	0.4	1.0	0.1	2.3
West Midlands RHA	**84.1**	**1.5**	**4.9**	**0.5**	**1.1**	**1.9**	**4.4**	**1.5**
Hereford and Worcester AHA	95.0	0.7	0.3	0.2	0.2	0.9	0.9	1.8
Hereford HD	96.9	0.4	0.1	-	0.1	0.5	0.1	1.9
Bromsgrove and Redditch HD	93.8	1.2	0.1	0.1	0.3	1.3	1.8	1.5
Kidderminster HD	95.8	0.8	0.3	0.6	0.1	0.8	-	1.6
Worcester HD	94.5	0.5	0.5	0.2	0.2	0.8	1.0	2.2
Salop AHA	95.0	0.5	0.7	0.1	0.4	0.9	0.6	1.8
Staffordshire AHA	94.6	0.5	0.5	0.1	0.2	0.7	2.0	1.3
Mid Staffordshire HD	96.0	0.5	0.6	0.0	0.2	0.7	0.1	1.9
North Staffordshire HD	94.8	0.3	0.4	0.1	0.2	0.6	2.4	1.2
South East Staffordshire HD	92.9	0.9	0.4	0.1	0.3	0.9	3.2	1.3

Table A5.15 Live births by mother's country of birth by area of residence, England and Wales, 1980 - *continued*

Area of residence	Mother's country of birth							
	United Kingdom	Irish Republic	India	Bangladesh	African Common-wealth	Rest of New Common-wealth	Pakistan	Elsewhere
West Midlands RHA - continued								
Warwickshire AHA	90.3	1.6	3.2	-	1.2	1.1	0.4	2.2
North Warwickshire HD	93.1	1.1	2.3	-	1.1	0.9	0.2	1.2
Rugby HD	88.1	2.4	1.6	-	2.8	1.6	1.3	2.2
South Warwickshire HD	88.7	1.7	4.6	-	0.6	1.0	0.1	3.3
Birmingham AHA	66.7	3.4	7.1	1.5	2.4	4.5	12.2	1.9
Central HD	52.3	4.6	6.2	2.4	4.5	4.9	23.1	2.0
East HD	69.3	2.4	1.1	0.8	0.6	2.0	22.9	0.9
North HD	87.9	3.4	1.2	0.1	0.5	2.7	1.9	2.2
South HD	86.1	3.7	1.5	0.2	1.2	2.6	2.2	2.5
West HD	50.0	2.4	20.6	2.9	3.3	8.3	10.9	1.6
Coventry AHA	77.6	3.8	9.8	0.4	2.7	1.4	2.9	1.5
Dudley AHA	90.8	0.6	2.0	0.2	0.6	1.1	4.0	0.8
Sandwell AHA	76.1	0.7	12.2	1.6	1.3	2.4	4.5	1.2
Solihull AHA	94.6	2.1	0.3	-	0.4	1.3	0.2	1.1
Walsall AHA	81.2	0.4	8.2	0.9	1.0	1.2	6.3	0.7
Wolverhampton AHA	73.1	0.7	19.2	0.1	1.4	3.0	1.5	1.0
Mersey RHA	**96.1**	**1.0**	**0.2**	**0.1**	**0.3**	**0.6**	**0.1**	**1.5**
Cheshire AHA	96.0	0.9	0.3	0.1	0.3	0.5	0.2	1.7
Chester HD	95.3	1.2	0.4	0.1	0.2	0.7	0.1	2.0
Crewe HD	97.2	0.7	0.1	0.0	0.4	0.5	0.2	0.9
Halton HD	96.9	0.8	0.1	0.1	0.2	0.4	-	1.5
Macclesfield HD	94.8	0.6	0.3	-	0.3	0.4	0.3	3.1
Warrington HD	95.4	0.9	0.4	-	0.1	0.6	0.5	2.0

Table A5.15 Live births by mother's country of birth by area of residence, England and Wales, 1980 - continued

Area of residence	Mother's country of birth							
	United Kingdom	Irish Republic	India	Bangladesh	African Common-wealth	Rest of New Common-wealth	Pakistan	Elsewhere
Mersey RHA - continued								
Liverpool AHA	95.0	1.2	0.3	0.1	0.6	0.9	0.1	1.7
Central Southern HD } Eastern HD	95.0	1.2	0.3	0.1	0.6	0.9	0.1	1.8
St Helens with Knowsley AHA	97.3	0.8	0.2	0.0	0.1	0.4	0.1	1.0
Sefton AHA	96.6	1.3	0.1	0.0	0.1	0.6	-	1.3
Northern HD	94.8	1.5	-	0.1	0.2	1.0	-	2.5
Southern HD	97.5	1.2	0.2	-	0.1	0.3	-	0.7
Wirral AHA	96.0	1.1	0.2	0.1	0.2	0.8	0.0	1.5
Northern HD } Southern HD	96.0	1.1	0.2	0.1	0.2	0.7	0.0	1.6
North Western RHA	**87.1**	**1.7**	**2.3**	**0.6**	**1.1**	**0.9**	**4.6**	**1.6**
Lancashire AHA	86.6	0.9	3.3	0.3	1.1	0.6	5.6	1.5
Lancaster HD	93.3	0.6	2.0	-	0.4	0.7	0.2	2.7
Blackpool HD	96.1	0.9	0.3	0.0	0.3	0.9	0.0	1.5
Preston HD	87.6	1.0	5.6	0.1	1.8	0.7	1.9	1.5
Blackburn HD	75.0	0.9	7.5	0.1	2.2	0.5	12.2	1.7
Burnley HD	84.1	0.5	0.4	1.1	0.3	0.5	12.0	1.1
Ormskirk HD	95.6	1.3	0.1	-	0.5	0.6	0.2	1.8
Bolton AHA	80.8	0.9	8.7	0.1	3.2	0.6	4.2	1.5
Bury AHA	89.6	2.7	0.6	0.1	0.1	0.8	4.2	1.9
Manchester AHA	79.6	4.8	1.3	0.7	1.7	3.0	6.2	2.7
North HD	87.2	2.9	0.5	0.2	1.1	2.1	4.3	1.8
Central HD	68.7	6.7	2.2	1.8	2.9	5.0	10.2	2.5
South HD	81.8	5.1	1.4	0.1	1.4	2.1	4.5	3.7
Oldham AHA	81.8	1.0	1.1	3.5	0.8	0.8	9.8	1.1
Rochdale AHA	82.3	2.3	0.9	1.1	0.6	0.3	11.3	1.2

Table A5.15 Live births by mother's country of birth by area of residence, England and Wales, 1980 - *continued*

Area of residence	Mother's country of birth							
	United Kingdom	Irish Republic	India	Bangladesh	African Commonwealth	Rest of New Commonwealth	Pakistan	Elsewhere
North Western RHA - continued								
Salford AHA	93.7	2.3	0.3	0.2	0.2	0.6	0.6	2.2
Stockport AHA	93.9	1.6	0.6	0.1	0.4	0.6	0.6	2.2
Tameside AHA	90.7	1.1	1.5	1.0	1.8	0.4	2.3	1.2
Trafford AHA	89.6	2.7	1.8	0.2	0.6	2.2	0.7	2.1
Wigan AHA	97.6	0.8	0.1	0.0	0.2	0.3	0.2	0.6
Wales	**95.9**	**0.6**	**0.3**	**0.1**	**0.3**	**0.6**	**0.4**	**1.7**
Clwyd AHA	97.1	0.6	0.1	0.0	0.1	0.6	0.1	1.2
Rhyl HD	97.5	0.7	0.1	-	0.2	0.5	-	1.0
Wrexham HD	96.9	0.5	0.2	0.1	0.1	0.6	0.1	1.5
Dyfed AHA	95.5	0.5	0.3	-	0.3	0.5	0.0	2.7
Ceredigion HD	93.3	0.5	0.5	-	0.8	1.1	0.2	3.7
Carmarthen/Dinefwr HD	96.8	0.5	0.2	-	0.2	-	0.1	2.1
Preseli/South Pembs HD	93.4	0.9	0.1	-	0.3	0.7	-	4.5
Llanelli/Dinefwr HD	98.4	-	0.4	-	-	0.2	-	1.0
Gwent AHA	95.9	0.6	0.4	0.1	0.2	0.4	0.9	1.3
Abergavenny HD	97.8	0.2	0.7	-	-	0.2	0.1	1.0
Newport HD	95.3	0.7	0.3	0.2	0.3	0.4	1.2	1.6
Gwynedd AHA	95.9	0.9	0.2	0.1	0.2	0.6	0.1	2.0
Mid Glamorgan AHA	97.7	0.3	0.2	0.0	0.1	0.6	0.1	0.9
Ogwr HD	96.9	0.6	-	-	0.2	0.6	0.1	1.7
Rhymney Valley HD	97.7	0.3	0.2	0.1	0.2	0.6	0.1	0.9
East Glamorgan HD	97.9	0.2	0.1	-	0.1	0.7	0.1	0.9
Merthyr and Cynon Valley HD	98.0	0.3	0.5	-	0.1	0.4	0.1	0.6

Table A5.15 Live births by mother's country of birth by area of residence, England and Wales, 1980 – *continued*

Area of residence	Mother's country of birth							
	United Kingdom	Irish Republic	India	Bangladesh	African Common-wealth	Rest of New Common-wealth	Pakistan	Elsewhere
Wales – continued								
Powys AHA	97.8	0.2	0.1	-	0.1	0.3	-	1.6
South Glamorgan AHA	91.2	0.8	0.6	0.5	1.1	1.4	1.2	3.2
West Glamorgan AHA	96.8	0.6	0.2	0.2	0.2	0.6	0.1	1.2
Neath HD	97.9	0.3	0.2	0.1	0.2	0.5	-	0.8
Swansea HD	96.3	0.8	0.2	0.3	0.2	0.6	0.2	1.4

Total numbers of live births in each area are given in Table A3.24
Source: OPCS unpublished data

Table A5.16 Percentage distribution of birthweights of live births by mother's country of birth, England and Wales, 1980

Mother's country of birth	Birthweight g									Total stated birthweight (=100%)	Not stated	Total
	Under 1,000	1,001-1,499	1,500-1,990	2,000-2,499	Under 2,500	2,500-2,999	3,000-3,499	3,500-3,999	4,000 and over			
All countries	**0.2**	**0.5**	**1.3**	**4.8**	**6.7**	**19.2**	**39.1**	**26.8**	**8.1**	**569,315**	**86,918**	**656,233**
United Kingdom	0.2	0.5	1.2	4.5	6.4	18.3	39.1	27.8	8.4	490,252	78,816	569,068
Irish Republic	0.2	0.4	1.1	4.0	5.8	16.4	37.2	29.9	10.7	8,216	938	9,154
Australia, Canada and New Zealand	0.1	0.3	1.0	2.5	3.9	17.4	38.8	29.5	10.4	2,160	337	2,497
India and Bangladesh	0.3	0.6	1.8	9.2	11.9	33.4	38.6	13.6	2.5	15,191	1,003	16,194
African Commonwealth	0.4	0.7	1.9	9.5	12.4	30.1	37.0	16.7	3.8	9,222	818	10,040
West Indies	0.6	0.9	1.7	5.8	9.0	24.1	40.8	21.5	4.7	6,534	530	7,064
Malta, Gibraltar and Cyprus	0.3	0.5	1.1	4.0	5.9	20.9	42.2	24.9	6.1	2,836	383	3,219
Rest of New Commonwealth	0.0	0.4	1.4	4.8	6.7	25.7	41.9	20.9	4.8	4,618	499	5,117
Pakistan	0.3	0.6	1.7	7.9	10.5	30.1	38.7	17.0	3.6	13,017	827	13,844
Europe	0.1	0.5	1.1	3.4	5.1	16.7	39.8	29.1	9.3	8,172	1,352	9,524
Elsewhere	0.2	0.3	1.0	4.6	6.2	18.4	40.8	26.6	8.1	8,817	1,363	10,180
Not stated	0.7	0.7	1.8	3.2	6.4	14.6	42.5	21.8	14.6	280	52	332

Source: OPCS unpublished data

Table A5.17 Stillbirths and infant mortality by mother's country of birth, England and Wales, 1980

Mother's country of birth	Stillbirths		Perinatal deaths		Neonatal deaths		Postneonatal deaths		Infant deaths		Number of live births
	Number	Rate*	Number	Rate*	Number	Rate†	Number	Rate†	Number	Rate†	
All countries	**4,773**	**7.2**	**8,796**	**13.3**	**4,987**	**7.6**	**2,803**	**4.3**	**7,790**	**11.9**	**656,234**
United Kingdom	4,001	7.0	7,390	12.9	4,186	7.4	2,393	4.2	6,579	11.6	569,069
Irish Republic	60	6.5	125	13.6	74	8.1	43	4.7	117	12.8	9,154
Australia, Canada, New Zealand	12	4.8	20	8.0	15	6.0	9	3.6	24	9.6	2,497
New Commonwealth and Pakistan	566	10.1	1,018	18.2	577	10.4	289	5.2	866	15.6	55,478
New Commonwealth											
Bangladesh, India	160	9.8	257	15.7	135	8.3	72	4.4	207	12.8	16,194
Africa	93	9.2	159	15.7	92	9.2	49	4.9	141	14.0	10,040
West Indies	70	9.8	128	17.9	71	10.1	38	5.4	109	15.4	7,064
Malta, Gibraltar, Cyprus	15	4.6	46	14.2	36	11.2	15	4.7	51	15.8	3,219
Rest of New Commonwealth	33	6.4	59	11.5	33	6.4	21	4.1	54	10.6	5,117
Pakistan	195	13.9	369	26.3	210	15.2	94	6.8	304	22.0	13,844
Remainder of Europe	54	5.6	104	10.9	58	6.1	36	3.8	94	9.9	9,524
Other	55	5.4	105	10.3	66	6.5	31	3.0	97	9.5	10,180
Not stated or at sea	25	7C.0	34	95.2	11	33.1	2	6.0	13	39.2	332

* Per 1,000 total births
† Per 1,000 live births

Source: OPCS Mortality statistics: perinatal and infant, Series DH3 No. 9.

161

Table A5.18 Teenage pregnancies, England and Wales
(a) maternities by age of mother, 1939-80

Year	Age of mother									Total aged 16-19	Rate (per 1,000 women aged 16-19)
	11	12	13	14	15	16	17	18	19		
1939	-	-	4	34	161	833	3,282	8,802	16,045	28,962	
1940	-	1	6	30	153	777	2,964	8,010	15,737	27,488	19.7
1941	-	-	7	43	168	799	2,786	6,996	14,080	24,661	18.9
1942	-	1	3	39	197	884	2,821	6,958	13,534	24,197	19.9
1943	-	-	5	36	219	852	2,891	6,971	13,623	24,337	20.6
1944	-	-	7	29	214	1,001	2,936	7,166	13,704	24,807	21.2
1945	-	-	12	34	246	1,089	3,321	7,355	13,659	25,424	22.1
1946	-	-	4	38	239	969	3,070	7,063	13,776	24,878	24.4
1947	-	-	9	37	158	871	3,135	8,012	15,829	27,847	26.5
1948	-	2	1	37	176	954	3,466	8,795	17,322	30,537	28.0
1949	-	3	3	31	169	960	3,926	9,354	17,694	31,934	27.6
1950	-	-	6	39	176	890	3,686	9,039	17,312	30,927	
1951	-	-	4	25	167	821	3,359	8,674	16,397	29,251	26.7
1952	-	-	5	36	176	959	3,562	8,767	16,090	29,378	26.9
1953	-	-	10	46	170	961	3,738	9,144	16,740	30,583	27.8
1954	-	-	5	33	155	981	3,926	9,786	17,289	31,982	
1955	-	-	8	40	185	1,027	4,414	9,836	17,945	33,222	
1956	-	-	5	56	208	1,313	5,164	11,632	20,115	38,224	33.9
1957	-	2	9	45	243	1,441	5,606	12,635	21,776	41,458	37.4
1958	1	1	10	62	309	1,666	5,936	13,442	23,021	44,065	39.9
1959	-	4	10	78	393	2,099	6,729	13,808	23,516	46,152	40.7
1960	-	-	15	98	601	2,784	8,505	15,491	24,744	51,524	43.2
1961	-	-	23	133	731	3,789	10,390	18,470	26,929	59,578	47.0
1962	-	1	19	192	929	3,892	11,482	20,876	30,595	66,845	51.0
1963	-	3	22	174	984	4,854	11,871	21,764	32,578	71,067	50.9
1964	-	5	15	172	901	4,952	14,902	22,434	34,037	76,325	52.8
1965	-	1	23	170	970	4,722	14,399	27,521	34,478	81,120	55.6
1966	1	7	27	193	1,068	4,744	13,673	25,970	41,733	86,120	58.0
1967	1	6	30	194	1,009	4,932	13,929	25,697	39,423	83,981	59.8
1968	-	4	25	194	1,100	5,206	14,263	25,216	36,738	81,423	60.5
1969	4	11	32	207	1,253	5,506	14,569	25,296	35,382	80,753	61.4
1970	4	9	25	219	1,184	5,652	14,980	24,876	34,634	80,142	61.5

Table A5.18 Teenage pregnancies, England and Wales

(a) maternities by age of mother, 1939-80 - continued

Year	Age of mother									Total aged 16-19	Rate (per 1,000 women aged 16-19
	11	12	13	14	15	16	17	18	19		
1971	2	4	35	233	1,267	5,894	15,614	25,871	34,298	81,677	63.1
1972	1	4	28	241	1,336	6,290	15,160	24,282	32,184	77,916	59.9
1973	1	7	39	272	1,377	6,102	14,135	21,941	29,869	72,047	54.7
1974	-	6	26	264	1,299	5,587	14,008	20,842	27,132	67,569	50.4
1975	1	3	37	230	1,272	4,755	12,345	19,587	25,575	62,262	45.1
1976	1	3	35	215	1,174	4,389	10,752	17,684	23,966	56,791	40.2
1977	1	3	23	212	1,088	4,415	10,222	16,465	22,381	53,483	37.0
1978	2	1	22	197	1,175	4,458	10,549	16,796	23,072	54,875	37.0
1979	2	2	27	212	1,143	4,327	11,062	18,087	24,510	57,986	37.6
1980	9	8	18	191	1,057	4,321	10,938	18,661	25,711	59,631	38.1

Sources: *Registrar General's Statistical Review*, 1939-73
OPCS, *Birth statistics, Series FM1*, 1974-80

(b) Abortions by age, 1968-80

Year Age	11	12	13	14	15	Total 11-15	Rate (per 1,000) 11-15	16	17	18	19	Total 16-19	Rate (per 1,000) 16-19
1968	3	6	21	150	363	543	2.4	559	693	945	1,088	3,285	14.7
1969	2	7	38	279	848	1,174	2.4	1,445	1,816	2,255	2,543	8,057	16.2
1970	3	20	85	391	1,233	1,732	2.3	2,530	3,188	3,864	3,936	13,518	17.8
1971	3	16	77	529	1,671	2,296	2.4	3,465	4,426	5,193	5,092	18,176	19.2
1972	-	7	98	586	2,113	2,804	2.6	4,318	5,395	6,038	6,035	21,786	20.1
1973	5*	14	108	693	2,270	3,089	2.8	5,082	5,775	6,374	6,249	23,480	21.2
1974	1	9	117	718	2,490	3,335	3.0	5,348	6,225	6,564	6,060	24,197	22.1
1975	-	12	120	747	2,691	3,570	3.4	5,411	6,394	6,389	5,928	24,122	22.7
1976	6	14	122	738	2,545	3,425	3.4	5,429	6,285	6,282	5,967	23,963	23.5
1977	1	13	105	804	2,701	3,624	3.5	5,510	6,367	6,576	6,139	24,592	24.0
1978	3	20	113	708	2,454	3,298	2.9	5,675	6,733	7,276	6,679	26,363	23.6
1979	9	18	116	698	2,693	3,534	2.9	6,030	7,412	8,028	7,722	29,192	24.2
1980	5	17	141	770	2,717	3,650	2.8	6,370	8,108	8,756	8,644	31,878	24.7

* Includes 1 10 year old

Source: OPCS *Abortion statistics, Series AB*

163

Table A5.19 Maternal height by social class, singleton births, Scotland, 1979

Mother's height cm	Social class of father						Total
	I	II	III	IV	V	Not known	
	Numbers						
Less than 150	66	163	852	348	349	615	2,393
150-154	353	731	3,461	1,396	1,024	2,005	8,970
155-159	933	1,718	6,602	2,597	1,528	3,518	16,896
160-164	1,437	2,351	7,269	2,767	1,486	3,801	19,111
165-169	962	1,495	3,944	1,515	637	2,116	10,669
170-174	350	545	1,149	512	181	700	3,437
175 and over	98	115	274	94	44	180	805
Total known	4,199	7,118	23,551	9,229	5,249	12,935	62,281
Not known	228	425	1,240	569	328	1,168	3,958
Total	4,427	7,543	24,791	9,798	5,577	14,103	66,239
	Percentages of births with known maternal height						
Less than 150	1.6	2.3	3.6	3.8	6.6	4.8	3.8
150-154	8.4	10.3	14.7	15.1	19.5	15.5	14.4
155-159	22.2	24.1	28.0	28.1	29.1	27.2	27.1
160-164	34.2	33.0	30.9	30.0	28.3	29.4	30.7
165-169	22.9	21.0	16.7	16.4	12.1	16.4	17.1
170-174	8.3	7.7	4.9	5.5	3.4	5.4	5.5
175 and over	2.3	1.6	1.2	1.0	0.8	1.4	1.3
Total known	100	100	100	100	100	100	100
Not known as a percentage of total	5.2	5.6	5.0	5.8	5.9	8.3	6.0

Source: Information Services Division, SMR2

Table A5.20 Birthweight by maternal height, singletons born to primiparae, Scotland, 1979

Mother's height cm	Birthweight g										Total, stated birthweight	Not stated*	Total	Mean birthweight g
	Under 500	500-999	1,000-1,499	1,500-1,999	2,000-2,499	2,500-2,999	3,000-3,499	3,500-3,999	4,000-4,499	4,500 and over				
Numbers														
Less than 150	0	2	15	33	109	306	371	145	19	1	1,001	6	1,007	2,987.1
150-154	0	11	37	66	251	995	1,492	661	115	15	3,643	22	3,665	3,111.4
155-159	0	17	51	83	426	1,606	2,933	1,580	324	45	7,065	36	7,101	3,194.0
160-164	1	16	53	94	323	1,523	3,383	2,179	555	53	8,180	30	8,210	3,283.4
165-169	1	7	24	31	121	705	1,901	1,439	360	51	4,640	19	4,659	3,363.7
170-174	0	2	7	12	45	197	601	476	160	32	1,532	6	1,538	3,415.9
175 and over	0	1	0	1	4	32	135	137	57	7	374	1	375	3,538.0
Not known	0	10	36	34	98	319	601	331	77	9	1,515	24	1,539	3,142.2
Total	2	66	223	354	1,377	5,683	11,417	6,948	1,667	213	27,950	144	28,094	3,244.1
Percentages of babies with stated birthweights														
Less than 150	—	0.2	1.5	3.3	10.9	30.6	37.1	14.5	1.9	0.1	100	0.6		
150-154	—	0.3	1.0	1.8	6.9	27.3	41.0	18.1	3.2	0.4	100	0.6		
155-159	—	0.2	0.7	1.2	6.0	22.7	41.5	22.4	4.6	0.6	100	0.5		
160-164	0.0	0.2	0.6	1.1	3.9	18.6	41.4	26.6	6.8	0.6	100	0.4		
165-169	0.0	0.2	0.5	0.7	2.6	15.2	41.0	31.0	7.8	1.1	100	0.4		
170-174	—	0.1	0.5	0.8	2.9	12.9	39.2	31.1	10.4	2.1	100	0.4		
175 and over	—	0.3	—	0.3	1.1	8.6	36.1	36.6	15.2	1.9	100	0.3		
Not known	—	0.7	2.4	2.2	6.5	21.1	39.7	21.8	5.1	0.6	100	1.6		
Total	0.0	0.2	0.8	1.3	4.9	20.3	40.8	24.9	6.0	0.8	100	0.5		

* *Proportion 'not stated' is given as a percentage of 'total'*
Source: Information Services Division, SMR2

Table A5.21   Stillbirths and infant deaths of babies born to women in the OPCS longitudinal study 1971-75, age standardised ratio by household tenure and woman's family status

Family status at 1971 Census		Tenure of woman's household at 1971 census				
		All tenures	Owner occupier	Privately rented	Council tenant	Other
Stillbirths						
All women	Observed	262	108	55	93	6
	Expected	262.0	126.0	56.1	75.3	4.4
	SMR	100	86	98	124	136
Dependent children	Observed	17	4	1	12	
	Expected	14.9	5.3	1.8	7.8	
	SMR	114	75	56	154	
Other children	Observed	57	23	9	25	
	Expected	48.1	15.3	6.3	26.5	
	SMR	119	150	143	94	
Married couple without children	Observed	58	29	18	11	
	Expected	67.3	41.3	18.4	7.6	
	SMR	86	70	98	145	
Married couple with children	Observed	103	44	20	39	
	Expected	105.8	58.0	20.6	27.2	
	SMR	97	76	97	143	
Other	Observed	27	8	13	6	
	Expected	25.9	6.1	13.6	6.2	
	SMR	104	131	96	97	
Infant deaths						
All women	Observed	407	172	97	128	8
	Expected	407.0	189.6	89.8	120.1	7.2
	SMR	100	91	108	107	111
Dependent children	Observed	33	13	6	14	
	Expected	25.9	9.2	3.4	13.3	
	SMR	127	141	176	105	
Other children	Observed	75	27	10	38	
	Expected	83.0	26.1	10.9	46.0	
	SMR	90	103	92	83	
Married couple without children	Observed	105	66	27	12	
	Expected	109.1	65.7	30.9	12.5	
	SMR	96	100	87	96	
Married couple with children	Observed	149	57	43	49	
	Expected	149.7	79.5	31.1	39.1	
	SMR	100	72	138	125	
Other	Observed	45	9	21	15	
	Expected	39.3	9.1	21.0	9.2	
	SMR	115	99	100	163	

Source: Unpublished data from the OPCS Longitudinal Study

Table A5.22 Housing profile of families with dependent children, Great Britain, 1979-80

	One-parent families			Other families with dependent children*
	No others in household	Other persons in household	Total	
Tenure	%	%	%	%
Owner occupied, owned outright	10	10	10	9
Owner occupied, with mortgage	19	18	19	53
Rented with job or business	1	1	1	4
Rented from local authority/New Town	63	63	63	30
Rented privately unfurnished, or from housing association or co-operative	6	7	6	3
Rented privately furnished	2	1	1	1
Base = 100%	*759*	*227*	*986*	*7,521*
Age of building				
Before 1919	16	17	16	20
1919-1944	23	30	25	24
1945-1964	34	33	34	27
1965 or later	27	20	25	29
Base = 100%	*752*	*225*	*977*	*7,457*
Type of accommodation†				
Detached house	7	7	7	20
Semi-detached house	29	27	29	38
Terraced house	36	42	37	32
Purpose-built flat or maisonette	23	19	22	7
Converted flat or maisonette/rooms	5	4	5	2
With business premises/Other	1	0	1	1
Base = 100%	*759*	*226*	*985*	*7,504*

* *5% of these families lived in a household with other persons, compared with 23% of non-parent families.*
† *Households sharing a house or a purpose-built flat are attributed to the category 'converted flat or maisonette/rooms'.*

Table A5.22 Housing profile of families with dependent children, Great Britain, 1979-80 - *continued*

	One-parent families			Other families with dependent children*
	No others in household	Other persons in household	Total	
Amenities				
Bath - sole use	98	99	98	99
- shared	1	-	1	0
- none	1	1	1	1
WC - sole use, inside accommodation	97	97	97	98
- sole use, outside accommodation	2	3	2	2
- shared or none	1	-	1	1
Base = 100%	*755*	*225*	*980*	*7,478*
Central heating				
Yes	51	45	50	66
No	49	55	50	34
Base = 100%	*762*	*227*	*989*	*7,549*
Bedroom standard (bedrooms)	%	%	%	%
2 or more below standard	1	11	3	1
1 below standard	12	42	19	8
Equals standard	55	41	52	41
1 above standard	29	4	23	41
2 or more above standard	4	0	3	8
Base = 100%	*763*	*227*	*990*	*7,548*
Persons per room				
Under 0.5	18	1	14	3
0.5 to 0.65	47	15	40	23
0.66 to 0.99	25	44	29	50
1	6	21	9	16
Over 1 to 1.5	3	15	6	6
Over 1.5	0	4	1	1
Base = 100%	*763*	*227*	*990*	*7,548*

* *5% of these families lived in a household with other persons, compared with 23% of non-parent families.*
† *Households sharing a house or a purpose-built flat are attributed to the category 'converted flat or maisonette/rooms'.*

Source: OPCS *General Household Survey 1980*

Table A5.23 Percentage of women working by age of their youngest dependent child, Great Britain, 1978-80

Age of youngest dependent child and whether woman working full-time or part-time	Lone mothers					Married* women with dependent children
	Single	Widowed	Divorced	Separated	All lone mothers	
	%	%	%	%	%	%
Under 5 years:						
Working full-time	20	1	8	10	14	5
Working part-time	8	3	18	12	12	23
All working†	28	4	26	22	26	29
*Base = 100%***	*152*	*12*	*99*	*118*	*381*	*4,192*
5 years or over:						
Working full-time	30	18	30	24	26	21
Working part-time	20	31	30	33	30	45
All working†	50	49	61	58	56	67
*Base = 100%***	*92*	*231*	*410*	*199*	*932*	*7,269*
All ages						
Working full-time	24	18	26	19	22	16
Working part-time	12	31	28	25	25	37
All working†	36	49	54	45	48	53
*Base = 100%***	*244*	*243*	*509*	*317*	*1,313*	*11,461*

*   *Including married women whose husbands were not defined as resident in the household*
†   *Including, in 1979 and 1980, a few women whose hours of work were not known*
** *Including some women whose economic activity status was not known*

Source: OPCS *General Household Survey 1980*

Table A5.24 Selected social and economic indices, constituent countries of the UK and standard regions

Area	Household income and unemployment			Government expenditure on benefits, year ending March 1980	
	Mean weekly household income £ 1979-80	Percentage of households with income less than £50 1979-80	Percentage unemployment 1981	Maternity benefits (£ per live birth)	Unemployment and supplementary benefit (£ per head)
ENGLAND	136.05	18.4			
North	119.33	25.4	15.3	168	68
Yorkshire and Humberside	116.68	23.7	12.3	176	53
East Midlands	135.36	17.5	10.2	183	45
East Anglia	131.04	18.7	9.2	168	40
South East	153.21	14.8	8.1	177	48
South West	124.23	18.6	10.0	158	51
West Midlands	133.49	16.6	13.7	161	52
North West	128.04	20.7	13.9	176	66
WALES	123.98	21.6	14.8	171	67
SCOTLAND	126.46	22.1	13.8		
N. IRELAND	112.97	27.3	18.4		

Source: DE, *Family Expenditure Survey 1980*
DHSS, *Social Security Statistics 1981*
CSO, *Regional Trends 1981*
MAFF, *Household food consumption and expenditure 1980.* Annual report of the National Food Survey.

Housing

Average weekly household expenditure and consumption

Percentage of dwellings owner occupied 1980	Percentage of houses in 1977 lacking:			Expenditure 1980-81 (£)		Consumption, 1980 (oz per person)		
	Indoor WC	Bath/ shower	Hot water	Alcohol	Tobacco	Fresh fruit	Fresh vegetables	Sugar and preserves
57	7.1	5.7	4.3		2.97	21.1	69.2	13.2
46	5.0	3.3	2.0	6.47	4.03	15.5	73.6	13.0
55	7.4	4.9	3.6	6.13	3.96	17.5	69.0	12.5
58	6.6	4.2	3.1	4.89	3.34	20.1	65.6	14.1
59	6.0	5.3	5.2	4.52	2.92	25.2	67.8	12.1
57	7.3	7.0	5.1	5.89	3.20			
64	5.6	5.4	4.9	4.79	2.71	21.0	71.9	14.3
57	7.2	4.6	4.4	5.63	3.47	18.8	70.5	15.2
59	9.2	6.0	4.4	6.19	3.77	18.4	69.3	13.8
60	8.2	6.0	5.1	5.27	3.53	21.9	82.1	13.9
36	..	..	..	6.08	4.51	17.4	65.5	13.5
48	..	..	..	4.02	4.56	..	..	..

Table A6.1 Live births and stillbirths by birthweight, England and Wales, 1980

Previous weight ranges			ICD 9th Revision weight ranges		
Birthweight g	Number	Percentage*	Number	Percentage*	Birthweight g
Live birth					
Under 1,001	1,213	0.21	1,132	0.20	Under 1,000
1,001-1,500	3,007	0.53	2,932	0.52	1,000-1,499
1,501-2,000	7,376	1.30	7,119	1.25	1,500-1,999
2,001-2,500	28,753	5.05	27,176	4.77	2,000-2,499
Under 2,501	40,349	7.09	38,359	6.74	Under 2,500
2,501-3,000	114,047	20.03	109,518	19.24	2,500-2,999
3,001-3,500	223,040	39.18	222,578	39.10	3,000-3,499
3,501-4,000	148,824	26.14	152,835	26.85	3,500-3,999
4,001 and over	43,056	7.56	46,026	8.08	4,000 and over
Total stated	**469,316**	**100.00**	**569,316**	**100.00**	**Total stated**
Not stated	86,918	—	86,918	—	Not stated
All birthweights	**656,234**	—	**656,234**	—	**Total**
Stillbirths					
Under 1,001	587	14.51	561	13.87	Under 1,000
1,001-1,500	780	19.28	785	19.40	1,000-1,499
1,501-2,000	696	17.20	701	17.33	1,500-1,999
2,001-2,500	632	15.62	623	15.40	2,000-2,499
Under 2,501	2,695	66.61	2,670	65.99	Under 2,500
2,501-3,000	594	14.68	598	14.78	2,500-2,999
3,001-3,500	437	10.80	446	11.02	3,000-3,499
3,501-4,000	213	5.26	224	5.54	3,500-3,999
4,001 and over	107	2.64	108	2.67	4,000 and over
Total stated	**4,046**	**100.00**	**4,046**	**100.00**	**Total stated**
Not stated	727	—	727	—	Not stated
All birthweights	**4,773**	—	**4,773**	—	**All birthweights**

* Expressed as a percentage of births with stated birthweight.
Source: OPCS Monitor DH3 81/4.

Table A6.2 Singleton and multiple births by birthweight, England and Wales, 1980

	Birthweight g									Total stated	Not stated	All birthweights
	Under 1,000	1,000-1,499	1,500-1,999	2,000-2,499	Under 2,500	2,500-2,999	3,000-3,499	2,500-3,999	4,000 and over			
LIVE BIRTHS												
Number												
Singleton	924	2,335	5,613	23,907	32,779	105,962	221,127	182,618	46,012	558,498	85,162	643,660
Multiple	208	597	1,506	3,269	5,580	3,556	1,451	217	14	10,818	1,756	12,594
Percentage												
Singleton	0.2	0.4	1.0	4.3	5.9	19.0	39.6	32.7	8.2	100.0	—	—
Multiple	1.9	5.5	13.9	30.2	51.6	32.9	13.4	2.0	0.1	100.0	—	—
STILLBIRTHS												
Number												
Singleton	496	714	646	577	2,433	572	440	222	108	3,775	662	4,437
Multiple	65	71	55	46	237	26	6	2	0	271	65	336
Percentage												
Singleton	13.1	18.9	17.1	15.3	64.5	15.2	11.9	5.9	2.9	100.0	—	—
Multiple	24.0	26.2	20.3	17.0	87.5	9.6	2.2	0.7	—	100.0	—	—

Source: *OPCS Monitor DH3 81/4*

Table A6.3 Mortality and estimated numbers of live births by birthweight, England and Wales, 1980

	Birthweight g (ICD 9th Revision groupings)								All birthweights
	Under 1,500	1,500- 1,999	2,000- 2,499	Under 2,500	2,500- 2,999	3,000- 3,499	3,500- 3,999	4,000 and over	
Numbers									
Stillbirths	1,517	787	701	3,005	668	502	252	115	4,542
Perinatal deaths	3,188	1,311	1,122	5,621	1,118	904	464	210	8,317
Neonatal deaths	1,922	601	522	3,045	624	606	317	121	4,713
Postneonatal deaths	153	129	312	594	656	908	484	124	2,766
Infant deaths	2,075	730	834	3,639	1,280	1,514	801	245	7,479
Estimated numbers of live births	4,856	8,072	29,465	42,393	126,653	257,309	176,658	53,221	656,234
Rates									
Stillbirths*	238.0	88.8	23.2	66.2	5.2	1.9	1.4	2.2	6.9
Perinatal deaths*	500.2	148.0	37.2	123.8	8.8	3.5	2.6	3.9	12.6
Neonatal deaths†	395.8	74.5	17.7	71.8	4.9	2.4	1.8	2.3	7.2
Postneonatal deaths†	31.5	16.0	10.6	14.0	5.2	3.5	2.7	2.3	4.2
Infant deaths†	427.3	90.4	28.3	85.8	10.1	5.9	4.5	4.6	11.4

* Per 1,000 total births
† Per 1,000 live births

Table A6.3 Mortality and estimated numbers of live births by birthweight, England and Wales, 1980 - *continued*

	Birthweight g (Previous birthweight groupings)								All birthweights
	Up to 1,500	1,501-2,000	2,001-2,500	Up to 2,500	2,501-3,000	3,001-3,500	3,501-4,000	Over 4,000	
Numbers									
Stillbirths	1,543	783	714	3,040	661	488	240	113	4,542
Perinatal deaths	3,239	1,309	1,132	5,680	1,116	875	447	199	8,317
Neonatal deaths	1,949	503	521	3,073	634	586	311	109	4,713
Postneonatal deaths	155	137	313	605	678	896	473	114	2,766
Infant deaths	2,104	740	834	3,678	1,312	1,482	784	223	7,479
Estimated numbers of live births	5,185	8,597	32,090	45,872	131,575	257,374	171,736	49,677	656,234
Rates									
Stillbirths*	229.3	33.5	21.8	62.2	5.0	1.9	1.4	2.3	6.9
Perinatal deaths*	481.4	139.6	34.5	116.1	8.4	3.4	2.6	4.0	12.6
Neonatal deaths†	375.9	70.1	16.2	67.0	4.8	2.3	1.8	2.2	7.2
Postneonatal deaths†	29.9	15.9	9.8	13.2	5.2	3.5	2.8	2.3	4.2
Infant deaths†	405.8	86.1	26.0	80.2	10.0	5.8	4.6	4.5	11.4

* *Per 1,000 total births*

†*Per 1,000 live births*

Source: *OPCS Monitor DH3 83/1* and unpublished data

175

Table A6.4 Perinatal mortality by birthweight and cause, England and Wales, 1980

(a) Birthweights grouped according to ICD Ninth Revision

ICD code	Cause of death	Birthweight g								All birth-weights
		Under 1,500	1,500-1,999	2,000-2,499	Under 2,500	2,500-2,999	3,000-3,499	3,500-3,999	4,000 and over	
		Numbers								
000-999	All causes	3,188	1,311	1,122	5,621	1,118	904	464	210	8,317
000-139	Infections	2	3	1	6	2	1	0	2	11
460-519	Diseases of respiratory system	7	5	7	19	7	11	4	4	45
480-487	Pneumonia and influenza	6	4	7	17	5	9	4	3	38
740-759	Congenital anomalies	483	318	296	1,097	323	238	116	44	1,818
740	Anencephalus	235	73	44	352	12	13	4	0	381
741	Spina bifida	32	21	32	85	71	51	24	11	242
742	Other congenital anomalies of nervous system	43	37	32	112	46	27	21	8	214
745-747	Congenital anomalies of circulatory system	11	28	39	78	70	81	44	14	287
760-779	Certain conditions arising in the perinatal period	2,667	967	794	4,428	761	621	329	156	6,295
760, 761	Maternal conditions	428	125	92	645	59	35	15	9	763
762	Fetus or newborn affected by complications of placenta, cord and membranes	578	361	334	1,273	330	241	112	31	1,987
763	Fetus or newborn affected by other complications of labour and delivery	12	16	17	45	15	31	19	27	137
765	Disorders relating to short gestation and unspecified low birthweight	433	26	6	465	4	4	2	3	478
767	Birth trauma	34	18	16	68	27	24	17	5	141
768	Intra uterine hypoxia and birth asphyxia	135	58	79	272	115	117	68	34	606
769	Respiratory distress syndrome	429	138	54	621	21	20	7	4	673
770	Other respiratory conditions of fetus and newborn	198	37	30	265	46	43	23	12	389
771	Infections specific to perinatal period	18	16	14	48	15	4	2	3	72
772	Fetal and neonatal haemorrhage	113	30	8	151	6	6	8	3	174
773	Haemolytic disease of fetus or newborn, due to isoimmunization	18	15	16	49	10	13	6	1	79
E800-E999	External causes of infant poisoning	0	2	5	7	4	5	4	0	20

Table A6.4 Perinatal mortality by birthweight and cause, England and Wales, 1980-*continued*

(a) Birthweights grouped according to ICD Ninth Revision-*continued*

ICD code	Cause of death	Birthweight g								All birthweights
		Under 1,500	1,500-1,999	2,000-2,499	Under 2,500	2,500-2,999	3,000-3,499	3,500-3,999	4,000 and over	
		Rates (per 1,000 total births)								
000-999	All causes	500.2	148.0	37.2	123.8	8.8	3.5	2.6	3.9	12.6
000-139	Infections	0.3	0.3	0.0	0.1	0.0	0.0	—	0.0	0.0
460-519	Diseases of respiratory system	1.1	0.6	0.2	0.4	0.1	0.0	0.0	0.1	0.1
480-487	Pneumonia and influenza	0.9	0.5	0.2	0.4	0.0	0.0	0.0	0.1	0.1
740-759	Congenital anomalies	75.8	35.9	9.8	24.2	2.5	0.9	0.7	0.8	2.8
740	Anencephalus	36.9	8.2	1.5	7.8	0.1	0.1	0.0	—	0.6
741	Spina bifida	5.0	2.4	1.1	1.9	0.6	0.2	0.1	0.2	0.4
742	Other congenital anomalies of nervous system	6.7	4.2	1.1	2.5	0.4	0.1	0.1	0.1	0.3
745-747	Congenital anomalies of circulatory system	1.7	3.2	1.3	1.7	0.5	0.3	0.2	0.3	0.4
760-779	Certain conditions arising in the perinatal period	418.5	109.2	26.3	97.5	6.0	2.4	1.9	2.9	9.5
760, 761 762	Maternal conditions	67.2	14.1	3.0	14.2	0.5	0.1	0.1	0.2	1.2
	Fetus or newborn affected by complications of placenta, cord and membranes	90.7	40.7	11.1	28.0	2.6	0.9	0.6	0.6	3.0
763	Fetus or newborn affected by other complications of labour and delivery	1.9	1.8	0.6	1.0	0.1	0.1	0.1	0.5	0.2
765	Disorders relating to short gestation and unspecified low birthweight	67.9	2.9	0.2	10.2	0.0	0.0	0.0	0.1	0.7
767	Birth trauma	5.3	2.0	0.5	1.5	0.2	0.1	0.1	0.1	0.2
768	Intra uterine hypoxia and birth asphyxia	21.2	6.5	2.6	6.0	0.9	0.5	0.4	0.6	0.9
769	Respiratory distress syndrome	67.3	15.6	1.8	13.7	0.2	0.1	0.0	0.1	1.0
770	Other respiratory conditions of fetus and newborn	31.1	4.2	1.0	5.8	0.4	0.2	0.1	0.2	0.6
771	Infections specific to perinatal period	2.8	1.8	0.5	1.1	0.1	0.0	0.0	0.1	0.1
772	Fetal and neonatal haemorrhage	17.7	3.4	0.3	3.3	0.0	0.0	0.0	0.1	0.3
773	Haemolytic disease of fetus or newborn, due to isoimmunization	2.3	1.7	0.5	1.1	0.1	0.1	0.0	0.0	0.1
E800-E999	External causes of infant poisoning	—	0.2	0.2	0.2	0.0	0.0	0.0	—	0.0

Table A6.4 Perinatal mortality by birthweight and cause, England and Wales, 1980-*continued*

(b) Birthweights grouped according to previous groupings

ICD code	Cause of death	Birthweight g								All birth-weights
		Up to 1,500	1,501-2,000	2,001-2,500	Up to 2,500	2,501-3,000	3,001-3,500	3,501-4,000	Over 4,000	
		Numbers								
000-999	All causes	3,239	1,309	1,132	5,680	1,116	875	447	199	8,317
000-139	Infections	2	3	1	6	3	0	0	2	11
460-519	Diseases of respiratory system	7	5	7	19	7	11	4	4	45
480-487	Pneumonia and influenza	6	4	7	17	5	9	4	3	38
740-759	Congenital anomalies	497	319	298	1,114	319	231	111	43	1,818
740	Anencephalus	238	73	42	353	12	12	4	0	381
741	Spina bifida	32	22	35	89	70	49	23	11	242
742	Other congenital anomalies of nervous system	45	35	34	114	46	27	19	8	214
745-747	Congenital anomalies of circulatory system	13	28	40	81	70	81	41	14	287
760-779	Certain conditions arising in the perinatal period	2,703	964	799	4,466	763	600	320	146	6,295
760, 761	Maternal conditions	432	124	94	650	58	32	14	9	763
762	Fetus or newborn affected by complications of placenta, cord and membranes	587	365	338	1,290	324	236	106	31	1,987
763	Fetus or newborn affected by other complications of labour and delivery	12	16	19	47	16	29	19	26	137
765	Disorders relating to short gestation and unspecified low birthweight	434	25	6	465	4	4	2	3	478
767	Birth trauma	34	18	17	69	27	23	18	4	141
768	Intra uterine hypoxia and birth asphyxia	140	55	82	277	116	116	67	30	606
769	Respiratory distress syndrome	439	133	49	621	23	18	7	4	673
770	Other respiratory conditions of fetus and newborn	200	39	28	267	45	43	25	9	389
771	Infections specific to perinatal period	18	17	13	48	15	4	2	3	72
772	Fetal and neonatal haemorrhage	114	29	8	151	7	5	8	3	174
773	Haemolytic disease of fetus or newborn, due to isoimmunization	19	15	15	49	11	13	5	1	79
E800-E999	External causes of infant poisoning	0	2	5	7	4	5	4	0	20

Table A6.4 Perinatal mortality by birthweight and cause, England and Wales, 1980-*continued*

(b) Birthweights grouped according to previous groupings-*continued*

ICD code	Cause of death	Birthweight g								All birth-weights
		Up to 1,500	1,501-2,000	2,001-2,500	Up to 2,500	2,501-3,000	3,001-3,500	3,501-4,000	Over 4,000	
		Rates (per 1,000 total births)								
000-999	All causes	481.4	139.6	34.5	116.1	8.4	3.4	2.6	4.0	12.6
000-139	Infections	0.3	0.3	0.0	0.1	0.0	–	–	0.0	0.0
460-519	Diseases of respiratory system	1.0	0.5	0.2	0.4	0.1	0.0	0.0	0.1	0.1
480-487	Pneumonia and influenza	0.9	0.4	0.2	0.3	0.0	0.0	0.0	0.1	0.1
740-759	Congenital anomalies	73.9	34.0	9.1	22.8	2.4	0.9	0.6	0.9	2.8
740	Anencephalus	35.4	7.8	1.3	7.2	0.1	0.0	0.0	–	0.6
741	Spina bifida	4.8	2.3	1.1	1.8	0.5	0.2	0.1	0.2	0.4
742	Other congenital anomalies of nervous system	6.7	3.7	1.0	2.3	0.3	0.1	0.1	0.2	0.3
745-747	Congenital anomalies of circulatory system	1.9	3.0	1.2	1.7	0.5	0.3	0.2	0.3	0.4
760-779	Certain conditions arising in the perinatal period	401.8	102.8	24.4	91.3	5.8	2.3	1.9	2.9	9.5
760, 761 762	Maternal conditions	64.2	13.2	2.9	13.3	0.4	0.1	0.1	0.2	1.2
	Fetus or newborn affected by complications of placenta, cord and membranes	87.2	38.9	10.3	26.4	2.5	0.9	0.6	0.6	3.0
763	Fetus or newborn affected by other complications of labour and delivery	1.8	1.7	0.6	1.0	0.1	0.1	0.1	0.5	0.2
765	Disorders relating to short gestation and unspecified low birthweight	64.5	2.7	0.2	9.5	0.0	0.0	0.0	0.1	0.7
767	Birth trauma	5.1	1.9	0.5	1.4	0.2	0.1	0.1	0.1	0.2
768	Intra uterine hypoxia and birth asphyxia	20.8	5.9	2.5	5.7	0.9	0.4	0.4	0.6	0.9
769	Respiratory distress syndrome	65.2	14.2	1.5	12.7	0.2	0.1	0.0	0.1	1.0
770	Other respiratory conditions of fetus and newborn	29.7	4.2	0.9	5.5	0.3	0.2	0.1	0.2	0.6
771	Infections specific to perinatal period	2.7	1.8	0.4	1.0	0.1	0.0	0.0	0.1	0.1
772	Fetal and neonatal haemorrhage	16.9	3.1	0.2	3.1	0.1	0.0	0.0	0.1	0.3
773	Haemolytic disease of fetus or newborn, due to isoimmunization	2.8	1.6	0.5	1.0	0.1	0.1	0.0	0.0	0.1
E800-E999	External causes of infant poisoning	–	0.2	0.2	0.1	0.0	0.0	0.0	–	0.0

Source: OPCS *Monitor DH3 83/1* (for ICD 9th Revision groupings) and OPCS unpublished data (for previous groupings)

Table A6.5 Neonatal mortality by birthweight and cause, England and Wales, 1980

(a) Birthweights grouped according to ICD Ninth Revision

ICD code	Cause of death	Birthweight g								All birth-weights
		Under 1,500	1,500-1,999	2,000-2,499	Under 2,500	2,500-2,999	3,000-3,499	3,500-3,999	4,000 and over	
		Numbers								
000-999	All causes	1,922	601	522	3,045	624	606	317	121	4,713
000-139	Infections	3	3	2	8	4	5	0	3	20
460-519	Diseases of respiratory system	24	10	15	49	18	26	15	7	115
480-487	Pneumonia and influenza	22	9	13	44	13	20	10	4	91
740-759	Congenital anomalies	177	216	266	659	338	295	142	49	1,483
740	Anencephalus	28	10	18	56	3	7	1	0	67
741	Spina bifida	11	18	30	59	71	74	42	16	262
742	Other congenital anomalies of nervous system	15	15	17	47	21	16	11	4	99
745-747	Congenital anomalies of circulatory system	18	32	56	106	117	127	70	22	442
760-779	Certain conditions arising in the perinatal period	1,687	344	208	2,239	210	201	120	55	2,825
760, 761	Maternal conditions	140	10	7	157	4	3	2	1	167
762	Fetus or newborn affected by complications of placenta, cord and membranes	30	11	12	53	16	15	12	3	99
763	Fetus or newborn affected by other complications of labour and delivery	4	4	4	12	3	12	9	6	42
765	Disorders relating to short gestation and unspecified low birthweight	440	16	5	461	4	4	2	3	474
767	Birth trauma	39	17	17	73	28	23	12	5	141
768	Intra uterine hypoxia and birth asphyxia	54	30	28	112	43	56	36	15	262
769	Respiratory distress syndrome	475	149	57	681	21	20	7	4	733
770	Other respiratory conditions of fetus and newborn	231	40	30	301	46	37	19	10	413
771	Infections specific to perinatal period	26	15	15	56	14	8	2	4	84
772	Fetal and neonatal haemorrhage	143	31	11	185	7	5	7	3	207
773	Haemolytic disease of fetus or newborn, due to isoimmunization	7	5	6	18	3	6	1	0	28
E800-E999	External causes of infant poisoning	1	6	6	13	9	7	4	0	33

Table A6.5 Neonatal mortality by birthweight and cause, England and Wales, 1980-*continued*

(a) Birthweights grouped according to ICD Ninth Revision-*continued*

Rates per 1,000 live births

ICD code	Cause of death	Birthweight g								All birthweights
		Under 1,500	1,500-1,999	2,000-2,499	Under 2,500	2,500-2,999	3,000-3,499	3,500-3,999	4,000 and over	
000-999	All causes	395.8	74.5	17.7	71.8	4.9	2.4	1.8	2.3	7.2
000-139	Infections	0.6	0.4	0.1	0.2	0.0	0.0	–	0.1	0.0
460-519	Diseases of respiratory system	4.9	1.2	0.5	1.2	0.1	0.1	0.1	0.1	0.2
480-487	Pneumonia and influenza	4.5	1.1	0.4	1.0	0.1	0.1	0.1	0.1	0.1
740-759	Congenital anomalies	36.4	26.8	9.0	15.5	2.7	1.1	0.8	0.9	2.3
740	Anencephalus	5.8	1.2	0.6	1.3	0.0	0.0	0.0	–	0.1
741	Spina bifida	2.3	2.2	1.0	1.4	0.6	0.3	0.2	0.3	0.4
742	Other congenital anomalies of nervous system	3.1	1.9	0.6	1.1	0.2	0.1	0.1	0.1	0.2
745-747	Congenital anomalies of circulatory system	3.7	4.0	1.9	2.5	0.9	0.5	0.4	0.4	0.7
760-779	Certain conditions arising in the perinatal period	347.4	42.6	7.1	52.8	1.7	0.8	0.7	1.0	4.3
760, 761	Maternal conditions	28.8	1.2	0.2	3.7	0.0	0.0	0.0	0.0	0.3
762	Fetus or newborn affected by complications of placenta, cord and membranes	6.2	1.4	0.4	1.3	0.1	0.1	0.1	0.1	0.2
763	Fetus or newborn affected by other complications of labour and delivery	0.8	0.5	0.1	0.3	0.0	0.0	0.1	0.1	0.1
765	Disorders relating to short gestation and unspecified low birthweight	90.6	2.0	0.2	10.9	0.0	0.0	0.0	0.1	0.7
767	Birth trauma	8.0	2.1	0.6	1.7	0.2	0.1	0.1	0.1	0.2
768	Intra uterine hypoxia and birth asphyxia	11.1	3.7	1.0	2.6	0.3	0.2	0.2	0.3	0.4
769	Respiratory distress syndrome	97.8	18.5	1.9	16.1	0.2	0.1	0.0	0.1	1.1
770	Other respiratory conditions of fetus and newborn	47.6	5.0	1.0	7.1	0.4	0.1	0.1	0.2	0.6
771	Infections specific to perinatal period	5.4	1.9	0.5	1.3	0.1	0.0	0.0	0.1	0.1
772	Fetal and neonatal haemorrhage	29.4	3.8	0.4	4.4	0.1	0.0	0.0	0.1	0.3
773	Haemolytic disease of fetus or newborn, due to isoimmunization	1.4	0.6	0.2	0.4	0.0	0.0	0.0	–	0.0
E800-E999	External causes of infant poisoning	0.2	0.7	0.2	0.3	0.1	0.0	0.0	–	0.1

Table A6.5 Neonatal mortality by birthweight and cause, England and Wales, 1980-*continued*

(b) Birthweights grouped according to previous groupings

ICD code	Cause of death	Birthweight g								All birth-weights
		Up to 1,500	1,501-2,000	2,001-2,500	Up to 2,500	2,501-3,000	3,001-3,500	3,501-4,000	Over 4,000	
		Numbers								
000-999	All causes	1,949	603	521	3,073	634	586	311	109	4,713
000-139	Infections	3	3	2	8	5	4	0	3	20
460-519	Diseases of respiratory system	24	10	15	49	19	25	15	7	115
480-487	Pneumonia and influenza	22	9	13	44	14	19	10	4	91
740-759	Congenital anomalies	183	226	264	673	339	288	137	46	1,483
740	Anencephalus	28	13	16	57	3	6	1	0	67
741	Spina bifida	11	19	32	62	73	71	40	16	262
742	Other congenital anomalies of nervous system	16	14	18	48	21	16	10	4	99
745-747	Congenital anomalies of circulatory system	20	32	57	109	118	127	68	20	442
760-779	Certain conditions arising in the perinatal period	1,708	335	205	2,248	219	190	121	47	2,825
760, 761	Maternal conditions	140	10	7	157	5	2	2	1	167
762	Fetus or newborn affected by complications of placenta, cord and membranes	30	11	13	54	17	14	11	3	99
763	Fetus or newborn affected by other complications of labour and delivery	4	4	4	12	5	11	9	5	42
765	Disorders relating to short gestation and unspecified low birthweight	441	15	5	461	4	4	2	3	474
767	Birth trauma	39	17	18	74	28	22	13	4	141
768	Intra uterine hypoxia and birth asphyxia	57	28	31	116	44	54	37	11	262
769	Respiratory distress syndrome	487	142	52	681	23	18	7	4	733
770	Other respiratory conditions of fetus and newborn	233	41	29	303	44	38	20	8	413
771	Infections specific to perinatal period	26	17	13	56	14	8	2	4	84
772	Fetal and neonatal haemorrhage	144	30	11	185	8	4	7	3	207
773	Haemolytic disease of fetus or newborn, due to isoimmunization	8	5	5	18	3	6	1	0	28
E800-E999	External causes of infant poisoning	1	6	7	14	8	7	4	0	33

Table A6.5 Neonatal mortality by birthweight and cause, England and Wales, 1980-*continued*

(b) Birthweights grouped according to previous groupings-*continued*

ICD code	Cause of death	Birthweight g								All birthweights
		Up to 1,500	1,501-2,000	2,001-2,500	Up to 2,500	2,501-3,000	3,001-3,500	3,501-4,000	Over 4,000	
		Rates per 1,000 live births								
000-999	All causes	375.9	70.1	16.2	67.0	4.8	2.3	1.8	2.2	7.2
000-139	Infections	0.6	0.3	0.1	0.2	0.0	0.0	–	0.1	0.0
460-519	Diseases of respiratory system	4.6	1.2	0.5	1.1	0.1	0.1	0.1	0.1	0.2
480-487	Pneumonia and influenza	4.2	1.0	0.4	1.0	0.1	0.1	0.1	0.1	0.1
740-759	Congenital anomalies	35.3	26.3	8.2	14.7	2.6	1.1	0.8	0.9	2.3
740	Anencephalus	5.4	1.5	0.5	1.2	0.0	0.0	0.0	–	0.1
741	Spina bifida	2.1	2.2	1.0	1.4	0.6	0.3	0.2	0.3	0.4
742	Other congenital anomalies of nervous system	3.1	1.6	0.6	1.0	0.2	0.1	0.1	0.1	0.2
745-747	Congenital anomalies of circulatory system	3.9	3.7	1.8	2.4	0.9	0.5	0.4	0.4	0.7
760-779	Certain conditions arising in the perinatal period	329.4	39.0	6.4	49.0	1.7	0.7	0.7	0.9	4.3
760, 761	Maternal conditions	27.0	1.2	0.2	3.4	0.0	0.0	0.0	0.0	0.3
762	Fetus or newborn affected by complications of placenta, cord and membranes	5.8	1.3	0.4	1.2	0.1	0.1	0.1	0.1	0.2
763	Fetus or newborn affected by other complications of labour and delivery	0.8	0.5	0.1	0.3	0.0	0.0	0.1	0.1	0.1
765	Disorders relating to short gestation and unspecified low birthweight	85.1	1.7	0.2	10.0	0.0	0.0	0.0	0.1	0.7
767	Birth trauma	7.5	2.0	0.6	1.6	0.2	0.1	0.1	0.1	0.2
768	Intra uterine hypoxia and birth asphyxia	11.0	3.3	1.0	2.5	0.3	0.2	0.2	0.2	0.4
769	Respiratory distress syndrome	93.9	16.5	1.6	14.8	0.2	0.1	0.0	0.1	1.1
770	Other respiratory conditions of fetus and newborn	44.9	4.8	0.9	6.6	0.3	0.1	0.1	0.2	0.6
771	Infections specific to perinatal period	5.0	2.0	0.4	1.2	0.1	0.0	0.0	0.1	0.1
772	Fetal and neonatal haemorrhage	27.8	3.5	0.3	4.0	0.1	0.0	0.0	0.1	0.3
773	Haemolytic disease of fetus or newborn, due to isoimmunization	1.5	0.6	0.2	0.4	0.0	0.0	0.0	–	0.0
E800-E999	External causes of infant poisoning	0.2	0.7	0.2	0.3	0.1	0.0	0.0	–	0.1

Source: OPCS *Monitor DH3 83/1* (for ICD 9th Revision groupings) and OPCS unpublished data (for previous groupings)

Table A6.6 Infant mortality by birthweight and cause, England and Wales, 1980

(a) Birthweights grouped according to ICD Ninth Revision

ICD code	Cause of death	Birthweight g								All birthweights
		Under 1,500	1,500-1,999	2,000-2,499	Under 2,500	2,500-2,999	3,000-3,499	3,500-3,999	4,000 and over	
		Numbers								
000-999	All causes	2,075	730	834	3,639	1,280	1,514	801	245	7,479
000-139	Infections	11	8	11	30	24	38	23	6	121
460-519	Diseases of respiratory system	56	38	78	172	176	262	141	32	783
460-466	Acute respiratory infections	4	10	18	32	56	80	47	7	222
480-487	Pneumonia and influenza	46	25	49	120	97	140	70	17	444
740-759	Congenital anomalies	197	254	351	802	460	441	216	62	1,981
740	Anencephalus	28	10	18	56	3	7	1	1	68
741	Spina bifida	11	18	36	65	92	104	66	18	345
742	Other congenital anomalies of nervous system	22	16	25	63	30	26	11	4	134
745-747	Congenital anomalies of circulatory system	29	51	98	178	173	212	111	31	705
760-779	Certain conditions arising in the perinatal period	1,745	355	222	2,322	216	209	125	59	2,931
798.0	Sudden infant death (cause unknown)	18	39	96	153	248	350	196	52	999
E800-E999	External causes of infant poisoning	3	8	25	36	45	57	32	7	177
		Rates per 1,000 live births								
000-999	All causes	427.3	90.4	28.3	85.8	10.1	5.9	4.5	4.6	11.4
000-139	Infections	2.3	1.0	0.4	0.7	0.2	0.1	0.1	0.1	0.2
460-519	Diseases of respiratory system	11.5	4.7	2.6	4.1	1.4	1.0	0.8	0.6	1.2
460-466	Acute respiratory infections	0.8	1.2	0.6	0.8	0.4	0.3	0.3	0.1	0.3
480-487	Pneumonia and influenza	9.5	3.1	1.7	2.8	0.8	0.5	0.4	0.3	0.7
740-759	Congenital anomalies	40.6	31.5	11.9	18.9	3.6	1.7	1.2	1.2	3.0
740	Anencephalus	5.8	1.2	0.6	1.3	0.0	0.0	0.0	0.0	0.1
741	Spina bifida	2.3	2.2	1.2	1.5	0.7	0.4	0.4	0.3	0.5
742	Other congenital anomalies of nervous system	4.5	2.0	0.8	1.5	0.2	0.1	0.1	0.1	0.2
745-747	Congenital anomalies of circulatory system	6.0	6.3	3.3	4.2	1.4	0.8	0.6	0.6	1.1
760-779	Certain conditions arising in the perinatal period	359.3	44.0	7.5	54.8	1.7	0.8	0.7	1.1	4.5
798.0	Sudden infant death (cause unknown)	3.7	4.8	3.3	3.6	2.0	1.4	1.1	1.0	1.5
E800-E999	External causes of infant poisoning	0.6	1.0	0.8	0.8	0.4	0.2	0.2	0.1	0.3

(b) Birthweights grouped according to previous groupings-*continued*

ICD code	Cause of death	Birthweight g								All birth-weights
		Up to 1,500	1,501-2,000	2,001-2,500	Up to 2,500	2,501-3,000	3,001-3,500	3,501-4,000	Over 4,000	
		Numbers								
000-999	All causes	2,104	740	834	3,678	1,312	1,482	784	223	7,479
000-139	Infections	12	8	11	31	25	37	22	6	121
460-519	Diseases of respiratory system	56	39	78	173	182	262	136	30	783
460-466	Acute respiratory infections	4	10	19	33	56	79	47	7	222
480-487	Pneumonia and influenza	46	26	48	120	101	141	66	16	444
740-759	Congenital anomalies	204	266	349	819	465	431	211	55	1,981
740	Anencephalus	28	13	16	57	3	6	1	1	68
741	Spina bifida	11	19	38	68	95	100	65	17	345
742	Other congenital anomalies of nervous system	23	15	27	65	30	25	10	4	134
745-747	Congenital anomalies of circulatory system	31	51	101	183	177	209	110	26	705
760-779	Certain conditions arising in the perinatal period	1,766	346	219	2,331	225	198	126	51	2,931
798.0	Sudden infant death (cause unknown)	18	42	97	157	255	346	191	50	999
E800-E999	External causes of infant poisoning	3	9	26	38	46	55	31	7	177
		Rates per 1,000 live births								
000-999	All causes	405.8	86.1	26.0	80.2	10.0	5.8	4.6	4.5	11.4
000-139	Infections	2.3	0.9	0.3	0.7	0.2	0.1	0.1	0.1	0.2
460-519	Diseases of respiratory system	10.8	4.5	2.4	3.8	1.4	1.0	0.8	0.6	1.2
460-466	Acute respiratory infections	0.8	1.2	0.6	0.7	0.4	0.3	0.3	0.1	0.3
480-487	Pneumonia and influenza	8.9	3.0	1.5	2.6	0.8	0.5	0.4	0.3	0.7
740-759	Congenital anomalies	39.3	30.9	10.9	17.9	3.5	1.7	1.2	1.1	3.0
740	Anencephalus	5.4	1.5	0.5	1.2	0.0	0.0	0.0	0.0	0.1
741	Spina bifida	2.1	2.2	1.2	1.5	0.7	0.4	0.4	0.3	0.5
742	Other congenital anomalies of nervous system	4.4	1.7	0.8	1.4	0.2	0.1	0.1	0.1	0.2
745-747	Congenital anomalies of circulatory system	6.0	5.9	3.1	4.0	1.3	0.8	0.6	0.5	1.1
760-779	Certain conditions arising in the perinatal period	340.6	40.2	6.8	50.8	1.7	0.8	0.7	1.0	4.5
798.0	Sudden infant death (cause unknown)	3.5	4.9	3.0	3.4	1.9	1.3	1.1	1.0	1.5
E800-E999	External causes of infant poisoning	0.6	1.0	0.8	0.8	0.3	0.2	0.2	0.1	0.3

Source: OPCS *Monitor DH3 83/1* (for ICD 9th Revision groupings) and OPCS unpublished data (for previous groupings)

Table A6.7   Perinatal and infant mortality by birthweight and social class, England and Wales, 1980

Social class	Birthweight g								All birth weights
	Under 1,500	1,500- 1,999	2,000- 2,499	Under 2,500	2,500- 2,999	3,000- 3,499	3,500- 3,999	4,000 and over	
Perinatal deaths									
	Numbers								
I-V	2,556	1,080	940	4,576	905	749	397	179	6,806
I	135	60	52	247	43	50	25	9	374
II	441	203	183	827	187	164	89	24	1,291
IIIN	253	114	92	459	93	73	52	23	700
IIIM	1,029	418	364	1,811	354	287	141	76	2,669
IV	498	190	167	855	159	129	66	36	1,245
V	200	95	82	377	69	46	24	11	527
	Rates per 1,000 total births								
I-V	577.8	179.4	42.5	140.6	10.2	3.9	3.0	4.4	12.1
I	403.0	193.5	38.5	123.7	7.6	3.5	2.3	3.0	9.1
II	551.9	158.1	45.8	136.0	11.0	3.9	2.7	2.3	10.4
IIIN	546.4	189.4	42.5	142.1	10.2	3.5	3.4	4.9	11.2
IIIM	582.7	181.3	41.3	140.6	10.1	4.0	2.9	5.0	12.5
IV	631.2	170.9	41.9	145.3	10.1	4.3	3.5	6.8	14.1
V	735.3	234.0	45.6	152.3	10.5	4.1	3.7	6.7	16.0
Infant deaths									
	Numbers								
I-V	1,604	612	654	2,870	989	1,182	651	200	5,892
I	89	30	42	161	52	77	49	13	352
II	269	117	123	509	184	237	147	41	1,118
IIIN	176	67	58	301	99	111	76	23	610
IIIM	626	238	218	1,082	357	426	238	70	2,173
IV	315	107	146	568	199	227	99	41	1,134
V	129	53	67	249	98	104	42	12	505
	Rates per 1,000 live births								
I-V	485.6	112.3	30.3	94.6	11.2	6.2	4.9	5.0	10.5
I	317.9	107.1	31.8	85.5	9.3	5.4	4.5	4.3	8.6
II	447.6	99.8	31.5	89.6	10.9	5.6	4.5	3.9	9.0
IIIN	488.9	121.6	27.4	99.5	10.9	5.4	5.0	4.9	9.9
IIIM	477.1	114.2	25.4	90.2	10.3	6.0	4.9	4.6	10.2
IV	552.6	105.8	37.6	103.9	12.7	7.6	5.3	7.8	12.9
V	716.7	151.0	38.2	109.0	15.0	9.2	6.5	7.3	15.5

Source: OPCS *Monitor DH3 83/1*

Table A6.8 **Perinatal and infant mortality of singleton and multiple births by birthweight, England and Wales, 1980**

Social class	Birthweight g								All birth weights
	Under 1,500	1,500-1,999	2,000-2,499	Under 2,500	2,500-2,999	3,000-3,499	3,500-3,999	4,000 and over	
Perinatal deaths									
Numbers									
Singleton births	2,701	1,207	1,040	4,948	1,068	890	459	210	7,575
Multiple births	487	104	82	673	50	14	5	0	742
Rates per 1,000 total births									
Singleton births	514.6	170.2	39.1	127.2	8.7	3.5	2.6	3.9	11.7
Multiple births	433.3	58.9	22.8	103.7	12.1	8.3	23.5	–	59.1
Infant deaths									
Numbers									
Singleton births	1,672	645	777	3,094	1,240	1,494	798	245	6,871
Multiple births	403	85	57	545	40	20	3	0	608
Rates per 1,000 live births									
Singleton births	429.4	101.4	30.0	85.5	10.1	5.8	4.5	4.6	10.7
Multiple births	418.9	49.8	16.1	87.7	9.7	11.9	14.3	–	49.7

Source: OPCS *Monitor DH3 83/1*

Table A6.9 Birthweight by period of gestation and sex, Scotland, 1973-79

Gestational age, weeks	Not measured, number	Measured Number	Weight range g	Percentiles of birthweight distribution g								
				3%	5%	10%	25%	50%	75%	90%	95%	97%
Males												
26	2	50	595-1930			700		960		1270		
27	1	47	600-3560			880		1080		1410		
28	1	104	630-3720	770	800	890	1010	1200	1360	1620	1680	1780
29	3	102	520-4000	1000	1000	1040	1180	1320	1480	1740	1930	3280
30	5	138	800-3180	1000	1030	1200	1340	1510	1700	1930	2200	2400
31	3	138	860-3620	1020	1160	1230	1460	1680	1871	2040	2215	1406
32	5	277	737-3550	1100	1240	1360	1590	1800	2000	2310	2620	2720
33	0	290	1070-4280	1290	1446	1590	1800	2070	2370	2670	2980	3250
34	2	544	1040-4250	1460	1580	1740	1970	2240	2500	2835	3090	3220
35	1	785	850-4370	1670	1800	1970	2210	2490	2750	3050	3240	3400
36	1	1,991	980-4995	1920	2040	2210	2460	2740	3030	3320	3510	3690
37	1	3,488	900-4990	2140	2260	2430	2700	2980	3280	3590	3790	3940
38	2	9,618	1280-5875	2360	2495	2630	2920	3210	3500	3760	3940	4060
39	4	18,467	945-5780	2560	2660	2820	3090	3370	3660	3950	4120	4240
40	3	33,106	760-9100	2670	2770	2940	3200	3480	3780	4060	4240	4360
41	10	15,461	1920-7314	2774	2870	3020	3280	3597	3880	4180	4340	4460
42 and over	1	3,351	1840-9460	2775	2870	3015	3271	3580	3900	4171	4360	4490

Table A6.9   Birthweight by period of gestation and sex, Scotland, 1973-79 - *continued*

Gestational age, weeks	Not measured, number	Measured Number	Weight range g	Percentiles of birthweight distribution g 3%	5%	10%	25%	50%	75%	90%	95%	97%
Females												
26	1	47	480-2320			610		860		1090		
27	0	24	750-3200			830		1020		1190		
28	5	85	530-3660			840		1110		1410		
29	0	68	480-3000			960		1250		1620		
30	3	97	840-3180	970	1020	1106	1270	1410	1580	1820	1890	2560
31	1	122	510-3401	1000	1150	1250	1400	1575	1760	2320	2780	3200
32	0	220	840-4180	1160	1250	1330	1474	1800	1976	2290	2800	3140
33	1	235	960-3300	1300	1320	1440	1740	1970	2210	2430	2785	2880
34	4	476	660-4030	1300	1365	1640	1900	2140	2400	2720	2910	3000
35	1	683	920-4070	1600	1700	1850	2120	2410	2680	3000	3250	3390
36.	2	1,674	1100-4900	1860	1960	2100	2365	2640	2950	3220	3440	3580
37	6	2,904	1093-6140	2050	2180	2340	2600	2890	3175	3460	3650	3730
38	1	8,261	608-5320	2300	2410	2551	2800	3080	3380	3640	3810	3950
39	7	16,792	1040-5240	2480	2570	2720	2960	3240	3520	3800	3970	4080
40	20	31,652	1300-6090	2580	2680	2820	3070	3340	3630	3900	4070	4190
41	8	15,292	1360-6150	2680	2770	2910	3150	3430	3714	4000	4160	4276
42 and over	2	3,042	1920-6050	2660	2761	2911	3160	3440	3740	3980	4150	4260

Source: Information Services Division

Table A6.10   Certified causes of stillbirths and infant deaths, by sex, England and Wales, 1980

ICD code	Cause of death	Males		Females	
		Number	Rate*	Number	Rate*
Stillbirths					
000-999	All causes	2,483	7.34	3,290	7.10
740-759	Congenital anomalies	349	1.03	460	1.43
740	Anencephalus	110	0.32	232	0.72
741	Spina bifida	37	0.11	77	0.24
742	Other congenital anomalies of nervous system	88	0.26	61	0.19
743-759	Other congenital anomalies	114	0.34	90	0.28
760-779	Certain conditions originating in the perinatal period	2,131	6.30	1,821	5.65
760	Maternal conditions, possibly unrelated to present pregnancy	263	0.78	223	0.69
762	Complications of placenta cord and membranes	1,056	3.12	899	2.79
768	Intrauterine hypoxia and birth asphyxia	201	0.59	187	0.58
761, 763-767, 769-779	Other conditions originating in the perinatal period	611	1.81	512	1.59
000-739, 780-999	Other causes of stillbirth	3	0.00	9	0.00
Infant deaths					
000-999	All causes	4,471	13.31	3,428	10.70
460-519	Diseases of the respiratory system	449	1.34	353	1.10
740-759	Congenital anomalies	1,103	3.28	1,010	3.15
740-742	All anomalies of the central nervous system	243	0.72	327	1.02
745-747	Congenital anomalies of the heart and circulatory system	409	1.22	354	1.11
743, 744, 748-759	Other congenital anomalies	451	1.34	329	1.03
760-779	Certain conditions originating in the perinatal period	1,854	5.52	1,279	3.99
761-763	Obstetric complications affecting fetus or newborn	170	0.51	128	0.40
764, 765	Slow fetal growth, fetal malnutrition and immaturity	291	0.87	229	0.71
768	Intrauterine hypoxia and birth asphyxia	185	0.55	120	0.37
769	Respiratory distress syndrome	498	1.48	299	0.93
770	Other respiratory conditions of fetus and newborn	264	0.79	196	0.61
772	Fetal and neonatal haemhorrage	141	0.42	84	0.26
760, 766, 767, 771, 773-779	Other conditions originating in the perinatal period	305	0.91	223	0.70
780-799	Signs, symptoms and ill-defined conditions	650	1.87	418	1.27
798	Sudden death, cause unknown	622	1.85	401	1.25
780-797, 799	Other signs, symptoms and ill-defined conditions	28	0.08	17	0.05
800-999	External causes of injury and poisoning	96	0.29	95	0.30

Rates are per 1,000 total births for stillbirths and per 1,000 live births for infant deaths

Source: OPCS *Mortality Statistics: Childhood, 1980 Series DH3 No. 8* Tables 5 (Stillbirths) and 16 (Infant deaths)

Table A6.11 Live births, stillbirths and infant deaths, by sex, England and Wales, 1928-81

Year	Live births		Stillbirths				Infant deaths	
	Number		Number		Rate*		Rate†	
	Males	Females	Males	Females	Males	Females	Males	Females
1928	337,182	323,085	15,099	12,481	42.86	37.19	74	56
1929	328,642	315,031	14,961	11,886	43.54	36.36	83	65
1930	331,380	317,431	15,241	12,336	43.97	37.41	68	51
1931	323,565	308,516	14,951	11,982	44.17	37.39	74	57
1932	314,407	299,565	14,523	11,948	44.15	38.35	73	56
1933	296,729	283,684	13,576	11,508	43.75	38.98	71	54
1934	306,874	290,768	13,690	11,519	42.71	38.11	66	52
1935	307,552	291,204	13,790	11,645	42.91	38.45	64	50
1936	310,605	294,687	13,639	11,406	42.06	37.26	66	51
1937	313,618	296,939	13,479	11,327	41.21	36.74	65	50
1938	318,387	302,817	13,349	11,380	40.24	36.22	60	46
1939	315,606	298,873	13,088	11,232	39.82	36.22	56	44
1940	302,615	287,505	12,296	10,483	39.05	35.18	64	49
1941	297,054	282,037	11,268	9,608	36.55	32.94	67	52
1942	335,760	315,743	11,868	10,515	34.14	32.23	57	44
1943	352,798	331,536	11,469	9,793	31.49	28.69	55	43
1944	387,638	363,840	11,493	9,813	28.80	26.26	50	40
1945	350,072	329,865	10,367	8,966	28.76	26.46	51	40
1946	422,299	398,420	12,357	10,558	28.43	25.82	48	37
1947	453,590	427,436	11,792	10,003	25.34	22.87	46	36
1948	399,112	376,194	9,937	8,462	24.29	22.00	38	30
1949	376,064	354,454	9,129	7,818	23.70	21.58	36	28
1950	358,715	338,382	8,693	7,391	23.66	21.38	34	26
1951	348,604	328,925	8,669	7,316	24.26	21.76	34	26
1952	345,878	327,857	8,368	7,268	23.62	21.69	31	24
1953	352,037	332,335	8,311	7,370	23.06	21.70	30	24
1954	346,455	327,196	8,467	7,733	23.86	23.09	29	22
1955	343,673	324,138	8,303	7,526	23.59	22.69	28	21
1956	359,881	340,454	8,609	7,796	23.36	22.39	27	20
1957	372,298	351,083	8,613	8,002	22.61	22.28	26	20
1958	380,944	359,771	8,486	7,802	21.79	21.23	25	20
1959	385,689	362,812	8,242	7,659	20.92	20.67	25	20
1960	404,150	380,855	8,098	7,721	19.64	19.87	25	19
1961	417,768	393,513	8,076	7,651	18.96	19.07	24	19
1962	431,633	407,103	7,957	7,507	18.10	18.11	24	18
1963	438,476	415,579	7,884	7,105	17.66	16.81	24	18
1964	451,072	424,900	7,566	6,980	16.50	16.16	22	17
1965	443,190	419,535	7,200	6,641	15.99	15.58	21	16

*Per 1,000 total births
†Per 1,000 live births

Table A6.11 Live births, stillbirths and infant deaths, by sex, England and Wales, 1928-81 - *continued*

Year	Live births		Stillbirths				Infant deaths	
	Number		Number		Rate*		Rate†	
	Males	Females	Males	Females	Males	Females	Males	Females
1966	437,262	412,561	6,857	6,386	15.44	15.24	21	16
1967	427,901	404,263	6,520	6,008	15.01	14.64	20	16
1968	421,130	398,142	6,109	5,739	14.30	14.21	21	16
1969	410,052	387,486	5,620	5,034	13.52	12.82	20	16
1970	403,371	381,115	5,288	5,057	12.94	13.10	20	16
1971	403,223	379,932	5,036	4,863	12.34	12.64	20	15
1972	373,982	351,458	4,413	4,386	11.66	12.33	19	15
1973	348,678	327,275	4,036	3,900	11.44	11.78	19	15
1974	329,459	310,426	3,579	3,596	10.75	11.45	19	14
1975	310,751	292,694	3,115	3,180	9.92	10.75	18	14
1976	300,313	283,957	2,950	2,759	9.73	9.62	16	12
1977	292,957	276,302	2,813	2,592	9.51	9.29	15	12
1978	307,088	289,330	2,634	2,474	8.50	8.48	15	12
1979	328,308	309,720	2,656	2,469	8.03	7.91	14	11
1980	335,954	320,280	2,483	2,290	7.34	7.10	13	11
1981	325,700	308,756	2,184	2,019	6.66	6.50	13	9

*Per 1,000 total births
†Per 1,000 live births
Source: OPCS *Birth Statistics Series FM1* and *Registrar General's Statistical Reviews*

Table A6.12 Sex ratio of live births by month of occurrence of birth, England and Wales, 1980

Month of birth	Live births		Sex ratio males/females
	Males	Females	
Total	335,954	320,280	1.050
January	27,799	26,608	1.045
February	26,346	25,163	1.047
March	28,823	27,595	1.045
April	28,550	26,990	1.058
May	29,794	28,055	1.062
June	28,098	26,647	1.054
July	29,752	28,186	1.056
August	28,170	26,635	1,058
September	28,345	27,234	1.041
October	28,177	27,182	1.037
November	25,725	24,743	1.040
December	26,375	25,242	1.045

Source: OPCS *Birth Statistics 1980, Series FM1 No. 7* (Table 2.4)

Table A6.13 Maternities with multiple births, England and Wales, 1939-1980

Year	All maternities	Total multiple maternities	Rate (per 1,000 maternities)	Twins	Triplets	Quadruplets	Quintuplets	Sextuplets
1939	631,282	7,539	11.9	7,477	61	1	-	-
1940	605,534	7,319	12.1	7,254	65	-	-	-
1941	592,813	7,087	12.0	7,020	67	-	-	-
1942	665,838	7,976	12.0	7,904	72	-	-	-
1943	697,267	8,259	11.8	8,193	62	4	-	-
1944	763,092	9,604	12.6	9,520	80	4	-	-
1945	690,934	8,274	12.0	8,212	62	-	-	-
1946	832,761	10,788	13.0	10,703	85	-	-	-
1947	891,504	11,221	12.6	11,130	86	5	-	-
1948	783,926	9,687	12.4	9,597	88	2	-	-
1949	738,050	9,328	12.6	9,241	87	-	-	-
1950	704,102	8,979	12.8	8,880	98	1	-	-
1951	684,407	9,005	13.2	8,905	98	2	-	-
1952	680,715	8,590	12.6	8,525	64	1	-	-
1953	691,180	8,787	12.7	8,703	83	-	1	-
1954	681,058	8,724	12.8	8,655	69	-	-	-
1955	675,026	8,525	12.6	8,437	87	1	-	-
1956	707,921	8,739	12.3	8,660	78	1	-	-
1957	730,524	9,371	12.8	9,273	95	3	-	-
1958	747,536	9,377	12.5	9,287	90	-	-	-
1959	755,294	9,021	11.9	8,934	87	-	-	-
1960	791,584	9,163	11.6	9,086	77	-	-	-
1961	817,271	9,653	11.8	9,570	82	1	-	-
1962	844,265	9,845	11.7	9,756	88	1	-	-
1963	858,884	10,060	11.7	9,960	100	-	-	-
1964	880,173	10,238	11.6	10,135	99	4	-	-
1965	866,713	9,774	11.3	9,695	79	-	-	-
1966	853,481	9,501	11.1	9,418	82	1	-	-
1967	835,433	9,187	11.0	9,117	68	2	-	-
1968	822,247	8,783	10.7	8,697	84	1	-	1
1969	799,763	8,341	10.4	8,259	79	1	1	1
1970	786,587	8,143	10 4	8,042	100	1	-	-
1971	784,899	8,074	10.2	8,000	69	3	2	-
1972	726,715	7,431	10.2	7,345	81	3	2	-
1973	677,125	6,688	9.9	6,615	71	2	-	-
1974	640,777	6,215	9.7	6,151	60	4	-	-
1975	603,666	5,988	9.9	5,909	72	7	-	-
1976	584,263	5,621	9.6	5,538	76	4	2	1
1977	569,073	5,519	9.7	5,449	68	2	-	-
1978	595,515	5,930	10.0	5,859	62	8	1	-
1979	636,884	6,181	9.7	6,099	76	6	-	-
1980	654,501	6,404	9.8	6,308	91	4	1	-

Source: OPCS *Birth statistics Series FM1*

Table A6.14 Mortality among singleton and multiple births in the first year of life, England and Wales 1949/50, 1975-78

Year	Deaths among multiple births		Deaths among singleton births	
	Number	Rate*	Number	Rate*
Stillbirths				
1949/50	2,008	54.4	31,023	21.8
1975	353	29.3	5,942	9.9
1976	321	28.3	5,388	9.3
1977	324	29.2	5,081	9.0
1978	341	28.6	4,767	8.1
Perinatal deaths				
1949/50	..	..	..	..
1975	1,067	88.5	10,640	17.8
1976	880	77.6	9,532	16.5
1977	795	71.6	8,942	15.9
1978	878	73.5	8,452	14.3
Neonatal deaths				
1949/50	3,423	98.1	23,291	16.7
1975	774	66.1	5,612	9.5
1976	616	55.9	4,970	8.7
1977	528	49.0	4,722	8.5
1978	588	50.7	4,572	7.8
Postneonatal deaths				
1949/50	874	25.1	15,588	11.2
1975	106	9.1	2,776	4.7
1976	91	8.3	2,404	4.2
1977	84	7.8	2,435	4.4
1978	112	9.7	2,600	4.4
Infant deaths				
1949/50	4,297	123.2	38,879	27.9
1975	880	75.2	8,388	14.2
1976	707	64.2	7,374	12.9
1977	612	56.7	7,157	12.8
1978	700	60.3	7,172	12.3
Live births				
1949/50	34,879		1,392,505	
1975	11,709		591,736	
1976	11,015		573,254	
1977	10,786		558,473	
1978	11,600		584,818	

* *Rates are per 1,000 total births for stillbirths and perinatal deaths and per 1,000 live births for neonatal, postneonatal and infant deaths.*
Source: OPCS unpublished data

Table A6.15 Mortality among twins, England and Wales, 1975-78

Year	All twins		Two males		One male, one female		Two females	
	Number	Rate*	Number	Rate*	Number	Rate*	Number	Rate*
Stillbirths								
1975	343	29.0	157	38.8	44	11.8	142	35.2
1976	309	27.9	128	32.8	59	17.9	122	31.5
1977	307	28.2	154	37.8	40	12.7	113	30.6
1978	327	27.9	140	32.2	63	19.0	124	30.5
Perinatal deaths								
1975	1,005	85.0	406	100.4	244	65.2	355	88.0
1976	835	75.4	383	98.0	175	53.1	277	71.5
1977	753	69.1	341	83.8	143	45.6	269	72.9
1978	819	69.9	343	79.0	179	54.0	297	73.2
Neonatal deaths								
1975	720	62.7	266	68.5	217	58.6	237	60.9
1976	578	53.7	275	72.8	127	39.2	176	46.9
1977	502	47.4	217	55.4	111	35.8	174	48.6
1978	539	47.3	228	54.3	131	40.3	180	45.7
Postneonatal deaths								
1975	104	9.1	32	8.2	41	11.1	31	8.0
1976	87	8.1	35	9.3	27	8.3	25	6.7
1977	84	7.9	38	9.7	26	8.4	20	5.6
1978	109	9.6	47	11.2	32	9.8	30	7.6
Infant deaths								
1975	824	71.8	298	76.7	258	69.7	268	68.9
1976	665	61.8	310	82.0	154	47.6	201	53.6
1977	586	55.3	255	65.1	137	44.2	194	54.2
1978	648	56.9	275	65.4	163	50.1	210	53.4
Live births								
1975	11,475		3,885		3,700		3,890	
1976	10,767		3,780		3,237		3,750	
1977	10,591		3,916		3,098		3,577	
1978	11,391		4,202		3,253		3,936	

* *Rates are per 1,000 total births for stillbirths and perinatal deaths and per 1,000 live births for neonatal, postneonatal and infant deaths.*
Source: OPCS unpublished data

Table A6.16 Mortality among triplets, England and Wales, 1975-79

Year	Stillbirths		Perinatal deaths		Neonatal deaths		Postneonatal deaths		Infant deaths	
	Number	Rate*	Number	Rate*	Number	Rate*	Number	Rate*	Number	Rate*
1975-79	55	51.8	206	194.0	162	160.9	10	9.9	172	170.8
1975	8	37.0	52	240.7	45	216.4	1	4.8	46	221.2
1976	11	48.2	39	171.1	31	142.9	3	13.8	34	156.7
1977	16	78.4	38	186.3	23	122.3	0	–	23	122.3
1978	13	69.9	42	225.8	33	190.8	3	17.3	36	208.1
1979	7	30.7	35	153.5	30	135.7	3	13.6	33	149.3

*Rates are per 1,000 total births for stillbirths and perinatal deaths and per 1,000 live births for neonatal, postneonatal and infant deaths.
Source: OPCS unpublished data

Table A7.1 Sizes of maternity units and numbers of births, England, 1973, 1978, 1980

Size of unit, number of births each year	All units		Units with GP beds only		Units with GP and consultant beds		Units with consultant beds only	
	Number of units	Number of births*	Number of units	Number of births*	Number of units	Number of births*	Number of units	Number of births*
1973								
Less than 200	85	9,785	76	9,503	2	77	7	205
200-999	225	111,080	144	58,908	20	11,661	61	40,511
1,000-1,999	121	180,477	1	1,352	27	41,754	93	137,371
2,000-2,999	58	140,365	0	0	21	52,576	37	87,789
3,000-3,999	25	84,618	0	0	9	30,363	16	54,255
4,000 and over	13	65,344	0	0	8	39,605	5	25,739
All units	527	591,669	221	69,763	87	176,036	219	345,870
1978								
Less than 200	93	9,373	82	8,067	3	463	8	843
200-999	119	56,992	66	22,573	10	6,028	43	28,391
1,000-1,999	104	158,907	0	0	39	61,750	65	97,157
2,000-2,999	63	154,105	0	0	33	78,340	30	75,765
3,000-3,999	28	95,856	0	0	11	36,844	17	59,012
4,000 and over	16	75,061	0	0	10	46,928	6	29,133
All units	423	551,294	148	30,640	106	230,353	169	290,301
1980								
Less than 200	91	8,438	78	7,549	5	283	8	606
200-999	89	41,684	53	18,074	13	7,923	23	15,687
1,000-1,999	82	127,191	1	1,088	29	46,921	52	79,182
2,000-2,999	81	198,984	0	0	41	101,374	40	97,610
3,000-3,999	32	108,696	0	0	14	47,738	18	60,958
4,000 and over	25	122,886	0	0	13	66,844	12	56,042
All units	400	607,879	132	26,711	115	271,083	153	310,085

* *Births occurring in NHS maternity units*
Source: DHSS, SH3 Hospital Return

Table A7.2 Sizes of maternity units and numbers of births, Regional Health Authorities and constituent countries of the United Kingdom, 1980

Area	All units	Size of unit, number of births in 1980					
		Less than 200	200-999	1,000-1,999	2,000-2,999	3,000-3,999	4,000 and over
Numbers of units							
ENGLAND★	**400**	**91**	**89**	**82**	**81**	**32**	**25**
Regional Health Authorities							
Northern	31	4	8	12	6	1	0
Yorkshire	33	8	8	5	7	4	1
Trent	40	11	13	3	8	2	3
East Anglia	19	7	5	1	2	2	2
North West Thames	23	1	4	9	6	2	1
North East Thames	28	1	5	9	10	3	0
South East Thames	29	3	5	13	5	3	0
South West Thames	19	2	1	8	8	0	0
Wessex	33	16	6	5	3	1	2
Oxford	23	8	6	1	5	0	3
South Western	39	18	10	5	1	2	3
West Midlands	37	5	11	4	8	4	5
Mersey	17	4	2	3	3	4	1
North Western	28	3	5	4	9	4	3
WALES	**40**	**19**	**5**	**9**	**6**	**1**	**0**
SCOTLAND	**82**	**45**	**12**	**12**	**6**	**3**	**4**
NORTHERN IRELAND	**33**	**8**	**14**	**7**	**2**	**2**	**0**
Numbers of total births occurring in maternity units							
ENGLAND	**607,879**	**8,438**	**41,684**	**127,191**	**198,984**	**108,696**	**122,886**
Regional Health Authorities★							
Northern	41,403	306	3,555	18,247	15,653	3,642	0
Yorkshire	47,112	823	3,700	7,586	16,350	14,071	4,582
Trent	55,922	1,036	6,965	4,593	20,113	7,340	15,875
East Anglia	24,372	671	2,481	1,526	4,010	7,049	8,635
North West Thames	40,443	81	1,937	13,162	14,755	6,263	4,245
North East Thames	52,874	187	2,682	14,489	25,344	10,172	0
South East Thames	45,342	203	3,222	20,825	11,462	9,630	0
South West Thames	33,197	255	652	13,392	18,898	0	0
Wessex	33,385	1,848	3,068	7,362	6,872	3,089	11,139
Oxford	32,551	553	2,015	1,161	13,000	0	15,822
South Western	36,488	1,501	3,440	8,225	2,268	6,503	14,551
West Midlands	72,510	648	4,762	6,510	20,657	13,483	26,450

★ Includes London postgraduate teaching hospitals

Table A7.2   Sizes of maternity units and numbers of births, Regional Health Authorities and constituent countries of the United Kingdom, 1980 - *continued*

Area	All units	Size of unit, number of births in 1980					
		Less than 200	200-999	1,000-1,999	2,000-2,999	3,000-3,999	4,000 and over
Numbers of total births occurring in maternity units							
England-continued							
Mersey	31,644	284	1,120	4,182	7,168	14,411	4,479
North Western	56,162	42	2,085	5,931	22,427	13,043	12,634
WALES	**35,741**	**1,256**	**3,056**	**13,755**	**14,230**	**3,444**	**0**
SCOTLAND	**67,700**	**2,992**	**4,054**	**17,583**	**15,243**	**10,605**	**7,223**
NORTHERN IRELAND	**28,682**	**815**	**7,043**	**9,428**	**4,795**	**6,601**	**0**
Percentage of total births in region							
ENGLAND		**1.4**	**6.9**	**20.9**	**32.7**	**17.9**	**20.2**
Regional Health Authorities*							
Northern		0.7	8.6	44.1	37.8	8.8	—
Yorkshire		1.7	7.9	16.1	34.7	29.9	9.7
Trent		1.9	12.5	8.2	36.0	13.1	28.4
East Anglia		2.8	10.2	6.3	16.5	28.9	35.4
North West Thames		0.2	4.8	32.6	36.5	15.5	10.5
North East Thames		0.4	5.1	27.4	47.9	19.2	—
South East Thames		0.4	7.1	45.9	25.3	21.2	—
South West Thames		0.8	2.0	40.3	56.9	—	—
Wessex		5.5	9.2	22.1	20.6	9.3	33.4
Oxford		1.7	6.2	3.6	39.9	—	48.6
South Western		4.1	9.4	22.5	6.2	17.8	39.9
West Midlands		0.9	6.6	9.0	28.5	18.6	36.5
Mersey		0.9	3.5	13.2	22.7	45.5	14.2
North Western		0.1	3.7	10.6	39.9	23.2	22.5
WALES		**3.5**	**8.6**	**38.5**	**39.8**	**9.6**	**—**
SCOTLAND		**4.4**	**6.0**	**25.9**	**22.5**	**15.7**	**25.4**
NORTHERN IRELAND		**2.8**	**24.6**	**32.9**	**16.7**	**23.0**	**—**

* *Includes London postgraduate teaching hospitals*
Source: Hospital Returns for England, DHSS SH3; for Wales, Welsh Office; for Scotland, ISD/CSA, SMR2; for Northern Ireland, DHSS Northern Ireland

Table A7.3   Available maternity beds, constituent countries of the United Kingdom, 1975-80

	1975	1976	1977	1978	1979	1980
Daily average number of available beds						
England						
Total	21,257	20,659	19,735	19,075	18,640	18,406
Obstetric	16,984	16,662	16,098	15,810	15,541	15,490
GP maternity	4,273	3,997	3,637	3,265	3,099	2,916
Wales						
Total	1,269	1,234	1,224	1,193	1,169	1,149
Obstetric	998	976	984	977	982	952
GP maternity	271	258	240	216	187	197
Scotland						
Total	3,035	2,979	2,874	2,776	2,750	2,689
Obstetric	2,361	2,348	2,272	2,201	2,226	2,218
GP maternity	674	631	602	575	524	471
Northern Ireland						
Total	977	958	932	953	909	917
Total beds per 1,000 maternities						
England	37.3	37.5	36.7	33.9	31.0	29.8
Wales	37.3	36.9	38.5	35.8	32.4	30.8
Scotland	44.6	45.9	46.1	43.2	40.3	39.1
Northern Ireland	38.0	36.7	36.5	36.2	32.5	32.4

Source: DHSS, Welsh Office, ISD/CSA, DHSS Northern Ireland (bed data)
OPCS, GRO Scotland and Northern Ireland (maternities)

Table A7.4 Available maternity beds, Regional Health Authorities, England, 1980

| Area | Beds for antenatal and postnatal care | | | | Beds used for labour and delivery only | | | | | |
| | Consultant obstetric | | GP maternity | | First stage | | Second stage | | Combined | |
	Number	Rate*	Number	Rate*	Number	Rate*	Number	Rate*	Number	Rate*
ENGLAND	**15,490**	**25.1**	**2,916**	**4.7**	**1,215**	**2.0**	**945**	**1.5**	**456**	**0.7**
Regional Health Authorities										
Northern	1,124	27.3	160	3.9	97	2.3	61	1.4	13	0.3
Yorkshire	1,285	27.0	247	5.2	97	2.0	79	1.7	25	0.5
Trent	1,385	23.0	362	6.0	141	2.3	108	1.8	55	0.9
East Anglia	601	24.4	131	5.3	52	2.1	35	1.4	20	0.8
North West Thames	1,255	26.5	32	0.7	70	1.5	58	1.2	55	1.2
North East Thames	1,448	28.2	134	2.6	103	2.0	94	1.8	39	0.8
South East Thames	1,249	27.4	93	2.0	108	2.4	67	1.5	35	0.8
South West Thames	921	26.2	113	3.2	126	3.6	57	1.6	12	0.3
Wessex	752	22.1	306	9.0	38	1.1	54	1.6	27	0.8
Oxford	648	19.7	231	7.0	26	0.8	17	0.5	66	2.0
South Western	758	19.4	364	9.3	55	1.4	47	1.2	17	0.4
West Midlands	1,553	21.8	455	6.4	141	2.0	119	1.7	41	0.6
Mersey	898	27.9	81	2.5	53	1.6	38	1.2	14	0.4
North Western	1,476	27.2	206	3.8	108	2.0	111	2.0	24	0.4
London postgraduate hospitals	137		0		0		0		12	

*Per 1,000 maternities to residents of region, including maternities in London postgraduate maternity hospitals

Source: DHSS, SH3 Hospital Return, OPCS

Table A7.5 Available cots in Special Care Baby Units, Regional Health Authorities and constituent countries of the United Kingdom, 1974-80

Area	1974	1975	1976	1977	1978	1979	1980
	Numbers						
ENGLAND*	**3,932**	**3,978**	**4,018**	**4,007**	**3,972**	**3,945**	**3,959**
Regional Health Authorities							
Northern	344	333	335	336	332	324	323
Yorkshire	330	336	339	339	341	344	337
Trent	347	349	360	358	349	345	334
East Anglia	155	154	140	140	140	140	141
North West Thames	288	287	300	309	323	319	324
North East Thames	348	362	369	365	342	331	349
South East Thames	268	294	303	286	289	291	286
South West Thames	209	214	213	225	212	211	216
Wessex	194	199	197	195	191	190	191
Oxford	211	210	216	202	194	194	194
South Western	190	190	207	207	207	207	207
West Midlands	405	406	407	405	431	438	446
Mersey	246	247	245	236	234	207	203
North Western	377	377	367	364	367	385	388
WALES	**234**	**232**	**235**	**239**	**237**	**237**	**237**
SCOTLAND†	..	..	**634**	**625**	**635**	**628**	**626**
NORTHERN IRELAND‡	**194**	**191**	**191**	**193**	**193**	**195**	**195**
	Cots per 1,000 live births						
ENGLAND*	**6.5**	**7.0**	**7.3**	**7.5**	**7.1**	**6.6**	**6.4**
Regional Health Authorities							
Northern	8.6	8.8	9.1	9.4	8.7	7.8	7.8
Yorkshire	7.0	7.5	7.9	8.2	7.8	7.4	7.1
Trent	5.9	6.3	6.7	6.8	6.4	5.9	5.5
East Anglia	6.5	6.8	6.4	6.5	6.3	5.9	5.7
North West Thames	6.4	6.7	7.2	7.4	7.4	6.8	6.8
North East Thames	7.0	7.7	8.0	8.1	7.3	6.7	6.8
South East Thames	6.1	7.0	7.4	7.2	6.9	6.6	6.3
South West Thames	6.2	6.7	6.9	7.3	6.5	6.1	6.1
Wessex	5.7	6.2	6.4	6.6	6.2	5.8	5.6
Oxford	6.9	7.3	7.5	7.2	6.6	6.1	5.9
South Western	4.9	5.3	6.0	6.1	5.8	5.5	5.3
West Midlands	5.8	6.2	6.5	6.6	6.8	6.4	6.3
Mersey	7.6	7.9	8.2	8.3	7.8	6.4	6.3
North Western	6.9	7.4	7.5	7.7	7.4	7.3	7.1

Table A7.5 Available cots in Special Care Baby Units, Regional Health Authorities and constituent countries of the United Kingdom, 1974-80 - *continued*

Area	1974	1975	1976	1977	1978	1979	1980
Cots per 1,000 live births							
WALES	6.5	6.8	7.0	7.5	7.1	6.6	6.3
SCOTLAND†	..	..	9.8	10.0	9.9	9.2	9.1
NORTHERN IRELAND‡	7.1	7.3	7.2	7.6	7.4	6.9	6.8
Cots per 1,000 live births weighing 2,500 g or less							
ENGLAND*	**101.0**	**109.2**	**113.5**	**114.6**	**107.2**	**96.8**	**93.2**
Regional Health Authorities							
Northern	131.2	146.5	149.2	149.0	134.8	127.6	119.7
Yorkshire	104.8	111.7	118.0	117.3	109.4	99.0	95.2
Trent	91.7	97.2	99.2	101.5	95.4	87.8	79.3
East Anglia	119.7	126.4	112.6	117.6	107.4	94.2	91.0
North West Thames	99.1	102.1	106.0	108.8	108.5	96.1	94.9
North East Thames	103.8	119.9	128.8	118.1	107.3	99.2	94.7
South East Thames	99.1	110.4	108.7	113.4	105.5	95.5	93.7
South West Thames	118.8	109.9	122.8	128.8	110.6	97.4	105.5
Wessex	83.5	93.7	103.6	110.2	97.2	84.7	86.2
Oxford	124.2	129.1	122.9	116.6	104.7	99.3	93.5
South Western	87.0	92.1	108.1	110.2	105.6	95.9	92.9
West Midlands	79.8	84.4	88.7	88.4	94.1	84.5	84.3
Mersey	110.9	134.0	157.3	163.3	136.1	105.3	91.8
North Western	97.7	109.5	105.5	103.7	101.1	97.5	91.2
WALES	**97.4**	**109.9**	**114.4**	**123.3**	**114.1**	**104.0**	**103.5**
SCOTLAND†	..	..	..	..	..	..	..
NORTHERN IRELAND‡	..	..	..	..	..	..	..

* *Including London postgraduate hospitals*
† *Calculated for year ending 30 September and includes 'borrowed', 'lent' and temporary beds*
‡ *Beds for 'sick babies including premature'*
Source: *Health and Personal Social Services Statistics for England*
Health and Personal Social Services Statistics for Wales
Scottish Health Statistics
Health and Personal Social Services Statistics for Northern Ireland

Table A7.6   Combined special and intensive care units for neonatal care, Regional Health Authorities, March 1980

Area	Status of units*					All units
	A	B	B+C	C	D	
	Number of units					
Regional Health Authorities						
Northern		2				2
Yorkshire					1	1†
Trent	2		1			3
East Anglia	1					1
North West Thames			1		5	6
North East Thames	2					2
South East Thames	1				4	5
South West Thames				1‡	3	4
Wessex					1	1
Oxford	1					1
South Western					6	6
West Midlands		2		2		4
Mersey	1				2	3
North Western	1				1	2
London postgraduate hospital		1				1†
	Total cots					
Regional Health Authorities						
Northern		45				45
Yorkshire					35	35†
Trent	64		26			90
East Anglia	24					24
North West Thames			20		87	107
North East Thames	30					30
South East Thames	20				82	102
South West Thames				10‡	63	73
Wessex					20	20
Oxford	34					34
South Western					163	163
West Midlands		68		55		123

Table A7.6 Combined special and intensive care units for neonatal care, Regional Health Authorities, March 1980 - *continued*

Area	Status of units*					All units
	A	B	B+C	C	D	
Total cots						
Regional Health Authorities - continued						
Mersey	24				28	52
North Western	30				21	51
London postgraduate hospital		20				20†
Maximum number of intensive care cots available at any one time						
Regional Health Authorities						
Northern		5				5
Yorkshire					6	6†
Trent	10		5			15
East Anglia	4					4
North West Thames			4		17	21
North East Thames	11-13					11-13
South East Thames	4				12	16
South West Thames				2†	10	12
Wessex					4	4
Oxford	6					6
South Western					29	29
West Midlands		7		9		16
Mersey	4				10	14
North Western	10				2	12
London postgraduate hospitals		2-5				2-5

The combined special and intensive care units included are those which accept referrals of mother with high-risk pregnancies and are able to provide intensive care for their new born babies as required.

* *A denotes officially designated functioning Regional Units*
  B denotes units which are recognised as having a regional commitment but are not officially designated
  C denotes units which are being developed with a view to designation in due course.
  D denotes units which provide a local service

† *The Hospitals for Sick Children (London) and Leeds General Infirmary provide surgery and paediatric intensive care according to demand, and so a figure for available cots is variable.*

‡ *New unit opened February 1980 in South West Thames RHA.*

Source: Second Report from the Social Services Committee 1979-80 *Perinatal and Neonatal Mortality. Vol 5: 96-97*
    Hansard 2 July 1982

Table A7.7   Nurseries, child minders and mother and baby homes, England 1977-80

	1977	1978	1979	1980
Mother and baby homes*				
Number of beds	511	492	..	..
Number of women admitted	1,858	1,475	..	..
Day nurseries maintained by local authorities or by voluntary bodies under agency arrangements†				
Premises	582	592	609	613
Places	22,385	27,677	28,313	28,437
Children on register	28,919	28,885	28,858	29,928
Part-time nursery groups maintained by local authorities or by voluntary bodies under agency arrangements†				
Premises	100	138	129	112
Places	2,549	3,532	3,325	2,865
Children on register	2,473	2,507	5,256	2,455
Registered nurseries†				
Premises: all day care	875	853	804	806
sessional care	14,836	14,466	14,425	14,814
Places: all day care	24,916	23,498	22,381	22,017
sessional care	365,759	357,950	362,279	365,003
Registered child minders†				
Child minders: all day care	30,939	28,100	30,358	31,851
sessional care	2,574	9,627	12,060	11,113
Places: all day care	69,153	62,168	67,438	70,165
sessional care	17,553	32,392	36,525	37,066
Children receiving nursery education (at January)◊				
Full-time Thousands	285	258	268	266
Part-time Thousands	179	189	194	197

* Homes and hostels for unmarried mothers and their babies. Data not collected after 1978.
  Data about nursery facilities was collected in different format from 1978 onwards. This may affect comparability.

† Part-time nursery groups maintained by local authorities or by voluntary bodies under agency arrangements fall under section 22 of the National Health Services Act 1946. Registered nurseries and registered child minders are covered by the Nurseries and Child Minders Regulation Act 1948 (amended in Health Services and Public Health Act 1968).

◊ Nursery education includes children under 5 in maintained and non-maintained schools.

Source: DHSS Health and Personal Social Services Statistics 1982

Table A7.8   Qualified midwives and pupil midwives employed by Regional Health Authorities, 1975-80

Area	Number of whole time equivalent* staff in post on 30 September					
	1975	1976	1977	1978	1979	1980
England†						
Qualified	**14,335**	**14,940**	**15,183**	**14,774**	**15,382**	**15,705**
Hospital	**11,380**	**12,115**	**12,142**	**11,984**	**12,398**	**12,932**
Community‡	**2,955**	**2,825**	**3,041**	**2,790**	**2,984**	**2,773**
Pupils	**4,244**	**4,482**	**4,738**	**5,116**	**4,640**	**4,231**
Regional Health Authorities						
Northern						
Qualified	989	976	975	979	1,064	1,004
Hospital	748	786	789	836	869	848
Community‡	241	190	186	143	195	156
Pupils	254	280	273	227	286	285
Yorkshire						
Qualified	1,022	1,015	1,096	1,106	1,144	1,185
Hospital	828	850	885	913	947	1,006
Community‡	194	165	211	193	197	179
Pupils	301	332	333	339	320	299
Trent						
Qualified	1,435	1,407	1,373	1,294	1,457	1,520
Hospital	1,134	1,117	1,033	966	1,133	1,167
Community‡	301	290	340	328	324	353
Pupils	346	255	339	358	358	353
East Anglian						
Qualified	574	623	574	572	654	617
Hospital	378	478	406	430	474	461
Community‡	196	145	168	142	180	156
Pupils	163	146	208	303	264	178
North West Thames						
Qualified	1,028	1,030	1,060	1,059	1,089	1,097
Hospital	893	909	931	951	968	984
Community‡	135	121	129	108	121	113
Pupils	452	363	396	377	372	335
North East Thames						
Qualified	1,185	1,347	1,405	1,201	1,233	1,241
Hospital	1,010	1,171	1,182	1,050	1,010	1,067
Community‡	175	176	223	151	223	174
Pupils	417	416	421	707	503	371

* *Whole time equivalent is calculated by dividing the total number of contract hours by the number of full time-hours. Because full-time hours changed from 40 to 37.5 during 1980, the numbers of whole time equivalent part-time staff are artificially inflated for 1980. The numbers for 1980 may also overstate whole time equivalent staff because the 37.5 hour working week was not mandatory for midwives and nurses before 31 March 1981.*

† *Includes London postgraduate teaching hospitals.*

‡ *Community midwives are those employed solely in the district, excluding hospital midwives who also work in the district, and community nurses holding joint health visitor/district nurse/midwife posts.*

Table A7.8   Qualified midwives and pupil midwives employed by Regional Health Authorities, 1975-80 - *continued*

Regional Health Authority	Number of whole time equivalent* staff in post on 30 September					
	1975	1976	1977	1978	1979	1980
England† - continued						
South East Thames						
Qualified	1,140	1,208	1,196	1,154	1,180	1,264
Hospital	911	1,008	1,003	952	1,023	1,034
Community‡	229	200	193	202	157	230
Pupils	443	357	439	433	335	316
South West Thames						
Qualified	779	887	801	808	772	869
Hospital	724	814	751	758	722	752
Community‡	55	73	50	50	50	117
Pupils	226	217	203	225	280	249
Wessex						
Qualified	849	733	810	786	876	806
Hospital	668	528	620	591	651	674
Community‡	181	205	190	195	225	132
Pupils	146	178	340	290	227	277
Oxford						
Qualified	698	754	752	770	780	820
Hospital	652	670	647	675	678	678
Community‡	46	84	105	95	102	142
Pupil	205	178	133	212	211	184
South Western						
Qualified	870	907	937	981	998	880
Hospital	632	683	703	736	762	804
Community‡	238	224	234	245	236	76
Pupils	226	277	313	349	350	290
West Midlands						
Qualified	1,508	1,633	1,700	1,663	1,618	1,663
Hospital	1,016	1,171	1,202	1,210	1,218	1,287
Community‡	492	462	498	453	400	376
Pupils	425	668	517	499	420	370

Table A7.8   Qualified midwives and pupil midwives employed by Regional Health Authorities, 1975-80 - *continued*

Area	Number of whole time equivalent* staff in post on 30 September					
	1975	1976	1977	1978	1979	1980
England† - continued						
Mersey						
Qualified	702	860	844	807	875	921
Hospital	524	700	699	676	688	728
Community‡	178	160	145	131	187	193
Pupils	184	280	311	254	247	172
North Western						
Qualified	1,477	1,459	1,543	1,495	1,531	1,702
Hospital	1,182	1,129	1,171	1,141	1,142	1,327
Community‡	295	330	372	354	389	375
Pupils	414	484	470	499	422	500
Wales						
Qualified	**972**	**849**	**875**	**907**	**939**	**942**
Hospital	**681**	**743**	**775**	**723**	**746**	**748**
Community‡	**291**	**106**	**100**	**184**	**193**	**194**
Pupils	**181**	**171**	**218**	**214**	**203**	**205**

* *Whole time equivalent is calculated by dividing the total number of contract hours by the number of full time-hours. Because full-time hours changed from 40 to 37.5 during 1980, the numbers of whole time equivalent part-time staff are artificially inflated for 1980. The numbers for 1980 may also overstate whole time equivalent staff because the 37.5 hour working week was not mandatory for midwives and nurses before 31 March 1981.*

† *Includes London postgraduate teaching hospitals.*

‡ *Community midwives are those employed solely in the district, excluding hospital midwives who also work in the district, and community nurses holding joint health visitor/district nurse/midwife posts.*

Source: DHSS

Table A7.9   Qualified midwives (per 1,000 maternities) employed by Regional Health Authorities, 1975-80

Area	Qualified midwives per 1,000 maternities					
	1975	1976	1977	1978	1979	1980
England*	**25.2**	**27.1**	**28.3**	**26.3**	**25.6**	**25.4**
Regional Health Authorities						
Northern	26.0	26.4	27.1	25.6	25.5	24.4
Yorkshire	22.9	23.7	26.6	25.4	24.7	24.9
Trent	25.7	26.1	26.3	23.8	25.2	25.2
East Anglia	25.4	28.3	26.8	26.0	27.6	25.0
North West Thames	24.2	24.7	25.4	24.2	23.3	23.2
North East Thames	25.1	29.3	31.4	25.8	24.9	24.1
South East Thames	27.1	27.9	30.0	27.8	26.6	27.8
South West Thames	24.4	25.3	26.1	24.9	22.3	24.7
Wessex	26.5	27.5	27.3	25.6	26.7	23.7
Oxford	24.1	26.4	26.7	26.2	24.7	24.9
South Western	24.3	25.1	27.4	27.7	26.5	22.5
West Midlands	23.0	24.0	27.9	26.1	23.7	23.4
Mersey	22.4	23.5	29.7	27.0	27.2	28.6
North Western	29.1	29.9	32.6	30.2	28.8	31.3
Wales	**28.6**	**25.4**	**27.5**	**27.2**	**26.0**	**25.3**

Includes London postgraduate teaching hospitals
Source: DHSS

Table A7.10 Midwives employed in Scotland 1975-81

Grade	Number of whole time equivalent* staff in post on 30 September						
	1975	1976	1977	1978	1979	1980	1981
Hospital							
Total	1,839	1,980	1,944	1,830	1,852.6	1,930.3	2,049.9
Divisional nursing officer					9.0	9.0	10.0
Senior nursing officer	220	211	211	200	37.0	34.0	31.0
Nursing officer					138.0	137.9	136.7
Midwifery sister	712	720	715	683	701.7	718.3	742.2
Staff midwife	907	1,049	1,018	947	966.9	1,031.1	1,130.0
Community							
Total	998	916	888	934	899.1	859.0	840.5
Midwife	123	75	92	98	117.0	123.5	142.8
Triple duty	332	236	210	182	156.3	101.0	105.3
HV/Midwife	7	32	24	19	9.3	9.0	7.0
DN/Midwife	536	573	562	635	616.5	625.5	585.4
Teaching							
Total	45	48	53	56	57.1	49.7	48.4
Teacher	45	48	53	56	42.1	37.7	37.9
Clinical instructor					15.0	12.0	10.5
Student midwife	1,278	1,263	1,106	1,080	1,075.8	1,088.0	1,128.0
All grades	**4,160**	**4,207**	**3,991**	**3,900**	**3,884.6**	**3,927.0**	**4,066.8**
All midwives per 1,000 maternitics	61.1	64.8	64.1	60.7	57.0	57.2	59.1

Conditioned hours for nurses and midwives were reduced in the year ending March 1981 from 40.00 hours/week to 37.50 hours/week. In this table, whole time equivalent (wte) for 1975 to 1979 is calculated on a 40.00 hours/week base, and for 1980 and 1981 on a 37.50 hours/week base. This has the effect of increasing the whole time equivalent (wte) of part time staff by 6.7%

Source: Information Services Division.

Table A7.11 Midwives employed in Northern Ireland, 1978-80

	Numbers and whole time equivalent (wte)					
	1978		1979		1980	
	Number	wte	Number	wte	Number	wte
Total	1,460	1,304.4	1,535	1,359	1,558	1,363.5
Hospital	893	742	946	774	1,030	839
Community only	363	359.4	372	368.4	377	373.5
Pupils	204	203	217	217	151	151

	Midwives (wte) per 1,000 deliveries		
	1978	1979	1980
Total	49.6	48.5	48.1
Qualified midwives	41.9	40.8	42.8

	Nursing staff in hospital maternity departments in 1980		
	Number	wte	Per 1,000 deliveries
All grades	1,457	1,201.02	45.6

Source: DHSS Northern Ireland

Table A7.12   Nurses employed in hospital maternity departments, Regional Health Authorities, England and Wales, 1975-80

Area	Numbers of whole time equivalent* staff in post on 30 September					
	1975	1976	1977	1978	1979	1980
England						
All grades	**9,045**	**8,707**	**8,521**	**8,409**	**8,958**	**9,004**
SRN	**1,192**	**1,248**	**1,086**	**1,006**	**1,118**	**1,288**
SEN	**1,470**	**1,570**	**1,640**	**1,597**	**1,664**	**1,696**
Regional Health Authorities						
Northern						
All grades	688	646	668	642	581	607
SRN	81	83	84	58	64	..
SEN	134	160	161	159	145	..
Yorkshire						
All grades	805	827	780	765	790	336
SRN	126	111	92	76	76	..
SEN	166	174	169	161	163	..
Trent						
All grades	944	869	789	794	860	1,064
SRN	89	123	72	64	86	..
SEN	210	217	215	220	219	..
East Anglia						
All grades	336	453	417	365	329	374
SRN	36	133	111	84	47	..
SEN	45	51	44	40	45	..
North West Thames						
All grades	545	506	527	667	670	391
SRN	70	63	58	94	91	..
SEN	97	118	126	143	143	..
North East Thames						
All grades	827	900	841	521	566	714
SRN	77	167	163	74	95	..
SEN	152	135	151	103	103	..
South East Thames						
All grades	684	755	602	589	624	672
SRN	115	136	97	80	77	..
SEN	74	91	105	104	94	..
South West Thames						
All grades	389	470	462	419	461	443
SRN	46	59	55	48	78	..
SEN	51	63	58	59	71	..
Wessex						
All grades	440	462	430	461	493	497
SRN	52	74	56	74	67	..
SEN	54	56	50	52	54	..
Oxford						
All grades	538	498	431	342	479	548
SRN	88	84	91	66	101	..
SEN	62	75	68	62	63	..

The basis for calculation of whole time equivalent changed from 1980; see footnote to Table A7.8

* Excludes auxiliary staff

213

Table A7.12 Nurses employed in hospital maternity departments, Regional Health Authorities, England and Wales, 1975-80 - *continued*

Area	Numbers of whole time equivalent* staff in post on 30 September					
	1975	1976	1977	1978	1979	1980
Regional Health Authorities - continued						
South Western						
All grades	499	465	570	567	517	553
SRN	58	58	78	84	78	..
SEN	68	87	102	105	88	..
West Midlands						
All grades	932	476	680	973	1,057	1,157
SRN	104	9	0	66	87	..
SEN	132	78	109	114	128	..
Mersey						
All grades	538	519	502	524	524	578
SRN	172	62	56	61	54	..
SEN	102	128	136	150	145	..
North Western						
All grades	809	771	757	705	934	936
SRN	77	82	68	66	112	..
SEN	112	122	128	112	179	..
Wales						
All grades†	**151**	**306**	**299**	**286**	**300**	**318**
SRN	**48**	**100**	**89**	**77**	**87**	**92**
SEN	**103**	**206**	**210**	**209**	**213**	**226**

* *The basis for calculation of whole time equivalent changed from 1980; see footnote to Table A7.8*
† *Excludes auxiliary staff*
Sources: DHSS, Welsh Office

Table A7.13 Nurses (per 1,000 maternities) employed in hospital maternity departments, Regional Health Authorities, England and Wales, 1975-80

Area	Nurses per 1,000 maternities					
	1975	1976	1977	1978	1979	1980
England						
All grades	**15.9**	**15.8**	**15.9**	**15.0**	**14.9**	**14.6**
SRN and SEN	**4.7**	**5.1**	**5.1**	**4.6**	**4.6**	**4.8**
Northern						
All grades	18.1	17.5	18.6	16.8	14.0	14.8
SRN and SEN	5.6	6.6	6.8	5.7	5.0	..
Yorkshire						
All grades	18.0	19.3	18.9	17.6	17.1	7.0
SRN and SEN	6.5	6.7	6.3	5.4	5.2	..
Trent						
All grades	17.0	16.1	15.1	14.6	14.9	17.7
SRN and SEN	5.4	6.3	5.5	5.2	5.3	..
East Anglia						
All grades	14.9	20.6	19.5	16.6	13.9	15.2
SRN and SEN	3.6	8.4	7.2	5.6	3.9	..
North West Thames						
All grades	12.8	12.1	12.6	15.2	14.4	8.3
SRN and SEN	3.9	4.3	4.4	5.4	5.0	..
North East Thames						
All grades	17.5	19.6	18.8	11.2	11.4	13.9
SRN and SEN	4.9	6.6	7.0	3.8	4.0	..
South East Thames						
All grades	16.3	18.5	15.1	14.1	14.1	14.8
SRN and SEN	4.5	5.6	5.1	4.4	3.9	..
South West Thames						
All grades	12.2	15.3	15.1	12.9	13.3	12.6
SRN and SEN	3.0	4.0	3.7	3.3	4.3	..
Wessex						
All grades	13.7	15.0	14.5	15.0	15.0	14.6
SRN and SEN	3.3	4.2	3.6	4.1	3.7	..
Oxford						
All grades	18.6	17.4	15.3	11.6	15.1	16.7
SRN and SEN	5.2	5.6	5.6	4.3	5.2	..
South Western						
All grades	14.0	13.4	16.7	16.0	13.7	14.2
SRN and SEN	3.5	4.2	5.3	5.3	4.4	..
West Midlands						
All grades	14.2	7.6	11.1	15.2	15.5	16.3
SRN and SEN	3.6	1.4	1.8	2.8	3.2	..
Mersey						
All grades	17.2	17.4	17.6	17.5	16.3	18.0
SRN and SEN	8.8	6.4	6.7	7.1	6.2	..
North Western						
All grades	15.9	15.8	16.0	14.3	17.6	17.2
SRN and SEN	3.7	4.2	4.1	3.6	5.5	..
Wales						
All grades	..	..	..	..	..	..
SRN and SEN	**4.4**	**9.2**	**9.4**	**8.6**	**8.3**	**8.5**

Sources: DHSS, Welsh Office, OPCS

215

Table A7.14   Nurses in maternity units, Scotland, 1975-81

Grade	Number of whole time equivalent* staff in post on 30 September						
	1975	1976	1977	1978	1979	1980	1981
Qualified							
Total	313	323	263	286	282.5	307.2	334.9
Staff Nurse (not SCM)	144	144	119	151	132.2	141.9	141.6
Senior Enrolled Nurse	6	7	4	2	1.0	3.0	3.0
Enrolled Nurse	163	172	140	133	149.3	162.3	190.3
Unqualified							
Total	1,316	1,224	1,184	1,057	1,107.3	1,217.9	1,246.7
Nursing Auxiliary	1,151	1,086	1,032	941	974.8	1,011.5	1,032.0
Nursery Nurse	165	138	152	116	132.5	206.4	214.7
All grades	**1,629**	**1,547**	**1,447**	**1,343**	**1,389.8**	**1,525.1**	**1,581.6**
Per 1,000 maternities	23.9	23.8	23.2	20.9	20.4	22.2	23.0

* *Conditioned hours for nurses and midwives were reduced in the year ending March 1981 from 40.00 hours/week to 37.50 hours/week. In this table, whole time equivalent (wte) for 1975 to 1979 is calculated on a 40.00 hours/week base, and for 1980 and 1981 on a 37.50 hours/week base. This has the effect of increasing the whole time equivalent (wte) of part time staff by 6.7%.*

Source: ISD

Table A7.15 Health visitors*, Regional Health Authorities, England and Wales, 1976-80

Area	Numbers of whole time equivalent staff in post on 30 September					Per 10,000 population				
	1976	1977	1978	1979	1980†	1976	1977	1978	1979	1980
England	**8,059**	**8,477**	**8,674**	**9,010**	**8,797**	**1.7**	**1.8**	**1.9**	**1.9**	**1.9**
Regional Health Authorities										
Northern	532	562	551	559	575	1.7	1.8	1.8	1.8	1.9
Yorkshire	590	639	643	672	709	1.7	1.8	1.8	1.9	2.0
Trent	688	748	765	775	748	1.5	1.6	1.7	1.7	1.6
East Anglia	277	291	293	311	302	1.5	1.6	1.6	1.7	1.6
North West Thames	612	659	666	685	718	1.8	1.9	1.9	2.0	2.1
North East Thames	553	569	574	595	537	1.5	1.5	1.6	1.6	1.5
South East Thames	653	670	686	710	656	1.8	1.9	1.9	2.0	1.8
South West Thames	601	625	633	673	661	2.1	2.3	2.2	2.4	2.3
Wessex	487	511	497	525	477	1.8	1.9	1.9	2.0	1.8
Oxford	522	505	510	526	518	2.4	2.3	2.3	2.3	2.2
South Western	519	548	576	594	587	1.6	1.7	1.8	1.9	1.8
West Midlands	849	883	935	981	935	1.6	1.7	1.8	1.9	1.8
Mersey	411	428	470	487	484	1.7	1.7	1.9	2.0	2.0
North Western	755	840	876	915	890	1.9	2.1	2.2	2.3	2.2
Wales	**512**	**524**	**528**	**529**	**..**	**1.9**	**1.9**	**1.9**	**1.9**	**..**

* Includes school health staff and TB visitors with health visiting certificate, but excludes students, tutorial staff and health visitors holding dual or triple posts

† Statistics compiled from payroll data

Source: DHSS

217

Table A7.16   Hospital medical staff* in obstetric and paediatric specialties, constituent countries of the United Kingdom, 1975-81

Numbers in post at 30 September and whole time equivalent

	1975		1976		1977		1978		1979		1980		1981	
	Number	wte	Number	wte	Number	wte	Number	wte	Number	wte	Number	wte	Number	wte
England‡														
Obstetrics and gynaecology	2,349	2,168.1	2,348	2,175.9	2,374	2,195.3	2,396	2,216.6	2,422	2,243.6	2,460	2,312.9	2,507	2,359.1
Paediatrics†	1,394	1,246.1	1,464	1,313.6	1,506	1,336.4	1,552	1,390.1	1,653	1,484.7	1,736	1,568.5	1,872	1,690.0
Paediatric surgery	92	77.9	104	92.6	129	117.6	126	114.1	143	129.1	124	112.0	114	106.3
Wales														
Obstetrics and gynaecology	134	130.6	133	130.1	142	137.8	148	144.8	147	143.6	146	143.0	151	147.2
Paediatrics†	87	82.7	90	84.3	94	89.1	102	96.3	103	98.2	108	103.2	112	106.3
Paediatric surgery	4	3.1	3	2.1	4	3.1	5	4.1	6	4.1	5	5.1	6	5.0
Scotland														
Obstetrics and gynaecology	376	353.9	402	381.3	392	374.5	392	374.4	402	383.5	413	391.5	417	399.4
Medical paediatrics	185	172.1	197	181.5	193	179.7	206	194.4	220	209.0	221	207.2	212	200.7
Surgical paediatrics	40	38.2	40	39.5	37	36.1	38	37.1	40	38.7	40	38.9	38	36.9
Northern Ireland														
Obstetrics and gynaecology	..	..	114	106.5	123	115.6	136	127.9	124	117.2	129	121.5	131	125.1
Paediatrics	..	..	46	42.6	48	45.0	52	49.5	50	47.5	56	51.7	59	54.2
Paediatric surgery	..	..	7	6.8	12	12.0	13	13.0	11	11.0	11	11.0	11	11.0

* *Numbers and whole time equivalents exclude appointments under paragraph 94 of the terms and conditions of employment, and hospital practitioners—usually part-time appointments given to general practitioners who also do their work in hospitals*

† *Numbers of staff and whole time equivalents in paediatrics include staff in paediatric neurology, which from 1981 is classified as a separate specialty*

‡ *Staff who hold appointments in more than one region may be counted more than once*

Source: DHSS, ISD, DHSS Northern Ireland

218

Table A7.17 Rates of hospital medical staff in obstetric and paediatric specialties, constituent countries of the United Kingdom, 1975-80

	1975	1976	1977	1978	1979	1980
Staff in all grades (wte) per 1,000 maternities						
Obstetrics and gynaecology						
England	3.81	3.95	4.09	3.95	3.74	3.75
Wales	3.84	3.89	4.34	4.35	3.98	3.84
Scotland	5.20	5.87	6.01	5.83	5.62	5.70
Northern Ireland	..	4.08	4.53	4.86	4.19	4.29
Staff in all grades (wte) per 1,000 live births						
Paediatrics and paediatric neurology						
England	2.19	2.39	2.49	2.47	2.47	2.54
Wales	2.43	2.53	2.80	2.89	2.71	2.76
Scotland	2.53	2.80	2.88	3.02	3.06	3.01
Northern Ireland	..	1.62	1.77	1.89	1.69	1.81
Staff in all grades (wte) per 10,000 live births						
Paediatric surgery						
England	1.37	1.68	2.19	2.03	2.15	1.81
Wales	0.91	0.63	0.98	1.23	1.41	1.10
Scotland	5.62	6.09	5.79	5.77	5.66	5.65
Northern Ireland	..	2.58	4.72	4.95	3.90	3.85

Sources: DHSS, ISD, DHSS Northern Ireland

Table A7.18 Hospital medical staff by grade, Regional Health Authorities and constituent countries of the United Kingdom, 1980

(a) Obstetrics and gynaecology

Area	All grades*			Consultant†			Associate specialist		Senior registrar	
	Number	wte	wte per 1,000 maternities	Number	wte	wte per 1,000 maternities	Number	wte	Number	wte
England◊	2,460	2,312.9	3.8	699	612.4	1.0	38	28.3	122	100.5
RHAs										
Northern	199	189.4	4.6	58	53.8	1.3	5	2.5	7	5.0
Yorkshire	177	169.6	3.6	50	45.8	1.0	1	1.0	8	4.8
Trent	214	196.6	3.3	56	47.5	0.8	0	—	11	10.2
East Anglia	91	88.2	3.6	27	26.1	1.1	3	1.9	4	3.2
North West Thames	238	211.0	4.5	67	50.2	1.1	4	2.4	15	12.9
North East Thames	231	212.9	4.1	71	56.1	1.1	4	2.2	8	7.5
South East Thames	187	177.0	3.9	53	45.8	1.0	0	—	12	11.7
South West Thames	152	145.1	4.1	44	39.6	1.1	4	2.9	5	4.6
Wessex	111	106.1	3.1	36	32.7	1.0	1	1.0	10	8.4
Oxford	118	103.3	3.1	30	26.2	0.8	1	1.0	10	4.6
South Western	138	127.7	3.3	39	34.1	0.9	4	3.7	7	4.9
West Midlands	230	226.5	3.2	60	58.5	0.8	3	1.7	9	8.2
Mersey	126	123.6	3.8	36	33.6	1.0	3	3.0	3	3.0
North Western	223	217.7	4.0	61	57.6	1.1	5	5.0	9	8.0
London post-graduate teaching hospitals	25	18.2	—	11	4.7	—	0	—	4	3.5
Wales	**146**	**143.0**	**3.9**	**42**	**39.7**	**1.1**	**2**	**1.8**	**6**	**5.5**
Scotland	**413**	**391.5**	**5.7**	**120**	**108.3**	**1.6**	**6**	**5.5**	**29**	**23.9**
Northern Ireland	**129**	**121.5**	**4.3**	**38**	**32.0**	**1.2**	**0**	**—**	**7**	**6.0**

* *Except hospital practitioners and paragraph 94 appointments. Paragraph 94 appointments are those (mainly general practitioners) working in hospital as part-time medical officers.*

† *'Consultant' also includes senior hospital medical officers (SHMO). Associate specialists were formally known as medical assistants.*

‡ *'House Officer' includes senior house officer (SHO), house officer, post-registration, and house officer pre-registration.*

◊ *Duplication may occur where staff hold multiple appointments in more than one region.*

Registrar		House officers‡		Other		Hospital practitioner		Paragraph 94 appointments		Area
Number	wte	Number	wte	Number	wte	Number	wte	Number	wte	
419	**404.7**	**1,174**	**1,166.7**	**8**	**0.3**	**53**	**13.1**	**566**	**104.3**	**England**◊
										RHAs
32	31.1	97	97.0	0	—	3	0.4	29	5.2	Northern
23	23.0	95	95.0	0	—	3	1.1	48	12.0	Yorkshire
31	30.6	108	108.0	8	0.3	2	0.5	41	7.2	Trent
12	12.0	45	45.0	0	—	0	—	43	7.6	East Anglia
50	47.5	102	98.1	0	—	10	2.6	35	6.4	North West Thames
43	42.1	105	105.0	0	—	2	0.6	56	10.5	North East Thames
29	26.5	93	93.0	0	—	1	0.2	37	8.3	South East Thames
32	31.0	67	67.0	0	—	6	1.0	17	4.1	South West Thames
21	21.0	43	43.0	0	—	4	0.6	29	3.8	Wessex
22	18.7	55	52.8	0	—	7	2.3	37	7.0	Oxford
21	18.7	67	66.2	0	—	1	0.3	42	7.9	South Western
42	42.0	116	116.0	0	—	12	3.2	70	12.5	West Midlands
26	26.0	58	58.0	0	—	1	0.2	6	0.7	Mersey
35	34.5	113	112.6	0	—	0	—	65	9.4	North Western
0	—	10	10.0	0	—	1	0.0	11	1.7	London post-graduate teaching hospitals
30	**30.0**	**66**	**66.0**	**0**	**—**	**2**	**0.6**	**30**	**6.4**	**Wales**
99	**95.5**	**159**	**158.3**	**0**	**—**	..	..	..	..	**Scotland**
20	**20.0**	**62**	**61.5**	**0**	**—**	..	..	..	..	**Northern Ireland**

Table A7.18   Hospital medical staff by grade, Regional Health Authorities and constituent countries of the United Kingdom, 1980 – *continued*

(b) Paediatrics and paediatric neurology

Area	All grades*			Consultant†			Associate specialist		Senior registrar	
	Number	wte	wte per 1,000 live births	Number	wte	wte per 1,000 live births	Number	wte	Number	wte
England✦	**1,736**	**1,568.5**	**2.5**	**530**	**441.1**	**0.7**	**25**	**16.2**	**131**	**97.9**
RHAs										
Northern	126	114.0	2.8	41	36.1	0.9	1	1.0	7	4.4
Yorkshire	113	107.5	2.3	38	35.9	0.8	0	—	7	4.3
Trent	166	153.8	2.6	44	38.9	0.7	0	—	10	8.8
East Anglia	49	45.3	1.8	17	16.1	0.7	2	1.5	4	3.1
North West Thames	145	125.7	2.6	42	30.0	0.6	2	1.8	8	6.5
North East Thames	131	111.9	2.2	36	26.2	0.5	0	—	11	6.0
South East Thames	141	132.6	2.9	43	36.7	0.8	2	1.8	12	10.8
South West Thames	87	77.0	2.2	30	22.4	0.6	3	1.9	3	3.0
Wessex	67	62.4	1.8	24	21.1	0.6	2	1.5	4	3.6
Oxford	93	80.9	2.5	25	21.2	0.6	3	1.2	10	6.4
South Western	99	91.4	2.3	23	21.2	0.5	3	1.5	9	6.7
West Midlands	175	169.4	2.4	52	50.4	0.7	2	1.1	11	9.4
Mersey	98	91.9	2.9	28	22.2	0.7	1	1.0	3	3.0
North Western	146	137.9	2.5	48	44.6	0.8	1	1.0	9	6.7
London post-graduate teaching hospitals	100	66.9	—	39	18.2	—	3	0.9	23	15.2
Wales	**108**	**103.2**	**2.8**	**29**	**26.7**	**0.7**	**5**	**4.6**	**6**	**5.2**
Scotland	**221**	**207.2**	**3.0**	**69**	**63.6**	**0.9**	**0**	**—**	**20**	**16.4**
Northern Ireland	**56**	**51.7**	**1.8**	**17**	**13.7**	**0.5**	**0**	**—**	**3**	**2.5**

* *Except hospital practitioners and paragraph 94 appointments. Paragraph 94 appointments are those (mainly general practitioners) working in hospital as part-time medical officers.*

† *'Consultant' also includes senior hospital medical officers (SHMO). Associate specialists were formally known as medical assistants.*

‡ *'House Officer' includes senior house officer (SHO), house officer, post-registration, and house officer pre-registration.*

✦ *Duplication may occur where staff hold multiple appointments in more than one region.*

Registrar		House officers‡		Other		Hospital practitioner		Paragraph 94 appointments		Area
Number	wte	Number	wte	Number	wte	Number	wte	Number	wte	
234	208.9	811	811.0	5	0.5	28	6.4	171	34.9	**England**◊
										RHAs
22	18.0	55	54.5	0	—	2	0.5	7	1.5	Northern
8	8.0	60	59.3	0	—	2	0.5	16	5.1	Yorkshire
23	21.6	84	84.0	5	0.5	1	0.3	8	1.3	Trent
7	5.6	19	19.0	0	—	2	0.5	5	0.7	East Anglia
29	25.0	64	62.4	0	—	5	1.2	9	0.8	North West Thames
17	13.6	67	66.1	0	—	2	0.2	15	2.7	North East Thames
12	11.2	72	72.0	0	—	4	0.8	19	4.6	South East Thames
13	12.2	38	37.5	0	—	0	—	7	1.7	South West Thames
7	7.0	30	29.3	0	—	0	—	5	0.4	Wessex
15	12.8	40	39.3	0	—	5	0.8	25	4.0	Oxford
13	12.0	51	50.1	0	—	0	—	19	4.5	South Western
21	19.5	89	89.0	0	—	2	0.7	13	2.8	West Midlands
16	15.7	50	50.0	0	—	3	0.8	5	1.1	Mersey
18	16.1	70	69.5	0	—	0	—	17	3.5	North Western
										London post-graduate teaching hospitals
13	10.6	22	22.0	0	—	0	—	1	0.2	
9	9.0	58	57.5	1	0.2	0	—	10	3.7	**Wales**
63	60.0	69	67.2	0	—	..	..	..	..	**Scotland**
6	6.0	29	29	0	—	..	..	..	..	**Northern Ireland**

Table A7.18 Hospital medical staff by grade, Regional Health Authorities and constituent countries of the United Kingdom, 1980 – *continued*

(c) Paediatric surgery

Area	All grades*			Consultant†			Associate specialist		Senior registrar	
	Number	wte	wte per 10,000 live births	Number	wte	wte per 10,000 live births	Number	wte	Number	wte
England◊	124	112.0	1.8	47	35.9	0.6	0	—	6	6.0
RHAs										
Northern	7	6.6	1.6	2	1.6	0.4	0	—	0	—
Yorkshire	4	4.0	0.8	2	2.0	0.4	0	—	0	—
Trent	16	16.0	2.7	4	4.0	0.7	0	—	0	—
East Anglia	4	4.0	1.6	0	—	—	0	—	0	—
North West Thames	8	5.8	1.2	4	1.8	0.4	0	—	0	—
North East Thames	3	2.4	0.5	3	2.4	0.5	0	—	0	—
South East Thames	14	12.6	2.8	5	3.6	0.8	0	—	0	—
South West Thames	7	4.0	1.1	4	1.0	0.3	0	—	0	—
Wessex	4	4.0	1.2	2	2.0	0.6	0	—	1	1.0
Oxford	7	6.1	1.7	2	2.0	0.6	0	—	0	—
South Western	5	5.0	1.3	1	1.0	0.3	0	—	0	—
West Midlands	12	12.0	1.7	4	4.0	0.6	0	—	0	—
Mersey	11	10.0	3.1	5	4.0	1.2	0	—	1	1.0
North Western	8	7.7	1.4	4	3.7	0.7	0	—	1	1.0
London post-graduate teaching hospitals	14	11.8		5	2.8		0	—	3	3.0
Wales	5	4.1	1.1	2	1.1	0.3	0	—	0	—
Scotland	40	38.9	5.6	11	10.3	1.5	0	—	2	1.6
Northern Ireland	11	11.0	3.8	3	3.0	1.1	0	—	0	—

* *Except hospital practitioners and paragraph 94 appointments. Paragraph 94 appointments are those (mainly general practitioners) working in hospital as part-time medical officers.*

† *'Consultant' also includes senior hospital medical officers (SHMO). Associate specialists were formally known as medical assistants.*

‡ *'House Officer' includes senior house officer (SHO), house officer, post-registration, and house officer pre-registration.*

◊ *Duplication may occur where staff hold multiple appointments in more than one region.*

Source: DHSS; ISD; DHSS, Northern Ireland.

Registrar		House officers‡		Other		Hospital practitioner		Paragraph 94 appointments		Area
Number	wte	Number	wte	Number	wte	Number	wte	Number	wte	
19	19.0	52	51.1	0	—	2	0.3	4	0.9	**England**◊
										RHAs
2	2.0	3	3.0	0	—	0	—	1	0.1	Northern
1	1.0	1	1.0	0	—	0	—	0	—	Yorkshire
3	3.0	9	9.0	0	—	0	—	0	—	Trent
1	1.0	3	3.0	0	—	0	—	0	—	East Anglia
1	1.0	3	3.0	0	—	0	—	0	—	North West Thames
—	—	—	—	0	—	0	—	0	—	North East Thames
—	—	9	9.0	0	—	0	—	0	—	South East Thames
1	1.0	2	2.0	0	—	0	—	0	—	South West Thames
—	—	1	1.0	0	—	0	—	0	—	Wessex
1	1.0	4	3.1	0	—	1	0.1	0	—	Oxford
—	—	4	4.0	0	—	0	—	0	—	South Western
4	4.0	4	4.0	0	—	0	—	0	—	West Midlands
2	2.0	3	3.0	0	—	1	0.2	0	—	Mersey
1	1.0	2	2.0	0	—	0	—	1	0.1	North Western
2	2.0	4	4.0	0	—	0	—	2	0.7	London post-graduate teaching hospitals
1	**1.0**	**2**	**2.0**	**0**	**—**	**0**	**—**	**1**	**0.1**	**Wales**
7	**7.0**	**20**	**20.0**	**0**	**—**	..	..	..	..	**Scotland**
3	**3.0**	**5**	**5.0**	**0**	**—**	..	..	..	..	**Northern Ireland**

Table A7.19   Community health services medical staff, Regional Health Authorities, England and Wales 1975-80

	Number of whole time equivalent staff						Rate per 10,000 population	
	1975	1976	1977	1978	1979	1980	1975	1980
England	**2,564.9**	**2,680.7**	**2,734.5**	**2,782.2**	**2,794.5**	**2,820.8**	**0.55**	**0.61**
RHAs								
Northern	172.0	183.8	179.6	177.5	178.2	180.5	0.55	0.59
Yorkshire	195.6	207.0	210.0	201.3	205.3	209.4	0.55	0.58
Trent	202.8	214.9	226.2	237.0	228.8	225.8	0.45	0.50
East Anglia	65.6	67.7	70.3	79.9	80.9	84.4	0.37	0.45
North West Thames	227.4	231.3	243.3	236.4	246.5	243.3	0.66	0.71
North East Thames	241.0	248.5	240.3	242.7	238.5	238.2	0.65	0.64
South East Thames	226.6	246.0	248.2	269.1	253.7	247.6	0.63	0.70
South West Thames	184.9	204.5	225.8	223.3	227.0	218.8	0.64	0.77
Wessex	149.1	149.5	150.4	151.1	149.1	149.2	0.57	0.55
Oxford	103.7	106.4	111.0	111.3	118.3	123.9	0.47	0.54
South Western	137.5	142.3	143.8	156.5	158.0	162.5	0.44	0.50
West Midlands	259.8	273.0	270.7	276.0	285.5	302.0	0.50	0.59
Mersey	158.4	164.5	165.1	159.6	159.5	156.2	0.63	0.64
North Western	240.6	241.4	249.9	260.5	265.2	279.1	0.59	0.70
Wales	**187.3**	**204.6**	**208.7**	**204.2**	**214.9**	**218.4**	**0.68**	**0.79**

Source: DHSS

Table A7.20 General medical practitioners, Regional Health Authorities, England and Wales, 1 October 1981

| | All practitioners | Unrestricted principals | Principals providing: | | | |
| | | | Maternity services | | Contraceptive services | |
			Number	Per 1,000 maternities in region in 1980	Number	Per 1,000 women aged 15-44
England	**24,359**	**22,304**	**18,045**	**29.2**	**21,274**	**2.19**
RHAs						
Northern	1,537	1,432	1,199	29.1	1,296	2.02
Yorkshire	1,823	1,694	1,473	30.9	1,658	2.25
Trent	2,213	2,054	1,695	28.2	1,885	1.98
East Anglia	996	894	832	33.7	857	2.23
North West Thames	2,020	1,820	1,156	24.4	1,718	2.25
North East Thames	1,970	1,803	1,206	23.5	1,731	2.16
South East Thames	1,897	1,740	1,270	27.9	1,626	2.20
South West Thames	1,564	1,420	1,024	29.1	1,357	2.22
Wessex	1,462	1,325	1,195	35.1	1,289	2.31
Oxford	1,184	1,095	924	28.1	1,058	2.07
South Western	1,788	1,623	1,417	36.3	1,584	2.60
West Midlands	2,588	2,395	2,107	29.6	2,334	2.17
Mersey	1,270	1,158	964	30.0	1,105	2.17
North Western	2,047	1,851	1,583	29.1	1,776	2.16
Wales	**1,547**	**1,397**	**1,120**	**30.1**	**1,376**	**2.45**

Source: DHSS, *Health and personal social services statistics for England, 1982*
Welsh Office

Table A7.21   General practitioners' claims for fees for maternity medical services, England and Wales, 1978-80

	Total number of claims*	Services for which fees were paid†					
		Care including delivery			Care without delivery		Miscarriage
		Complete care	Partial antenatal or postnatal care	Other, including delivery only	Complete care	Partial antenatal or postnatal care	
1978							
Number	576,880	82,005	9,954	6,007	46,425	382,047	49,577
Percentage of total maternities	96.9	13.8	1.7	1.0	7.8	64.2	8.3
1979							
Number	636,102	85,054	9,148	5,492	53,830	430,590	53,988
Percentage of total maternities	99.9	13.4	1.4	0.9	8.5	67.6	8.5
1980							
Number	663,970	79,177	9,625	5,589	64,017	449,517	56,045
Percentage of total maternities	101.0	12.1	1.5	0.9	9.8	68.7	8.6

* *Paid during the year ending 31 December*
† *Estimates based on a 10 per cent sample of claims*

Source: DHSS

Table A7.22   General practitioners' claims for fees for maternity medical services, Regional Health Authorities, England and Wales, 1980

| | Total claims* | Services for which fees were paid† | | | | | Miscarriage |
| | | Care including delivery | | | Care without delivery | | |
		Complete care	Partial antenatal or postnatal care	Other including delivery only	Complete care	Partial antenatal or postnatal care	
	Numbers of claims						
England	**625,102**	**77,154**	**9,103**	**5,297**	**59,630**	**420,952**	**52,966**
RHAs							
Northern	40,848	3,914	693	362	3,092	29,635	3,152
Yorkshire	49,118	7,422	320	261	5,818	31,242	4,055
Trent	62,617	7,954	822	50	6,667	41,392	5,732
East Anglia	25,238	2,842	517	149	2,057	17,675	1,998
North West Thames	42,973	1,861	241	301	4,875	31,477	4,218
North East Thames	49,027	4,521	751	181	4,802	34,077	4,695
South East Thames	40,929	3,617	201	141	4,272	29,361	3,337
South West Thames	33,145	3,813	110	1,001	3,363	22,204	2,654
Wessex	36,922	4,766	980	0	3,604	24,447	3,125
Oxford	35,566	5,386	1,140	10	5,281	20,628	3,121
South Western	42,982	7,360	1,335	665	2,937	27,360	3,325
West Midlands	76,612	11,955	1,102	1,132	6,192	50,490	5,741
Mersey	33,652	4,697	320	431	2,193	29,935	3,076
North Western	55,473	7,046	571	613	4,477	38,029	4,737
Wales	**38,868**	**2,023**	**522**	**292**	**4,387**	**28,565**	**3,079**

Table A7.22 General practitioners' claims for fees for maternity medical services, Regional Health Authorities, England and Wales, 1980
– *continued*

| | Total claims* | Services for which fees were paid† | | | | | Miscarriage |
| | | Care including delivery | | | Care without delivery | | |
		Complete care	Partial antenatal or postnatal care	Other including delivery only	Complete care	Partial antenatal or postnatal care	
	*Claims as a percentage of maternities in resident population**						
England	**101.3**	**12.5**	**1.5**	**0.9**	**9.7**	**68.2**	**8.6**
RHAs							
Northern	99.3	9.5	1.7	0.9	7.5	72.0	7.6
Yorkshire	103.0	15.6	0.7	0.5	12.2	65.5	8.5
Trent	104.0	13.2	1.4	0.1	11.1	68.8	9.5
East Anglia	102.2	11.5	2.0	0.6	8.3	71.6	8.1
North West Thames	90.7	3.9	0.5	0.6	10.3	66.5	8.9
North East Thames	95.3	8.8	1.4	0.4	9.3	66.3	9.1
South East Thames	89.9	7.9	0.4	0.3	9.4	64.5	7.3
South West Thames	94.3	10.8	0.3	2.8	9.6	63.2	7.6
Wessex	108.4	14.0	2.9	—	10.6	71.8	9.2
Oxford	108.2	16.3	3.5	—	16.1	62.8	9.5
South Western	110.1	18.9	3.4	1.7	7.5	70.1	8.5
West Midlands	107.8	16.8	1.5	1.6	8.7	71.0	8.1
Mersey	104.6	14.6	1.0	1.3	6.8	93.0	9.6
North Western	102.5	13.0	1.1	1.1	8.2	70.0	8.7
Wales	**104.3**	**5.4**	**1.4**	**0.8**	**11.8**	**76.7**	**8.3**

* *Paid during the year ending 31 December*

† *Estimates based on a 10 per cent sample of claims*

Source: DHSS

Table A7.23 Use of services for antenatal care, England and Wales, 1975-80

Year	Women attending hospital out-patient antenatal clinics*	Women attending community antenatal clinics†	Number of GP claims for care including antenatal careφ
England			
1975	511,105	234,383	484,967
1976	503,922	266,948	466,610
1977	518,345	241,782	454,855
1978	560,917	277,422	465,492
1979	589,686	..	516,575
1980	607,674	..	540,526
Wales			
1975	30,292	12,534	30,040
1976	29,753	15,733	30,294
1977	29,759	10,095	28,650
1978	32,922	10,906	29,759
1979	36,974	..	32,450
1980	37,101	..	33,928

Most women attend more than one type of antenatal clinic

* *Including GP obstetric clinics in hospitals*

† *Excluding women attending sessions held by their own general practitioner. (Data not collected after 1978)*

φ *Including either complete or partial antenatal care but excluding cases where partial antenatal care was included in claims for complete postnatal care. In 1980 those were less than 1.5 per cent of claims made in that year.*

Sources: DHSS, Welsh Office

Table A7.24 Maternity care, Scotland, 1975-80

Year	Hospital obstetric clinics			Domiciliary care (number of visits, thousands)				
	Specialist antenatal*	Specialist postnatal*	GP	Community midwives		Health visitors		
				Antenatal	Postnatal	Antenatal	Postnatal	Expectant women visited
1975	..	..	..	..	..	54.5	..	22.9
1976	76,255*	5,158*	4,022	..	..	55.5	..	24.6
1977	70,963	5,380	3,374	..	..	48.7	..	26.0
1978	71,103	6,386	3,264	29.2	287.4	46.6	171.2	25.7
1979	72,651	6,808	3,882	34.3	249.2	45.8	153.0	25.0†
1980	74,814	5,818	4,021	36.2	260.3	51.4	157.0	28.6†

* *A new system of hospital data collection was introduced in 1977 so that these data may be incompatible with those for later years*

† *Excluding Greater Glasgow Health Board*

Source: *Scottish Health Statistics* (Tables 6.6a, 8.11 and 8.14)

Table A7.25 In-patient maternity care, England and Wales, 1974-78

Type of care	Estimated number of in-patient episodes*				
	1974	1975	1976	1977	1978
Antenatal care only†	98,360	100,720	103,430	102,200	106,370
Antenatal care with delivery and postnatal careφ	293,850	266,320	209,120	197,100	199,170
Delivery and postnatal care only‡	308,510	307,720	351,590	332,620	354,120
Postnatal care only	22,770	21,810	23,160	24,200	26,370
Total	723,490	696,580	687,300	656,120	686,030

* *More than one episode of in-patient care may be recorded for a single maternity*
† *Discharged undelivered*
φ *Admitted before labour, discharged delivered*
‡ *Admitted in labour, discharged delivered*
Source: OPCS and DHSS, Hospital In-patient Enquiry (maternity)

Table A7.26 In-patient antenatal care in maternity hospitals: cases with selected complications, England and Wales, 1973-78

ICD code (8th Rev.)	Maternal complication	Estimated number of women with complications*					
		1973	1974	1975	1976	1977	1978
632	Haemorrhage of pregnancy	12,400	11,530	11,790	12,690	13,110	12,700
635, 636	Urinary infections and renal disease	7,850	7,580	7,030	7,090	7,110	7,420
637	Pre-eclampsia, eclampsia and toxaemia (unspecified)	49,490	41,160	38,360	38,890	37,830	37,650
Y60	Pre-natal care and observation	9,080	8,000	9,370	12,430	13,010	11,930
	All antenatal cases	145,050	144,070	143,800	146,310	142,540	146,570

Antenatal cases are counted as those women discharged undelivered and those admitted five or more days before delivery.
* *More than one complication may be recorded for each woman.*
Source: OPCS and DHSS, Hospital In-patient Enquiry (maternity)

Table A7.27   In-patient antenatal care, Scotland, 1980

	All antenatal episodes	ICD code (9th revision) and maternal complication		
		641 Haemorrhage	642 Hypertension	646.6 Genito-urinary infections
Number of antenatal episodes in which each diagnosis was mentioned	20,095	1,763	3,801	1,796

Antenatal episodes are all those where the patient is discharged still pregnant.
Source: Information Services Division (SMR2)

Table A7.28 Live births by legitimacy, parity, place of delivery and age of mother, England and Wales, 1980

Legitimacy/parity	Place of delivery	All ages Number	%	Under 20 Number	%	20-24 Number	%	25-29 Number	%	30-34 Number	%	35 and over Number	%
All live births	Total	656,234	100.0	60,754	100.0	201,541	100.0	223,438	100.0	129,908	100.0	40,593	100.0
	NHS hospital A	27,177	4.1	1,760	2.9	9,081	4.5	10,612	4.7	5,028	3.9	696	1.7
	NHS hospital B	612,934	93.4	58,070	95.6	188,283	93.4	206,969	92.6	120,818	93.0	38,794	95.6
	Other hospitals	7,537	1.1	460	0.8	2,235	1.1	2,613	1.2	1,662	1.3	567	1.4
	At home	8,056	1.2	379	0.6	1,749	0.9	3,103	1.4	2,324	1.8	501	1.2
	Elsewhere	530	0.1	85	0.1	193	0.1	141	0.1	76	0.1	35	0.1
All legitimate	Total	578,862	100.0	34,894	100.0	174,934	100.0	209,976	100.0	122,320	100.0	36,738	100.0
	NHS hospital A	25,254	4.4	1,259	3.6	8,308	4.7	10,206	4.9	4,837	4.0	644	1.8
	NHS hospital B	538,972	93.1	33,083	94.8	162,843	93.1	194,252	92.5	113,689	92.9	35,105	95.6
	Other hospitals	7,214	1.2	383	1.1	2,148	1.2	2,539	1.2	1,604	1.3	540	1.5
	At home	7,037	1.2	142	0.4	1,493	0.9	2,851	1.4	2,126	1.7	425	1.2
	Elsewhere	385	0.1	27	0.1	142	0.1	128	0.1	64	0.1	24	0.1
Number of previous liveborn children													
0	Total	240,975	100.0	28,189	100.0	96,393	100.0	81,554	100.0	28,907	100.0	5,932	100.0
	NHS hospital A	7,696	3.2	901	3.2	3,744	3.9	2,689	3.3	340	1.2	22	0.4
	NHS hospital B	229,629	95.3	26,907	95.5	91,209	94.6	77,657	95.2	28,061	97.1	5,795	97.7
	Other hospitals	3,106	1.3	320	1.1	1,244	1.3	1,007	1.2	430	1.5	105	1.8
	At home	491	0.2	51	0.2	171	0.2	189	0.2	71	0.2	9	0.2
	Elsewhere	53	0.0	10	0.0	25	0.0	12	0.0	5	0.0	1	0.0
1	Total	209,164	100.0	6,307	100.0	60,501	100.0	84,580	100.0	48,205	100.0	9,571	100.0
	NHS hospital A	11,570	5.5	346	5.5	3,668	6.1	5,210	6.2	2,195	4.6	151	1.6
	NHS hospital B	191,670	91.6	5,807	92.1	55,123	91.1	76,898	90.9	44,658	92.6	9,184	96.0
	Other hospitals	2,646	1.3	58	0.9	755	1.2	1,035	1.2	637	1.3	161	1.7
	At home	3,101	1.5	80	1.3	876	1.4	1,378	1.6	696	1.4	71	0.7
	Elsewhere	177	0.1	16	0.3	79	0.1	59	0.1	19	0.0	4	0.0

Table A7.28 Live births by legitimacy, parity, place of delivery and age of mother, England and Wales, 1980 - *continued*

Legitimacy/parity	Place of delivery	Age of mother											
		All ages		Under 20		20-24		25-29		30-34		35 and over	
		Number	%	Number	%	Number	%	Number	%	Number	%	Number	%
2	Total	86,336	100.0	386	100.0	14,830	100.0	31,416	100.0	30,052	100.0	9,607	100.0
	NHS hospital A	4,726	5.5	12	3.1	795	5.4	1,883	6.0	1,764	5.9	272	2.8
	NHS hospital B	78,140	90.5	357	92.5	13,523	91.2	28,200	89.6	27,012	89.9	9,048	94.2
	Other hospitals	1,028	1.2	5	1.3	129	0.9	389	1.2	363	1.2	142	1.5
	At home	2,348	2.7	11	2.8	356	2.4	953	3.0	894	3.0	134	1.4
	Elsewhere	94	0.1	1	0.3	27	0.2	36	0.1	19	0.1	11	0.1
3 and over	Total	42,387	100.0	12	100.0	3,210	100.0	12,381	100.0	15,155	100.0	11,628	100.0
	NHS hospital A	1,262	3.0	0	—	101	3.1	424	3.4	538	3.5	199	1.7
	NHS hospital B	39,533	93.3	12	100.0	2,988	93.1	11,497	92.9	13,958	92.1	11,078	95.3
	Other hospitals	434	1.0	0	—	20	0.6	108	0.9	174	1.1	132	1.1
	At home	1,097	2.6	0	—	90	2.8	331	2.7	465	3.1	211	1.8
	Elsewhere	61	0.1	0	—	11	0.3	21	0.2	21	0.1	8	0.1
Illegitimate	Total	77,372	100.0	25,860	100.0	26,607	100.0	13,462	100.0	7,588	100.0	3,855	100.0
	NHS hospital A	1,923	2.5	501	1.9	773	2.9	406	3.0	191	2.5	52	1.3
	NHS hospital B	73,962	95.6	24,987	96.6	25,440	95.6	12,717	94.5	7,129	94.0	3,689	95.7
	Other hospitals	323	0.4	77	0.3	87	0.3	74	0.5	58	0.8	27	0.7
	At home	1,019	1.3	237	0.9	256	1.0	252	1.9	198	2.6	76	2.0
	Elsewhere	145	0.2	58	0.2	51	0.2	13	0.1	12	0.2	11	0.3

Source: OPCS *Birth statistics, Series FM1*

Table A7.29 Maternities and total births by place of delivery, England and Wales, 1954-81

(a) Numbers and percentages of maternities 1964-80

Year		NHS A hospitals	NHS B hospitals	Other hospitals	At home	Elsewhere	Total maternities
1964	Number	588,206		25,945	252,114	13,908	880,173
	Percentage	66.8		2.9	28.6	1.6	100.0
1965	Number	603,159		23,581	227,884	12,089	866,713
	Percentage	69.6		2.7	26.3	1.4	100.0
1966	Number	616,187		22,117	204,403	10,774	853,481
	Percentage	72.2		2.6	23.9	1.3	100.0
1967	Number	628,506		19,901	178,039	8,987	835,433
	Percentage	75.2		2.4	21.3	1.1	100.0
1968	Number	644,757		16,992	153,245	7,254	822,248
	Percentage	78.4		2.1	18.6	0.9	100.0
1969	Number	98,454	554,591	15,089	126,247	5,382	799,763
	Percentage	12.3	69.3	1.9	15.8	0.7	100.0
1970	Number	92,934	572,759	14,100	102,698	4,095	786,586
	Percentage	11.8	72.8	1.8	13.1	0.5	100.0
1971	Number	91,708	592,328	14,480	83,387	2,996	784,899
	Percentage	11.7	75.5	1.8	10.6	0.4	100.0
1972	Number	79,682	571,201	13,229	60,473	2,128	726,715
	Percentage	11.0	78.6	1.8	8.3	0.3	100.0
1973	Number	67,127	556,482	11,854	40,301	1,362	677,126
	Percentage	9.9	82.2	1.8	6.0	0.2	100.0
1974	Number	49,970	552,357	10,909	26,558	983	640,777
	Percentage	7.8	86.2	1.7	4.1	0.2	100.0
1975	Number	43,156	530,284	9,403	19,441	782	603,666
	Percentage	7.2	87.8	1.6	3.2	0.1	100.0
1976	Number	45,366	515,365	8,284	14,623	625	584,263
	Percentage	7.8	88.2	1.4	2.5	0.1	100.0
1977	Number	38,918	511,505	7,263	10,899	488	569,073
	Percentage	6.8	89.9	1.3	1.9	0.1	100.0
1978	Number	35,562	542,954	6,862	9,586	551	595,515
	Percentage	6.0	91.2	1.2	1.6	0.1	100.0
1979	Number	32,647	587,853	6,976	8,869	539	636,884
	Percentage	5.1	92.3	1.1	1.4	0.1	100.0
1980	Number	27,185	611,125	7,508	8,131	552	654,501
	Percentage	4.2	93.4	1.1	1.2	0.1	100.0

Table A7.29   Maternities and total births by place of delivery, England and Wales, 1954-81 - *continued*

(b) Numbers and percentages of total births 1954-81

Year		Place of delivery						Total births
		All NHS hospitals	NHS A hospitals	NHS B hospitals	Other hospitals	At home	Elsewhere	
1954	Number	408,205			30,817	234,438	16,391	689,851
	Percentage	59.2			4.5	34.0	2.4	100.0
1955	Number	411,700			28,146	228,225	15,569	688,640
	Percentage	60.2			4.1	33.4	2.3	100.0
1956	Number	433,194			28,028	238,668	16,830	716,740
	Percentage	60.4			3.9	33.3	2.3	100.0
1957	Number	448,176			27,620	246,856	17,344	739,996
	Percentage	60.6			3.7	33.4	2.3	100.0
1958	Number	457,206			26,765	254,943	18,089	757,003
	Percentage	60.4			3.5	33.7	2.4	100.0
1959	Number	464,293			26,384	256,414	17,311	764,402
	Percentage	60.7			3.5	33.5	2.3	100.0
1960	Number	490,622			27,186	265,931	17,085	800,824
	Percentage	61.3			3.4	33.2	2.1	100.0
1961	Number	515,274			27,168	267,970	16,596	827,008
	Percentage	62.3			3.3	32.4	2.0	100.0
1962	Number	536,495			26,653	274,390	16,662	854,200
	Percentage	62.8			3.1	32.1	2.0	100.0
1963	Number	566,068			26,644	260,952	15,380	869,044
	Percentage	65.1			3.1	30.0	1.8	100.0
1964	Number	597,438			26,163	252,959	13,958	890,518
	Percentage	67.1			2.9	28.4	1.6	100.0
1965	Number	612,127			23,773	228,538	12,128	876,566
	Percentage	69.8			2.7	26.1	1.4	100.0
1966	Number	624,967			22,277	205,018	10,804	863,066
	Percentage	72.4			2.6	23.8	1.2	100.0
1967	Number	637,078			20,058	178,547	9,009	844,692
	Percentage	75.4			2.4	21.1	1.1	100.0
1968	Number	653,107			17,114	153,626	7,273	831,120
	Percentage	78.6			2.1	18.5	0.9	100.0
1969	Number	661,046	97,091	563,955	15,208	126,535	5,403	808,192
	Percentage	81.8	12.0	69.8	1.9	15.7	0.7	100.0

Table A7.29 Maternities and total births by place of delivery, England and Wales, 1954-81 - *continued*

(b) Numbers and percentages of total births 1954-81 - *continued*

Year		All NHS hospitals	NHS A hospitals	NHS B hospitals	Other hospitals	At home	Elsewhere	Total births
1970	Number	673,497	93,192	580,305	14,251	102,970	4,113	794,831
	Percentage	84.7	11.7	73.0	1.8	13.0	0.5	100.0
1971	Number	691,795	91,924	599,871	14,614	83,637	3,008	793,054
	Percentage	87.2	11.6	75.6	1.8	10.5	0.4	100.0
1972	Number	657,607	79,801	577,806	13,268	60,636	2,103	733,614
	Percentage	89.6	10.9	78.7	1.8	8.3	0.3	100.0
1973	Number	630,120	67,257	562,863	11,975	40,412	1,382	683,889
	Percentage	92.1	9.8	82.3	1.8	5.9	0.2	100.0
1974	Number	608,422	50,089	558,333	11,010	26,635	993	647,060
	Percentage	94.0	7.7	86.3	1.7	4.1	0.2	100.0
1975	Number	579,950	43,862	536,088	9,500	19,504	786	609,740
	Percentage	95.1	7.2	87.9	1.6	3.2	0.1	100.0
1976	Number	566,323	45,458	520,865	8,360	14,667	629	589,979
	Percentage	96.0	7.7	88.3	1.4	2.5	0.1	100.0
1977	Number	555,913	39,019	516,894	7,318	10,940	493	574,664
	Percentage	96.7	6.8	89.9	1.3	1.9	0.1	100.0
1978	Number	584,441	35,645	548,796	6,921	9,608	556	601,526
	Percentage	97.2	5.9	91.2	1.2	1.6	0.1	100.0
1979	Number	626,664	32,700	593,964	7,041	8,904	544	643,153
	Percentage	97.4	5.1	92.4	1.1	1.4	0.1	100.0
1980	Number	644,710	27,225	617,485	7,576	8,162	559	661,007
	Percentage	97.5	4.1	93.4	1.1	1.2	0.1	100.0
1981	Number	623,876	22,440	601,436	7,479	6,790	514	638,659
	Percentage	97.7	3.5	94.2	1.2	1.1	0.1	100.0

Source: OPCS *Birth Statistics, Series FM1, Registrar General's Statistical Reviews*

Table A7.30 Department of delivery in NHS hospitals, England and Wales, 1964-78

| Year | Estimated percentage of all deliveries in England and Wales | | | |
	Obstetric units	GP maternity unit	Other departments	All deliveries in NHS non-psychiatric hospitals
1964	52.2	14.3	0.3	66.8
1965	54.3	14.5	0.8	69.6
1966	56.0	15.7	0.4	72.2
1967	58.9	16.0	0.3	75.2
1968	61.9	16.3	0.2	78.4
1969	62.8	18.4	0.4	81.7
1970	66.7	17.8	0.1	84.6
1971	69.2	17.3	0.6	87.1
1972	71.6	17.6	0.3	89.6
1973	75.1	16.8	0.1	92.1
1974	77.8	16.1	0.1	94.0
1975	78.8	16.4	0.4	95.6
1976	80.2	15.6	0.2	96.0
1977	81.2	14.8	0.0	96.7
1978	83.9	13.5	0.0	97.1

Source: OPCS and DHSS, Hospital In-patient Enquiry (maternity) and OPCS *Birth Statistics Series FM1*

Table A7.31 Stillbirths, perinatal and neonatal mortality by legitimacy, parity, place of delivery and age of mother, England and Wales, 1980

Stillbirths

Legitimacy/ parity	Place of delivery	All ages Number	Rate*	Under 20 Number	Rate*	20-24 Number	Rate*	25-29 Number	Rate*	30-34 Number	Rate*	35 and over Number	Rate*
All deaths	Total	4,773	7.2	508	8.3	1,387	6.8	1,460	6.5	953	7.3	465	11.3
	NHS hospitals A	48	1.8	6	3.4	18	2.0	11	1.0	9	1.8	4	5.7
	NHS hospitals B	4,551	7.4	468	8.0	1,311	6.9	1,410	6.8	922	7.6	440	11.2
	Other hospitals	39	5.1	2	4.3	14	6.2	10	3.8	8	4.8	5	8.7
	At home	106	13.0	27	66.5	33	18.5	22	7.0	13	5.6	11	21.5
	Elsewhere	29	51.9	5	55.6	11	53.9	7	47.3	1	13.0	5	125.0
All legitimate	Total	4,077	7.0	257	7.3	1,147	6.5	1,359	6.4	894	7.3	420	11.3
	NHS hospitals A	40	1.6	3	2.4	16	1.9	10	1.0	8	1.7	3	4.6
	NHS hospitals B	3,920	7.2	244	7.3	1,096	6.7	1,316	6.7	865	7.6	399	11.2
	Other hospitals	38	5.2	2	5.2	13	6.0	10	3.9	8	5.0	5	9.2
	At home	62	8.7	7	47.0	16	10.6	18	6.3	12	5.6	9	20.7
	Elsewhere	17	42.3	1	35.7	6	40.5	5	37.6	1	15.4	4	142.9
0	Total	1,856	7.6	216	7.6	715	7.4	620	7.5	225	7.7	80	13.3
	NHS hospitals A	21	2.7	3	3.3	11	2.9	5	1.9	1	2.9	1	43.5
	NHS hospitals B	1,792	7.7	204	7.5	691	7.5	602	7.7	219	7.7	76	12.9
	Other hospitals	15	4.8	1	3.1	7	5.6	4	4.0	2	4.6	1	9.4
	At home	23	44.7	7	120.7	5	28.2	7	35.7	2	27.4	2	181.8
	Elsewhere	5	86.2	1	90.9	1	38.5	2	142.9	1	166.7	-	-
1	Total	1,130	5.4	38	6.0	301	5.0	411	4.8	293	6.0	87	9.0
	NHS hospitals A	11	0.9	-	-	5	1.4	2	0.4	4	1.8	-	-
	NHS hospitals B	1,085	5.6	37	6.3	280	5.1	399	5.2	285	6.3	84	9.1
	Other hospitals	10	3.8	1	16.9	4	5.3	3	2.9	1	1.6	1	6.2
	At home	17	5.5	-	-	8	9.1	5	3.6	3	4.3	1	13.9
	Elsewhere	7	38.0	-	-	4	48.2	2	32.8	-	-	1	200.0
2	Total	627	7.2	3	7.7	100	6.7	207	6.5	228	7.5	89	9.2
	NHS hospitals A	5	1.1	-	-	-	-	1	0.5	2	1.1	2	7.3
	NHS hospitals B	596	7.6	3	8.3	94	6.9	199	7.0	218	8.0	82	9.0
	Other hospitals	12	11.5	-	-	2	15.4	3	7.7	5	13.6	2	13.9
	At home	11	4.7	-	-	3	8.4	3	3.1	3	3.3	2	14.7
	Elsewhere	3	30.9	-	-	1	35.7	1	27.0	-	-	1	83.3

* Per 1,000 total births

Table A7.31 Stillbirths, perinatal and neonatal mortality by legitimacy, parity, place of delivery and age of mother, England and Wales, 1980 - *continued*

Legitimacy/ parity	Place of delivery	All ages Number	Rate*	Under 20 Number	Rate*	20-24 Number	Rate*	25-29 Number	Rate*	30-34 Number	Rate*	35 and over Number	Rate*
		Stillbirths - continued											
3 and over	Total	464	10.8	-	-	31	9.6	121	9.7	148	9.7	164	13.9
	NHS hospitals A	3	2.4	-	-	-	-	2	4.7	1	1.9	-	-
	NHS hospitals B	417	11.2	-	-	31	10.3	116	10.0	143	10.2	157	14.0
	Other hospitals	1	2.3	-	-	-	-	-	-	-	-	1	7.5
	At home	11	9.9	-	-	-	-	3	9.0	4	8.5	4	18.6
	Elsewhere	2	31.7	-	-	-	-	-	-	-	-	2	200.0
Illegitimate	Total	696	8.9	251	9.6	240	8.9	101	7.4	59	7.7	45	11.5
	NHS hospitals A	8	4.1	3	6.0	2	2.6	1	2.5	1	5.2	1	18.9
	NHS hospitals B	631	8.5	224	8.9	215	8.4	94	7.3	57	7.9	41	11.0
	Other hospitals	1	3.1	-	-	1	11.4	-	-	-	-	-	-
	At home	44	41.4	20	77.8	17	62.3	4	15.6	1	5.0	2	25.6
	Elsewhere	12	76.4	4	64.5	5	89.3	2	133.3	-	-	1	83.3
		Perinatal deaths											
All deaths	Total	8,796	13.3	1,015	16.6	2,698	13.3	2,700	12.0	1,655	12.6	728	17.7
	NHS hospitals A	101	3.7	14	7.9	38	4.2	27	2.5	17	3.4	5	7.1
	NHS hospitals B	8,381	13.6	932	15.9	2,563	13.5	2,596	12.5	1,598	13.1	692	17.6
	Other hospitals	68	9.0	2	4.3	23	10.2	19	7.2	13	7.8	11	19.2
	At home	204	25.0	59	145.3	58	32.5	48	15.4	25	10.7	14	27.3
	Elsewhere	42	75.1	8	88.9	16	78.4	10	67.6	2	26.0	6	150.0
All legitimate	Total	7,480	12.8	532	15.1	2,254	12.8	2,495	11.8	1,541	12.5	658	17.7
	NHS hospitals A	88	3.5	9	7.1	33	4.0	26	2.5	16	3.3	4	6.2
	NHS hospitals B	7,180	13.2	506	15.2	2,157	13.2	2,401	12.3	1,488	13.0	628	17.7
	Other hospitals	63	8.7	2	5.2	22	10.2	18	7.1	11	6.8	10	18.3
	At home	122	17.2	13	87.2	32	21.2	42	14.6	24	11.2	11	25.3
	Elsewhere	27	67.2	2	71.4	10	67.6	8	60.2	2	30.8	5	178.6

* Per 1,000 total births

Table A7.31 Stillbirths, perinatal and neonatal mortality by legitimacy, parity, place of delivery and age of mother, England and Wales, 1980 - *continued*

Legitimacy/ parity	Place of delivery	All ages		Under 20		20-24		25-29		30-34		35 and over	
		Number	Rate*	Number	Rate*	Number	Rate*	Number	Rate*	Number	Rate*	Number	Rate=
		Perinatal deaths - continued											
0	Total	3,384	13.9	436	15.3	1,312	13.5	1,090	13.3	419	14.4	127	21.1
	NHS hospitals A	38	4.9	8	8.8	17	4.5	10	3.7	2	5.9	1	43.5
	NHS hospitals B	3,262	14.1	414	15.3	1,268	13.8	1,051	13.4	408	14.4	121	20.6
	Other hospitals	31	9.9	1	3.1	13	10.4	10	9.9	5	11.6	2	18.9
	At home	45	81.4	11	189.7	13	73.4	15	76.5	3	41.1	3	272.7
	Elsewhere	8	137.9	2	181.8	1	38.5	4	285.7	1	166.7	-	-
1	Total	2,168	10.3	86	13.6	660	10.9	813	9.6	484	10.0	125	12.9
	NHS hospitals A	29	2.5	1	2.9	13	3.5	9	1.7	6	2.7	-	-
	NHS hospitals B	2,071	10.7	83	14.2	620	11.2	780	10.1	468	10.4	120	12.9
	Other hospitals	15	5.6	1	16.9	6	7.9	4	3.9	1	1.6	3	18.5
	At home	42	13.5	1	12.5	14	15.9	17	12.3	9	12.9	1	13.9
	Elsewhere	11	59.8	-	-	7	84.3	3	49.2	-	-	1	200.0
2	Total	1,155	13.3	10	25.7	222	14.9	384	12.1	388	12.8	151	15.6
	NHS hospitals A	16	3.4	-	-	3	3.8	4	2.1	7	4.0	2	7.3
	NHS hospitals B	1,100	14.0	9	25.0	209	15.4	368	13.0	371	13.6	143	15.7
	Other hospitals	14	13.5	-	-	3	23.1	4	10.2	5	13.6	2	13.9
	At home	20	8.5	1	90.9	5	13.9	7	7.3	5	5.6	2	14.7
	Elsewhere	5	51.5	-	-	2	71.4	1	27.0	-	-	2	166.7
3 and over	Total	773	18.1	-	-	60	18.5	208	16.7	250	16.4	255	21.6
	NHS hospitals A	5	4.0	-	-	-	-	3	7.0	1	1.9	1	5.0
	NHS hospitals B	747	18.7	-	-	60	19.9	202	17.4	241	17.1	244	21.7
	Other hospitals	3	6.9	-	-	-	-	-	-	-	-	3	22.6
	At home	15	13.6	-	-	-	-	3	9.0	7	15.0	5	23.3
	Elsewhere	3	47.6	-	-	-	-	-	-	1	47.6	2	200.0
Illegitimate	Total	1,316	16.9	483	18.5	444	16.5	205	15.1	114	14.9	70	17.9
	NHS hospitals A	13	6.7	5	9.9	5	6.5	1	2.5	1	5.2	1	18.9
	NHS hospitals B	1,201	16.1	426	16.9	406	15.8	195	15.2	110	15.3	64	17.2
	Other hospitals	5	15.4	-	-	1	11.4	1	13.5	2	34.5	1	37.0
	At home	82	77.1	46	179.0	26	95.2	6	23.4	1	5.0	3	38.5
	Elsewhere	15	95.5	6	96.8	6	107.1	2	133.3	-	-	1	83.3

* Per 1,000 total births for perinatal deaths
= Per 1,000 live births for neonatal deaths

Table A7.31 Stillbirths, perinatal and neonatal mortality by legitimacy, parity, place of delivery and age of mother, England and Wales, 1980 - continued

Neo-natal deaths

Legitimacy/parity	Place of delivery	All ages		Under 20		20-24		25-29		30-34		35 and over	
		Number	Rate*	Number	Rate*	Number	Rate*	Number	Rate*	Number	Rate*	Number	Rate*
All deaths	Total	4,987	7.6	618	10.2	1,625	8.1	1,546	6.9	874	6.7	324	8.0
	NHS hospitals A	71	2.6	9	5.1	29	3.2	21	2.0	10	2.0	2	2.9
	NHS hospitals B	4,749	7.7	570	9.8	1,550	8.2	1,479	7.1	840	7.0	310	8.0
	Other hospitals	38	5.0	1	2.2	11	4.9	11	4.2	8	4.8	7	12.3
	At home	115	14.3	35	92.3	29	16.6	32	10.3	15	6.5	4	8.0
	Elsewhere	14	26.4	3	35.3	6	31.1	3	21.3	1	13.2	1	28.6
All legitimate	Total	4,233	7.3	340	9.7	1,369	7.8	1,428	6.8	803	6.6	293	8.0
	NHS hospitals A	66	2.6	7	5.6	26	3.1	21	2.1	10	2.1	2	3.1
	NHS hospitals B	4,051	7.5	325	9.8	1,309	8.0	1,365	7.0	771	6.8	281	8.0
	Other hospitals	34	4.7	1	2.6	11	5.1	10	3.9	6	3.7	6	11.1
	At home	71	10.1	6	42.3	18	12.1	29	10.2	15	7.1	3	7.1
	Elsewhere	11	28.6	1	37.0	5	35.2	3	23.4	1	15.6	1	41.7
0	Total	1,889	7.8	270	9.6	739	7.7	592	7.3	232	8.0	56	9.4
	NHS hospitals A	21	2.7	5	5.5	9	2.4	6	2.2	1	2.9	-	-
	NHS hospitals B	1,823	7.9	259	9.6	714	7.8	569	7.3	227	8.1	54	9.3
	Other hospitals	19	6.1	1	3.1	7	5.6	7	7.0	3	7.0	1	9.5
	At home	23	46.8	4	78.4	9	52.6	8	42.3	1	14.1	1	111.1
	Elsewhere	3	56.6	1	100.0	-	-	2	166.7	-	-	-	-
1	Total	1,313	6.3	62	9.8	455	7.5	502	5.9	241	5.0	53	5.5
	NHS hospitals A	28	2.4	2	5.8	13	3.5	10	1.9	3	1.4	-	-
	NHS hospitals B	1,241	6.5	59	10.2	428	7.8	474	6.2	230	5.2	50	5.4
	Other hospitals	7	2.6	-	-	3	4.0	2	1.9	-	-	2	12.4
	At home	32	10.3	1	12.5	7	8.0	15	10.9	8	11.5	1	14.1
	Elsewhere	5	28.2	-	-	4	50.6	1	16.9	-	-	-	-
2	Total	642	7.4	8	20.7	142	9.6	229	7.3	190	6.3	73	7.6
	NHS hospitals A	13	2.8	-	-	4	5.0	4	2.1	5	2.8	-	-
	NHS hospitals B	611	7.8	7	19.6	134	9.9	218	7.7	180	6.7	72	8.0
	Other hospitals	5	4.9	-	-	1	7.8	1	2.6	3	8.3	-	-
	At home	11	4.7	1	90.0	2	5.6	6	6.3	2	2.2	-	-
	Elsewhere	2	21.3	-	-	1	37.0	-	-	-	-	1	90.9

* Per 1,000 live births

Table A7.31 Stillbirths, perinatal and neonatal mortality by legitimacy, parity, place of delivery and age of mother, England and Wales, 1980 - *continued*

Legitimacy/ parity	Place of delivery	Age of mother											
		All ages		Under 20		20-24		25-29		30-34		35 and over	
		Number	Rate*	Number	Rate*	Number	Rate*	Number	Rate*	Number	Rate*	Number	Rate*
		Neonatal deaths - continued											
3 and over	Total	389	9.2	-	-	33	10.3	105	8.5	140	9.2	111	9.5
	NHS hospitals A	4	3.2	-	-	-	-	1	2.4	1	1.9	2	10.1
	NHS hospitals B	376	9.5	-	-	33	11.0	104	9.0	134	9.6	105	9.5
	Other hospitals	3	6.9	-	-	-	-	-	-	-	-	3	22.7
	At home	5	4.6	-	-	-	-	-	-	4	8.6	1	4.7
	Elsewhere	1	16.4	-	-	-	-	-	-	1	47.6	-	-
Illegitimate	Total	754	9.7	278	10.8	256	9.6	118	8.8	71	9.4	31	8.0
	NHS hospitals A	5	2.6	2	4.0	3	3.9	-	-	-	-	-	-
	NHS hospitals B	698	9.4	245	9.8	241	9.5	114	9.0	69	9.7	29	7.9
	Other hospitals	4	12.4	-	-	-	-	1	13.5	2	34.5	1	37.0
	At home	44	43.2	29	122.4	11	43.0	3	11.9	-	-	1	13.2
	Elsewhere	4	20.7	2	34.5	1	19.6	-	-	-	-	-	-

* *Per 1,000 live births*
Source: OPCS unpublished data

Table A7.32   Trends in obstetric intervention, England and Wales, 1953-78

(a) Induction, caesarean section, instrumental delivery and episiotomy, 1953-78

Year	Estimated percentage of all deliveries in England and Wales§				
	Induction of labour or artificial rupture of membranes	Admitted before labour, discharged delivered	Caesarean section	Instrumental delivery*	Episiotomy
1953	..	..	2.2	3.7	..
1954	..	..	..	..	..
1955	..	..	2.2	4.4	..
1956	..	..	2.3	4.1	..
1957	..	..	2.2	4.1	..
1958	..	..	2.3	4.4	..
1959	..	..	2.6	4.4	..
1960	..	..	2.8	4.5	..
1961	..	..	2.8	4.9	..
1962	8.3	15.4	3.0	5.1	..
1963	8.9	16.1	3.1	5.3	..
1964	8.9	16.3	3.3	5.6	..
1965	10.2	18.2	3.5	5.8	..
1966	12.7	19.4	3.4	6.0	..
1967	16.8	23.4	3.8	7.5	25.0†
1968	18.0	25.5	4.0	7.9	..
1969	20.3	28.9	4.3	8.2	..
1970	23.2	31.5	4.3	8.8	..
1971	26.3	34.4	4.6	9.4	..
1972	29.2	36.6	4.9	10.5	..
1973	34.9	42.2	5.0	11.0	44.0
1974	38.9	45.9	5.3	12.0	47.4
1975	35.0	44.1	5.7	12.4	48.6
1976	35.5	35.8	6.3	13.0	50.6
1977	36.8	36.0	7.1	13.4	52.0
1978	36.3	35.0	7.3	13.3	53.4

* *Forceps or vacuum extraction*
† *Not recorded in Birmingham Region*
§ *Includes women resident outside England and Wales*

Table A7.32   Trends in obstetric intervention, England and Wales, 1953-78 - *continued*

(b) Induction, caesarean section and instrumental delivery by department, 1964-78

Year	Percentage of deliveries in consultant obstetric units with:			Percentage of deliveries in GP maternity units with:		
	Induction or artificial rupture of membranes	Caesarean section	Instrumental delivery*	Induction or artificial rupture of membranes	Caesarean section	Instrumental delivery*
1964	15.6	6.1	9.7	4.7	0.4	3.7
1965	17.0	6.2	8.6	5.6	0.5	3.4
1966	20.5	5.9	9.7	6.9	0.4	3.7
1967	23.0	6.4	11.6	9.8	0.3	4.2
1968	26.3	6.4	11.7	10.1	0.2	3.9
1969	28.6	6.6	11.8	13.0	0.8	4.5
1970	30.8	5.9	11.6	14.0	1.5	5.1
1971	33.8	6.4	12.0	13.2	0.6	4.1
1972	36.0	6.4	12.9	13.0	0.6	4.1
1973	41.9	6.3	13.7	16.2	0.6	4.1
1974	43.9	6.7	14.4	17.8	0.7	4.7
1975	41.4	7.1	14.6	16.4	1.0	5.6
1976	41.0	7.6	15.1	16.5	1.3	7.6
1977	41.0	8.6	15.3	19.8	1.0	6.2
1978	39.0	8.6	15.1	19.3	1.1	5.7

* *Forceps or vacuum extraction*

(c) Method used for instrumental delivery, 1973-78

Year	Estimated percentage of all deliveries in England and Wales§		
	Method		Total
	Forceps	Vacuum extraction	
1973	10.3	0.7	11.0
1974	11.3	0.7	12.0
1975	11.8	0.7	12.4
1976	12.4	0.6	13.0
1977	12.7	0.7	13.4
1978	12.7	0.6	13.3

§ *Includes women resident outside England and Wales*
Source: OPCS and DHSS, Hospital In-patient Enquiry (maternity)

Table A7.33 Trends in obstetric intervention, singleton births, Scotland, 1975-79

| Year | Number of singleton births | Induced singleton births | | Mode of delivery as a percentage of all singleton births | | | | | |
		Number	Percentage of all singleton births	Spontaneous	Forceps	Vacuum extraction	Breech	Caesarean section	Other
1975	64,139	31,138	48.5	75.8	13.1	0.5	1.6	8.5	0.4
1976	63,359	28,135	44.4	74.9	13.7	0.5	1.5	9.4	0.2
1977	61,044	26,831	44.0	75.0	13.1	0.4	1.4	10.0	0.1
1978	63,193	25,656	40.6	72.9	12.6	0.5	1.2	10.7	2.2
1979	66,239	25,208	38.1	73.7	13.4	0.5	1.2	11.1	0.1

Source: *Scottish Health Statistics* 1976-80

Table A7.34 Obstetric intervention, Regional Health Authorities, England and Wales, 1975-78

Area		Percentage of maternities to residents of area				
		Induction	Caesarean section	Instrumental delivery	Episiotomy	All deliveries i NHS hospitals
England and Wales*						
	1975	**35.2**	**5.7**	**12.4**	**48.5**	**94.9**
	1976	**35.3**	**6.2**	**12.9**	**50.4**	**95.5**
	1977	**36.4**	**7.1**	**13.4**	**52.0**	**96.5**
	1978	**35.2**	**7.3**	**13.3**	**53.3**	**97.1**
Regional Health Authorities						
Northern	1975	36.2	5.7	12.6	53.6	96.9
	1976	37.7	6.3	12.0	55.8	97.7
	1977	34.4	7.2	12.7	57.5	98.0
	1978	31.5	7.3	13.8	59.8	98.4
Yorkshire	1975	38.9	5.0	10.0	47.9	95.5
	1976	36.9	6.0	9.9	48.0	96.3
	1977	36.5	6.9	11.6	51.7	96.5
	1978	41.6	6.8	9.9	52.7	97.0
Trent	1975	32.9	5.1	12.4	45.6	94.8
	1976	31.2	5.4	13.5	48.8	96.1
	1977	33.2	6.3	14.6	51.4	96.9
	1978	36.8	7.3	14.9	53.0	97.2
East Anglia	1975	25.2	5.2	10.3	39.7	87.6
	1976	23.9	6.5	11.1	45.8	89.4
	1977	31.8	6.4	11.8	45.6	90.9
	1978	29.2	6.2	10.9	44.8	91.9
N. W. Thames	1975	37.6	6.2	14.4	49.6	94.6
	1976	39.6	7.0	14.6	52.8	95.6
	1977	38.2	6.9	15.1	54.2	96.2
	1978	37.8	7.3	15.9	57.4	96.4
N. E. Thames	1975	35.7	7.0	12.2	49.7	94.4
	1976	36.3	8.0	12.5	50.9	95.5
	1977	40.1	8.5	12.3	52.7	96.7
	1978	34.8	9.1	13.2	52.0	97.4
S. E. Thames	1975	36.6	6.3	12.6	50.6	94.6
	1976	36.9	5.8	13.4	53.1	95.5
	1977	40.4	6.7	13.5	53.7	97.0
	1978	39.7	7.1	14.0	54.0	97.7
S. W. Thames	1975	38.7	6.2	15.3	53.8	92.8
	1976	39.6	6.8	16.5	55.8	93.5
	1977	37.2	8.4	15.9	54.3	94.3
	1978	34.9	8.3	16.4	55.8	94.4

* *Excludes women resident outside England and Wales*

248

Area		Percentage of maternities to residents of area				
		Induction	Caesarean section	Instrumental delivery	Episiotomy	All deliveries in NHS hospitals
Regional Health Authorities - continued						
Wessex	1975	34.4	5.6	12.5	47.3	91.7
	1976	29.0	5.1	13.9	51.2	92.2
	1977	33.8	6.1	15.5	53.5	93.9
	1978	32.9	7.6	14.3	54.0	94.1
Oxford	1975	28.3	5.2	16.2	51.5	96.4
	1976	27.0	6.4	15.3	51.6	96.9
	1977	26.0	6.1	15.2	54.0	97.1
	1978	25.7	6.3	13.3	56.2	97.3
South Western	1975	40.7	6.5	13.3	51.0	97.7
	1976	42.5	7.2	15.7	51.1	98.1
	1977	45.1	7.1	14.7	53.3	98.3
	1978	41.8	7.7	16.0	55.3	98.5
West Midlands	1975	24.9	4.9	12.8	46.7	95.6
	1976	23.9	5.5	11.7	47.5	96.5
	1977	24.4	7.4	12.3	47.4	97.2
	1978	22.7	7.2	12.6	48.4	98.1
Mersey	1975	41.5	6.8	10.9	49.2	96.5
	1976	47.2	7.7	12.7	52.0	97.5
	1977	46.1	9.5	12.3	52.5	98.1
	1978	40.6	7.4	12.0	51.3	98.5
North Western	1975	34.0	5.0	10.0	43.9	96.4
	1976	34.2	5.9	11.1	47.2	97.3
	1977	33.9	7.6	10.8	48.2	98.0
	1978	34.8	7.6	10.1	49.6	98.5
Wales	1975	42.4	5.8	11.9	48.6	97.8
	1976	46.8	5.4	13.6	50.8	98.2
	1977	49.9	5.8	14.3	52.2	98.4
	1978	42.5	5.3	13.1	56.0	98.4

Source: OPCS and DHSS, Hospital In-patient Enquiry (maternity) unpublished data

Table A7.35   Obstetric intervention rates by maternal age and parity, England and Wales, 1978

Mother's age	Parity				All parities	
	0	1-3	4 or more	Not known		
Percentage of women delivered by forceps in each age group						
Under 25	18.5	4.8	(1.4)	17.9	13.5	
25-34	26.8	5.9	2.8	16.4	12.9	
35 and over	29.7	8.2	4.8	(23.3)	11.1	
All ages	22.1	5.7	3.5	17.3	13.1	
Percentage of women delivered by caesarean section in each age group						
Under 25	6.0	5.3	(2.7)	9.3	6.1	
25-34	10.2	6.4	6.7	9.5	7.7	
35 and over	31.5	13.1	12.7	(23.3)	16.1	
All ages	8.5	6.5	8.8	10.0	7.5	
Percentage of women having an episiotomy in each age group						
Under 25	69.5	42.1	(16.4)	72.5	59.5	
25-34	72.6	44.9	11.7	60.6	53.4	
35 and over	50.9	40.1	13.3	(43.3)	36.6	
All ages	70.3	43.8	12.5	64.9	55.0	
						Total maternities in NHS hospitals
Numbers of women in the sample						
Under 25	14,253	8,245	73	302	22,873	238,832
25-34	9,804	18,333	891	378	29,406	322,495
35 and over	499	1,914	607	30	3,050	34,188
All ages	24,556	28,492	1,571	710	55,329	595,515

Source: OPCS and DHSS, Hospital In-patient Enquiry (maternity) unpublished data

Table A7.36   Length of postnatal stay in NHS hospitals, England and Wales, 1970-78

	1970	1971	1974	1975	1976	1977	1978
Mean length of postnatal stay (days)	6.3	6.1	5.8	5.8	5.8	5.7	5.5
Estimated percent of women delivered in hospital whose stay was:—							
Less than 3 days	17.9	18.9	18.6	19.0	18.7	19.0	20.5
3-4 days	15.3	16.5	19.8	19.8	19.9	20.1	21.6
5-6 days	16.3	17.0	18.7	20.0	21.0	21.9	22.8
7-8 days	25.3	24.4	22.9	22.0	21.9	21.9	20.8
9-10 days	18.6	17.2	15.3	15.0	14.3	13.3	11.0
11 days or more	6.6	6.0	4.8	4.3	4.3	3.9	3.3
All durations	100	100	100	100	100	100	100

Source: OPCS and DHSS Hospital In-patient Enquiry (maternity)

Table A7.37   Use of services for postnatal care, England and Wales 1975-80

Year	Women attending hospital out-patient clinics	Community care		General Practitioners' claims for fees¢	
		Women attending postnatal clinics*	Women visited at home by midwife	Including some post-natal care†	For complete postnatal care‡
1975	135,624	60,249	475,586	545,186	160,422
1976	129,662	66,209	480,018	523,495	146,102
1977	126,196	70,810	483,632	509,933	138,122
1978	122,744	75,772	537,601	521,296	136,436
1979	124,805	..	583,812	576,622	146,277
1980	118,351	..	624,023	602,336	152,332

* Data not collected after 1978.
† All claims except those for delivery only or for miscarriage.
‡ Care of mother and baby for first 14 days and full postnatal examination at 6 weeks. May include women delivered in hospital but discharged within 48 hours.
¢ Estimates based on a ten per cent sample of claims.
Source: DHSS *Health and Personal Social Services Statistics, 1982,* Welsh Office *Health and Personal Social Services Statistics for Wales, 1979,* DHSS unpublished data

Table A7.38   Postnatal in-patient care, England and Wales, 1975-78

	Estimated number of women			
	1975	1976	1977	1978
Delivery in hospital	574,050	560,710	529,720	553,290
Transferred to other hospital	22,650	24,150	23,260	26,760
Other	551,400	536,560	506,460	526,530
Admitted after birth of baby	21,810	23,160	24,200	26,370
Transferred from other hospital	12,930	14,350	16,390	17,840
Other	8,880	8,810	7,810	8,530
All postnatal cases	595,860	583,880	553,920	579,660
Total maternities	603,666	584,263	569,073	595,515

Source: OPCS and DHSS Hospital In-patient Enquiry and OPCS *Birth Statistics Series FM1*

Table A7.39   Estimated number of discharges from and deaths in Special Care Baby Units, Regional Health Authorities, England and Wales, 1978

Area	Region of residence		Region of treatment
	Number	Percentage of live births	
England and Wales	**92,400**	**15.5**	**92,400**
England	**85,780**	**15.2**	**86,170**
Regional Health Authority			
Northern	5,500	14.4	5,510
Yorkshire	9,230	21.2	9,230
Trent	9,320	17.1	8,730
East Anglia	3,150	14.3	3,400
North West Thames	7,940	18.1	7,320
North East Thames	6,290	13.5	6,730
South East Thames	6,430	15.3	6,660
South West Thames	5,290	16.2	4,950
Wessex	3,970	12.9	3,980
Oxford	3,130	10.6	2,950
South Western	3,240	9.1	3,050
West Midlands	9,830	15.4	10,110
Mersey	5,980	20.0	6,040
North Western	6,480	13.1	6,800
Board of Governors			710
Wales	**6,460**	**19.4**	**6,230**
Outside England and Wales	160		

Source: OPCS and DHSS, *Hospital In-patient Enquiry*

Table A7.40 Infant and child health care by health visitors, England, Wales and Scotland, 1975-81

Year	Clinic attendances (number of children attending child health clinics)		Domiciliary visits by health visitors (number of children visited)	
	Born in year	Others aged under 5	Born in year	Others aged under 5
England				
1975	500.9	1,006.1	618.4	1,760.4
1976	495.9	1,005.0	609.1	1,723.7
1977	486.1	986.0	578.2	1,670.7
1978	470.2	972.0	605.4	1,654.3
1979	525.9	980.7	650.9	1,635.8
1980	550.9	1,017.0	678.5	1,650.9
1981	517.0	1,075.1	646.5	1,638.1
Wales				
1975	30.2	71.4	34.7	113.4
1976	30.7	69.2	35.7	117.2
1977	28.2	69.0	33.2	111.5
1978	29.6	63.5	34.8	108.6
1979	31.5	63.3	37.7	104.9
1980	32.6	67.5	38.7	108.2
1981	30.9	66.5	37.8	108.2
Scotland				
1975	..	..	309.0	
1976	..	..	303.1	
1977	..	..	328.9	
1978	..	..	290.8	
1979	58.5	91.2	280.8	
1980	61.4	96.9	281.0	
1981	59.9	100.8	288.5	

Sources: DHSS, *Health and Personal Social Services Statistics for England*
Welsh Office, *Health and Personal Social Services Statistics for Wales.*
Information Services Division, *Scottish Health Statistics*

Table A8.1 Registration of disabled persons in England, at 31 March 1980

Disability	Age 0-4	5-15	16-29	30-49	50-64	65-74	75 and over	All ages
Visual disability								
*Total on registers**								
Blind	254	1,781		24,630		19,499	61,601	107,765
Partially sighted	157	2,226		13,136		8,494	27,413	51,426
New cases								
Blind	66	147		1,875		2,457	8,069	12,614
Partially sighted	54	204		1,441		1,903	4,684	8,286
Persons with additional disability								
Total	..	..		..		..	..	24,113
Mentally ill	..	..		..		..	..	957
Mentally ill and other	..	..		..		..	..	300
Mentally handicapped	..	..		..		..	..	2,092
Mentally handicapped and other	..	..		..		..	..	888
Physically handicapped	..	..		..		..	..	12,753
Physically handicapped and other	..	..		..		..	..	1,493
Deaf without speech	..	..		..		..	..	290
Deaf with speech	..	..		..		..	..	1,630
Hard of hearing	..	..		..		..	..	3,710
Other disabilities								
*Total on registers**								
Deaf with speech	1,566		2,790	3,196	2,229	2,050	3,039	14,870
Deaf without speech	1,545		2,877	4,393	2,725	1,946	1,309	35,123
General classes †	19,484		25,161	73,970	204,113	252,137	325,804	900,669

* *Figures estimated includes previous year's figures for five authorities who could not provide the information required.*

† *Includes 'very severely handicapped', 'severely or appreciably handicapped', 'other classified persons' and 'unclassified persons'.*

Source: DHSS, *Personal Social Services, Local Authority Statistics A/F80/7* and *A/F80/14*

Table A8.2   Educational provision for handicapped pupils, England, January 1981

	Total	Blind	Partially sighted	Deaf	Partially hearing	Physically handi-capped	Delicate	Mal-adjusted	Educationally sub-normal		Epileptic	Speech defects	Autistic
									Moder-ate	Severe			
Assessment and placement during 1980													
Pupils newly assessed as requiring special educational treatment	22,243	67	288	163	516	1,549	1,049	4,978	10,772	2,042	108	605	106
Pupils newly placed in special schools or boarding homes	22,232	69	304	179	517	1,635	1,009	4,747	10,919	2,150	99	511	93
Handicapped pupils in January 1981													
Attending special schools													
Maintained													
Day pupils	98,601	99	1,003	1,135	660	9,176	2,611	5,523	52,443	24,517	364	706	364
Boarding pupils	12,531	129	261	367	318	758	1,127	3,894	4,943	537	64	74	59
Non-maintained													
Day pupils	1,523	89	152	233	96	413	23	24	349	21	10	82	31
Boarding pupils	5,876	574	374	860	344	951	295	1,160	623	120	341	198	36
Attending maintained and non-maintained hospital special schools	4,373	18	4	4	0	408	31	396	33	3,341	46	18	74
Attending designated special classes at maintained primary, middle and secondary schools	16,456	7	205	491	3,365	639	348	1,822	8,019	269	94	1,085	112

Table A8.2 Educational provision for handicapped pupils, England, January 1981 - *continued*

	Total	Blind	Partially sighted	Deaf	Partially hearing	Physically handicapped	Delicate	Mal-adjusted	Educationally sub-normal		Epileptic	Speech defects	Autistic
									Moderate	Severe			
Handicapped pupils in January 1981 - continued													
Boarded in homes	390	0	0	0	0	1	8	369	6	5	0	0	1
Attending independent schools under arrangements made by authorities	7,372	30	20	314	79	666	172	4,448	510	676	43	110	304
Receiving education otherwise than at school	4,483	10	12	43	72	688	245	2,415	256	534	19	144	45
Awaiting admission to special schools													
Day pupils													
aged 5 and over	2,985	1	22	4	40	109	59	447	2,103	132	3	60	5
under 5	617	4	13	11	27	119	4	6	112	285	3	27	6
Boarding pupils													
aged 5 and over	1,212	10	26	8	9	53	63	752	189	39	20	31	12
under 5	39	4	6	1	19	9	0	0	0	0	0	0	0
All pupils	156,458	975	2,098	3,471	5,029	13,990	4,986	21,256	69,586	30,476	1,007	2,535	1,049
Pupils awaiting admission for more than a year	1,184	7	20	5	40	71	17	146	729	121	4	22	2

Source: Department of Education and Science

Table A8.3 Notifications of selected congenital malformations, England and Wales, 1964-81

Numbers

Year	All	Anencephalus and similar anomalies	Spina bifida*	Congenital hydrocephalus*	Cleft palate*	Total cleft lip*	Oesophageal atresia	Atresia of large gut, rectum and anus	Hypospadias and epispadias	Total reduction deformities*	Exomphalus omphalocele (excluding umbilical hernia)	Down's syndrome
1964	14,564	1,331	2,199			1,236	117	176	672	150	244	667
1965	13,841	1,347	2,158			1,152	119	182	637	149	234	577
1966	13,665	1,233	2,130			1,198	125	195	689	157	236	616
1967	14,062	1,248	2,121			1,171	127	199	700	155	243	613
1968	13,954	1,148	2,062			1,175	107	193	749	154	233	644
1969	13,959	1,118	1,556	456	337	798	82	173	815	324	180	538
1970	14,019	1,137	1,453	401	298	805	120	216	781	335	214	579
1971	14,407	1,166	1,552	432	321	742	133	186	934	316	230	582
1972	14,412	1,084	1,537	364	302	695	102	190	1,016	297	207	560
1973	13,353	849	1,267	336	333	652	121	182	945	286	192	523
1974	12,729	849	1,185	313	274	700	95	199	912	378	208	419
1975	12,230	775	1,101	249	279	583	87	166	875	320	198	454
1976	12,384	644	880	267	283	586	107	185	887	294	196	399
1977	12,402	568	881	259	277	566	98	147	907	257	170	425
1978	12,767	525	841	244	277	558	113	172	953	284	182	444
1979	13,529	455	845	227	273	585	104	190	1,079	264	167	463
1980	14,134	342	756	222	291	627	108	179	1,000	302	150	481
1981	13,450	247	653	188	259	605	112	157	1,016	256	169	475

* Definition changed in 1969

257

Table A8.3 Notifications of selected congenital malformations, England and Wales, 1964-81 - *continued*

Rates per 10,000 total births

Year	All	Anencephalus and similar anomalies	Spina bifida*	Congenital hydrocephalus*	Cleft palate*	Total cleft lip*	Oesophageal atresia	Atresia of large gut, rectum and anus	Hypospadias and epispadius	Total reduction deformities*	Exomphalus omphalocele (excluding umbilical hernia)	Down's syndrome
1964	163.55	14.95	24.69		13.88		1.31	1.98	7.55	1.68	2.74	7.49
1965	157.90	15.37	24.62		13.14		1.36	2.08	7.27	1.70	2.67	6.58
1966	158.33	14.29	24.68		13.88		1.45	2.26	7.98	1.82	2.73	7.14
1967	166.47	14.77	25.11		13.86		1.50	2.36	8.29	1.83	2.88	7.26
1968	167.89	13.81	24.81		14.14		1.29	2.32	9.01	1.85	2.80	7.75
1969	172.72	13.83	19.25	5.64	4.17	9.87	1.01	2.14	10.08	4.01	2.23	6.66
1970	176.38	14.30	18.28	5.05	3.75	10.13	1.51	2.72	9.83	4.21	2.69	7.28
1971	181.66	14.70	19.57	5.45	4.05	9.36	1.68	2.35	11.78	3.98	2.90	7.34
1972	196.28	14.76	20.93	4.96	4.11	9.47	1.39	2.59	13.84	4.05	2.82	7.63
1973	195.25	12.41	18.53	4.91	4.87	9.53	1.77	2.66	13.82	4.18	2.81	7.65
1974	196.72	13.12	18.31	4.84	4.23	10.82	1.47	3.08	14.09	5.84	3.21	6.48
1975	200.58	12.71	18.06	4.08	4.58	9.56	1.43	2.72	14.35	5.25	3.25	7.45
1976	209.91	10.92	14.92	4.53	4.80	9.93	1.81	3.14	15.03	4.98	3.32	6.76
1977	215.81	9.88	15.33	4.51	4.82	9.85	1.71	2.56	15.78	4.47	2.96	7.40
1978	212.24	8.73	13.98	4.06	4.60	9.28	1.88	2.86	15.84	4.72	3.03	7.38
1979	210.35	7.07	13.14	3.53	4.24	9.10	1.62	2.95	16.78	4.10	2.60	7.20
1980	213.83	5.17	11.44	3.36	4.40	9.49	1.63	2.71	15.13	4.57	2.27	7.28
1981	210.60	3.87	10.38	2.94	4.06	9.47	1.75	2.46	15.91	4.01	2.65	7.44

* *Definition changed in 1969*

Table A8.3 Notifications of selected congenital malformations, England and Wales, 1964-81 - *continued*

Site of Malformation		1964	1965	1966	1967	1968
Hydrocephalus without spina bifida	Number	633	537	514	517	527
	Rate†	7.1	6.1	6.0	6.1	6.3
Spina bifida without hydrocephalus	Number	1,081	1,124	1,138	1,113	1,023
	Rate†	12.1	12.8	13.2	13.2	12.3
Hydrocephalus and spina bifida	Number	485	497	478	491	512
	Rate†	5.4	5.7	5.5	5.8	6.2
Cleft lip without cleft palate	Number	340	347	361	334	304
	Rate†	3.8	4.0	4.2	4.0	3.7
Cleft palate without cleft lip	Number	397	339	339	327	350
	Rate†	4.5	3.9	3.9	3.9	4.2
Cleft lip and cleft palate	Number	499	466	498	510	521
	Rate†	5.6	5.3	5.8	6.0	6.3

† *Per 10,000 total births*

Source: OPCS, congenital malformation notifications

Table A8.4 Stillbirths due to anencephaly, by age of mother, England and Wales, 1961-80

Rates per 1,000 total births

Year	Age of mother at birth							
	All ages	Under 20	20-24	25-29	30-34	35-39	40-44	45 and over
1961	2.0	2.6	2.1	1.9	1.9	2.1	2.4	4.1
1962	1.8	2.2	2.0	1.7	1.7	1.8	1.8	4.4
1963	1.8	2.2	1.9	1.5	1.7	2.1	1.9	2.4
1964	1.7	2.0	1.8	1.6	1.5	2.1	1.8	1.5
1965	1.7	2.0	1.7	1.5	1.6	1.7	1.9	2.8
1966	1.6	2.0	1.6	1.5	1.5	2.1	2.0	-
1967	1.6	2.2	1.5	1.4	1.4	1.7	1.8	1.5
1968	1.5	2.0	1.5	1.3	1.3	1.6	1.8	1.7
1969	1.5	1.9	1.7	1.3	1.3	1.5	1.0	1.9
1970	1.5	1.9	1.6	1.3	1.4	1.8	1.9	2.1
1971	1.6	1.8	1.7	1.4	1.4	1.5	2.7	1.2
1972	1.6	1.7	1.9	1.5	1.3	1.5	2.3	2.8
1973	1.4	1.7	1.5	1.3	1.3	1.5	2.1	1.6
1974	1.4	1.8	1.5	1.3	1.2	1.6	2.2	7.3
1975	1.4	1.6	1.5	1.3	1.2	0.9	2.1	5.3
1976	1.2	1.5	1.4	1.1	1.0	0.9	0.7	2.0
1977	1.1	1.4	1.2	1.0	0.9	1.2	0.2	-
1978	0.9	1.6	1.0	0.9	0.7	0.8	1.0	-
1979	0.7	1.1	0.7	0.7	0.7	0.5	0.5	3.9
1980	0.5	0.6	0.6	0.5	0.4	0.4	0.6	-

Source: OPCS, *Mortality statistics: childhood, Series DH3* and *Registrar General's Statistical Reviews*

Table A8.5 Central nervous system malformations, England and Wales, 1969-1980   *Numbers and rates*

Year	Notifications		Stillbirths and deaths		Abortions		Abortions and notifications		Abortions, stillbirths and deaths	
	Number	Rate*	Number	Rate*	Number	Rate†	Number	Rate†	Number	Rate†
1969	3,302	4.1	2,172	2.7	..	..	..	..	..	..
1970	3,183	4.0	2,143	2.7	..	..	..	..	..	..
1971	3,378	4.3	2,294	2.9	..	..	..	..	..	..
1972	3,129	4.3	2,117	2.9	51	0.07	3,180	4.3	2,168	3.0
1973	2,553	3.7	1,836	2.7	45	0.07	2,598	3.8	1,881	2.8
1974	2,452	3.8	1,755	2.7	34	0.05	2,486	3.8	1,789	2.8
1975	2,227	3.7	1,576	2.6	73	0.12	2,300	3.8	1,649	2.7
1976	1,915	3.3	1,364	2.3	81	0.14	1,996	3.4	1,445	2.4
1977	1,869	3.3	1,279	2.2	124	0.22	1,993	3.5	1,403	2.4
1978	1,757	2.9	1,142	1.9	..	..	..	..	..	..
1979	1,637	2.6	1,167	1.8	285	0.44	1,922	3.0	1,452	2.3
1980	1,476	2.2	1,052	1.6	418	0.63	1,894	2.9	1,470	2.2

* *Per 1,000 total births*
† *Per 1,000 total births and abortions*

Source: OPCS, *Mortality statistics, childhood, Series DH3* and *Abortion statistics, Series AB*

Table A8.6 Cases of confirmed or suspected congenital rubella reported to the National Congenital Rubella Surveillance Programme, Great Britain, 1971-81

Year of birth	Number of cases	Rate per 100,000 live births	Clinical manifestations—percentage of cases with:				Maternal history—percentage of cases with:		
			Multiple defects	Single defect	Neonatal manifestation	None	Rubella-like illness	Rubella contact only	No history of illness, contact or rash
Before 1970	96	..	40	57	0	3	51	10	26
1970	60	6.9	32	57	2	10	41	14	29
1971	64	7.4	33	47	8	13	45	15	28
1972	81	10.1	42	41	6	11	41	22	30
1973	89	11.7	34	43	7	17	47	23	21
1974	52	7.0	35	52	4	10	52	13	21
1975	56	7.2	46	25	7	21	36	18	27
1976	33	5.1	48	36	0	15	52	3	26
1977	16	2.5	68	25	0	6	40	13	40
1978	43	6.5	42	23	5	30	56	16	16
1979	62	8.8	63	13	2	23	63	12	13
1980	12	1.6	58	8	0	33	58	17	8
All notified cases	664		42	40	4	14	48	15	24

Source: National Congenital Rubella Surveillance Programme

Table A8.7 Legal abortions on grounds of rubella, England Wales, 1969-80

Year	Rubella	Rubella contact	Rubella immunization	Total
1969	..	..	..	907
1970	..	..	..	919
1971	791	229	43	1,063
1972	579	161	39	779
1973	681	136	23	840
1974	512	121	31	664
1975	406	98	27	531
1976	144	69	40	253
1977	118	66	37	221
1978	659	171	66	896
1979	431	144	156	731
1980	153	47	101	301

Source: OPCS, *Abortion statistics, Series AB*

Table A9.1 Notifications of whooping cough in children aged under one year, by sex, England and Wales†, 1944-81

Year	Male Number	Male Rate‡	Female Number	Female Rate‡	Total Number	Total Rate‡
1944	5,053	1,431.4	5,018	1,493.5	10,071	1,461.7
1945	3,312	933.0	3,337	996.1	6,649	963.6
1946	4,585	1,273.6	4,783	1,402.6	9,368	1,336.4
1947	5,426	1,213.9	5,574	1,311.5	11,000	1,261.5
1948	7,305	1,817.2	7,627	1,991.4	14,932	1,902.2
1949	4,809	1,282.4	4,915	1,380.6	9,724	1,330.2
1950	6,577	1,842.3	6,468	1,896.8	13,045	1,868.9
1951	7,333	2,119.4	7,463	2,275.3	14,796	2,195.3
1952	5,041	1,500.3	5,167	1,619.7	10,208	1,558.5
1953	6,928	2,037.6	7,050	2,175.9	13,978	2,105.1
1954	4,709	1,372.9	4,729	1,446.2	9,438	1,408.7
1955	3,517	1,049.9	3,576	1,124.5	7,093	1,086.2
1956	4,299	1,235.3	4,167	1,266.6	8,466	1,250.5
1957	3,753	1,051.3	3,851	1,136.0	7,604	1,092.5
1958	1,637	442.4	1,669	475.5	3,306	458.5
1959	1,683	445.2	1,636	457.0	3,319	451.0
1960	2,975	780.8	2,894	803.9	5,869	792.0
1961	1,257	312.4	1,179	309.9	2,436	311.2
1962	515	123.5	511	128.7	1,026	126.1
1963	2,013	475.5	2,104	519.1	4,117	496.9
1964	1,772	412.4	1,852	450.5	3,624	431.0
1965	710	164.3	723	174.6	1,433	169.3
1966	1,075	252.0	1,022	250.1	2,097	251.0
1967	1,456	345.8	1,568	389.3	3,024	367.0
1968	893	219.4	860	218.6	1,753	219.0
1969	335	82.7	293	75.0	628	78.9
1970	966	247.6	1,040	281.0	2,006	263.8
1971	1,082	270.7	1,073	282.9	2,155	276.6
1972	141	37.3	122	34.1	263	35.8
1973	167	47.0	163	48.6	330	47.7
1974	1,089	330.3	1,086	348.6	2,175	339.2
1975	706	222.9	688	230.7	1,394	226.7
1976	238	79.1	240	84.3	478	81.7
1977	959	333.8	985	362.7	1,944	347.8
1978	3,444	1,180.7	3,232	1,168.1	6,676	1,174.5
1979	1,611	507.6	1,587	528.5	3,198	517.7
1980	1,100	335.4	1,061	341.0	2,161	338.1
1981	962	296.1	954	308.2	1,916	302.0

Excluding port health districts
Rate per 100,000 population aged under one year

Source: OPCS Notifications of communicable diseases

Table A9.2 Notifications of measles in children aged under one year, by sex, England and Wales†, 1944-8

Year	Male		Female		Total	
	Number	Rate‡	Number	Rate‡	Number	Rate‡
1944	3,102	878.8	3,032	902.4	6,134	890.3
1945	9,724	2,739.2	9,422	2,812.5	19,146	2,774.8
1946	3,372	936.7	3,494	1,024.6	6,866	979.5
1947	8,405	1,880.3	8,481	1,955.5	16,886	1,936.5
1948	8,217	2,044.0	8,285	2,163.2	16,502	2,102.2
1949	7,445	1,985.3	7,487	2,103.1	14,932	2,042.7
1950	6,507	1,822.7	6,719	1,970.4	13,226	1,894.8
1951	10,545	3,047.7	10,445	3,184.5	20,990	3,114.2
1952	6,048	1,800.0	6,203	1,944.5	12,251	1,870.4
1953	8,654	2,545.3	8,737	2,696.6	17,391	2,619.1
1954	2,801	816.6	2,951	902.4	5,752	858.5
1955	9,917	2,960.3	10,109	3,178.9	20,026	3,066.8
1956	2,484	713.8	2,602	790.9	5,086	751.3
1957	9,294	2,603.4	9,360	2,761.1	18,654	2,680.2
1958	3,892	1,051.9	4,076	1,161.3	7,968	1,105.1
1959	8,185	2,165.3	8,323	2,324.9	16,508	2,242.9
1960	2,872	753.8	2,888	802.2	5,760	777.3
1961	12,540	3,116.3	12,618	3,317.0	25,158	3,213.8
1962	3,073	737.1	3,075	774.6	6,148	755.4
1963	10,467	2,472.7	10,604	2,616.3	21,071	2,543.0
1964	6,400	1,489.4	6,380	1,551.9	12,780	1,520.0
1965	10,090	2,334.6	9,766	2,357.8	19,856	2,345.9
1966	7,176	1,682.1	7,108	1,739.2	14,284	1,710.0
1967	9,378	2,227.0	9,154	2,272.6	18,532	2,249.3
1968	5,546	1,362.3	5,342	1,357.9	10,888	1,360.1
1969	3,556	877.6	3,403	871.4	6,959	874.6
1970	7,135	1,828.5	6,975	1,884.6	14,110	1,855.8
1971	3,493	873.9	3,259	859.2	6,752	866.8
1972	3,694	978.0	3,653	1,022.1	7,347	999.5
1973	3,432	965.1	3,354	999.7	6,786	981.9
1974	2,436	738.9	2,372	761.5	4,808	749.8
1975	2,875	907.8	2,829	948.7	5,704	927.6
1976	1,419	417.9	1,430	502.5	2,849	486.8
1977	3,498	1,217.5	3,371	1,241.2	6,869	1,229.0
1978	2,508	859.8	2,403	868.4	4,911	864.0
1979	2,081	655.6	2,010	669.3	4,091	662.3
1980	3,731	1,137.5	3,675	1,181.3	7,406	1,158.8
1981	2,050	631.0	1,987	642.0	4,037	636.3

† *Excluding port health districts*
‡ *Rate per 100,000 population aged under one year*

Source: OPCS, Notifications of communicable diseases

264

Table A9.3 Notifications of acute meningitis (known as meningococcal infection during 1956-67), in children aged under one year, by sex, England and Wales,† 1956-81

Year	Male		Female		Total	
	Number	Rate‡	Number	Rate‡	Number	Rate‡
1956	168	48.3	111	33.7	279	41.2
1957	177	49.6	125	36.9	302	43.4
1958	158	42.7	108	30.8	266	36.9
1959	126	33.3	103	28.8	229	31.1
1960	101	26.5	66	18.3	167	22.5
1961	111	27.6	77	20.2	188	24.0
1962	90	21.6	65	16.4	155	19.0
1963	101	23.9	65	16.0	166	20.0
1964	79	18.4	47	11.4	126	15.0
1965	72	16.7	42	10.1	114	13.5
1966	67	15.7	43	10.5	110	13.2
1967	51	12.1	29	7.2	80	9.7
1968	72	17.7	47	11.9	119	14.9
1969	124	30.6	96	24.6	220	27.6
1970 (1)	80	20.5	48	13.0	128	16.8
(2)	27	6.9	34	9.2	61	8.0
(3)	27	6.9	29	7.8	56	7.4
1971 (1)	80	20.0	42	11.1	122	15.7
(2)	36	9.0	33	8.7	69	8.9
(3)	28	7.0	17	4.5	45	5.8
1972 (1)	65	17.2	58	16.2	123	16.7
(2)	23	6.1	28	7.8	51	6.9
(3)	32	8.5	13	3.6	45	6.1
1973 (1)	145	40.8	95	28.3	240	34.7
(2)	34	9.6	27	8.0	61	8.8
(3)	34	9.6	28	8.3	62	9.0
1974 (1)	180	54.6	118	37.9	298	46.5
(2)	54	16.4	29	9.3	83	12.9
(3)	32	9.7	22	7.1	54	8.4

Excluding port health districts
Rate per 100,000 population aged under one year
(1) Meningococcus
(2) Other specified organisms
(3) Unspecified organisms

Table A9.3 Notifications of acute meningitis (known as meningococcal infection during 1956-67), in children aged under one year by sex, England Wales, 1956-81 - *continued*

Year		Male		Female		Total	
		Number	Rate‡	Number	Rate‡	Number	Rate‡
1975	(1)	103	32.5	77	25.8	180	29.3
	(2)	52	16.4	43	14.4	95	15.4
	(3)	39	12.3	27	9.1	66	10.7
1976	(1)	76	25.3	65	22.8	141	24.1
	(2)	38	12.6	31	10.9	69	11.8
	(3)	24	8.0	16	5.6	40	6.8
1977	(1)	52	18.1	34	12.5	86	15.4
	(2)	50	17.4	41	15.1	91	16.3
	(3)	23	8.0	21	7.7	44	7.9
1978	(1)	60	20.6	37	13.4	97	17.1
	(2)	49	16.8	50	18.1	99	17.4
	(3)	33	11.3	31	11.2	64	11.3
1979	(1)	70	22.1	34	11.3	104	16.8
	(2)	77	24.3	49	16.3	126	20.4
	(3)	38	12.0	26	8.7	64	10.4
1980	(1)	67	20.4	49	15.8	116	18.2
	(2)	69	21.0	55	17.7	124	19.4
	(3)	34	10.4	20	6.4	54	8.4
1981	(1)	63	19.4	35	11.3	98	15.4
	(2)	50	15.4	37	12.0	87	13.7
	(3)	28	8.6	9	2.9	37	5.8

‡ *Rate per 100,000 population aged under one year*

(1) Meningococcus
(2) Other specified organisms
(3) Unspecified organisms

Source: OPCS, Notifications of communicable diseases

Table A9.4 Notifications of dysentery in children aged under one year, by sex, England and Wales†, 1956-81

Year	Male		Female		Total	
	Number	Rate‡	Number	Rate‡	Number	Rate‡
1956	932	267.8	810	246.2	1,742	257.3
1957	663	185.7	551	162.5	1,214	174.4
1958	898	242.7	793	225.9	1,691	234.5
1959	812	214.8	746	208.4	1,558	211.7
1960	859	225.5	757	210.3	1,616	218.1
1961	523	130.0	473	124.3	996	127.2
1962	859	206.0	672	169.3	1,531	188.1
1963	704	166.3	645	159.1	1,349	162.8
1964	595	138.5	507	123.3	1,102	131.1
1965	668	154.6	569	137.4	1,237	146.1
1966	538	126.1	444	108.6	982	117.6
1967	551	130.8	447	111.0	998	121.1
1968	511	125.5	423	107.5	934	116.7
1969	556	137.2	522	133.7	1,078	135.5
1970	310	79.4	293	79.2	603	79.3
1971	360	90.1	284	74.9	644	82.7
1972	295	78.1	260	72.7	555	75.5
1973	266	74.8	211	62.9	477	69.0
1974	242	73.4	219	70.3	461	71.9
1975	223	70.4	191	64.1	414	67.3
1976	187	62.2	143	50.2	330	56.4
1977	144	50.1	110	40.5	254	45.4
1978	117	40.1	95	34.3	212	37.3
1979	88	27.7	69	23.0	157	25.4
1980	87	26.5	71	22.8	158	24.7
1981	103	31.7	80	25.8	183	28.8

† Excluding port health districts
‡ Rate per 100,000 population aged under one year

Source: OPCS, Notifications of communicable diseases

267

Table A9.5 Notifications of scarlet fever in children aged under one year, by sex, England and Wales†, 1944-81

Year	Male		Female		Total	
	Number	Rate‡	Number	Rate‡	Number	Rate‡
1944	194	55.0	158	47.0	352	51.1
1945	174	49.0	176	52.5	350	50.7
1946	150	41.7	114	33.4	264	37.7
1947	111	24.8	103	24.2	214	24.5
1948	144	35.8	123	32.1	267	34.0
1949	122	32.5	108	30.3	230	31.5
1950	133	37.3	125	36.7	258	37.0
1951	87	25.1	102	31.1	189	28.0
1952	105	31.2	87	27.3	192	29.3
1953	94	27.6	84	25.9	178	26.8
1954	71	20.7	70	21.4	141	21.0
1955	64	19.1	49	15.4	113	17.3
1956	55	15.8	58	17.6	113	16.7
1957	50	14.0	45	13.3	95	13.6
1958	67	18.1	77	21.9	144	20.0
1959	96	25.4	83	23.2	179	24.3
1960	86	22.6	82	22.8	168	22.7
1961	57	14.2	54	14.2	111	14.2
1962	34	8.2	24	6.0	58	7.1
1963	47	11.1	57	14.1	104	12.6
1964	52	12.1	38	9.2	90	10.7
1965	75	17.4	54	13.0	129	15.2
1966	63	14.8	71	17.4	134	16.0
1967	48	11.4	45	11.2	93	11.3
1968	64	15.7	42	10.7	106	13.2
1969	44	10.9	51	13.1	95	11.9
1970	45	11.5	45	12.2	90	11.8
1971	28	7.0	32	8.4	60	7.7
1972	40	10.6	37	10.4	77	10.5
1973	35	9.8	36	10.7	71	10.3
1974	43	13.0	38	12.2	81	12.6
1975	27	8.5	27	9.1	54	8.8
1976	34	11.3	34	11.9	68	11.6
1977	40	13.9	39	14.4	79	14.1
1978	42	14.4	33	11.9	75	13.2
1979	39	12.3	22	7.3	61	9.9
1980	55	16.8	38	12.2	93	14.6
1981	32	9.8	33	10.7	65	10.2

† *Excluding port health districts*
‡ *Rate per 100,000 population aged under one year*

Source: OPCS, Notifications of communicable diseases

Table A9.6   Notifications of opthalmia neonatorum, England and Wales†, 1915-81

Year	Number	Rate‡	Year	Number	Rate‡
1915	6,802	8.3	1951	1,762	2.6
1916	7,611	9.7	1952	1,788	2.7
1917	6,712	10.0	1953	1,772	2.6
1918	6,532	9.9	1954	1,684	2.5
1919	8,648	12.5	1955	1,771	2.7
1920	10,302	10.8	1956	1,515	2.2
			1957	1,483	2.1
1921	8,312	9.8	1958	1,304	1.8
1922	7,106	9.1	1959	1,179	1.6
1923	6,592	8.7	1960	1,063	1.4
1924	6,267	8.6			
1925	5,748	8.1	1961	932	1.1
1926	5,896	8.5	1962	1,017	1.2
1927	5,891	9.0	1963	970	1.1
1928	5,609	8.5	1964	832	0.9
1929	5,448	8.5	1965	727	0.8
1930	5,481	8.4	1966	612	0.7
			1967	606	0.7
1931	5,158	8.2	1968	588	0.7
1932	4,730	7.7	1969	434	0.5
1933	4,056	7.0	1970	464	0.6
1934	4,487	7.5			
1935	4,369	7.3	1971	428	0.5
1936	4,586	7.6	1972	358	0.5
1937	5,050	8.3	1973	366	0.5
1938	5,168	8.3	1974	316	0.5
1939	4,594	7.5	1975	265	0.4
1940	4,390	7.4	1976	222	0.4
			1977	239	0.4
1941	4,195	7.2	1978	228	0.4
1942	4,516	6.9	1979	235	0.4
1943	4,502	6.6	1980	278	0.4
1944	3,659	4.9			
1945	3,314	4.9	1981	201	0.3
1946	3,416	4.2			
1947	3,245	3.7			
1948	2,729	3.5			
1949	2,229	3.1			
1950	1,935	2.8			

† *Excluding port health districts.*
‡ *Rate per 1,000 live births.*
Source: OPCS, Notifications of communicable diseases

Table A9.7 Estimated hospital in-patient stays by children aged under one year, by sex, England and Wales, 1978

ICD code	Cause	Estimated total discharge rates per 100,000 population			Mean duration of stay, days	
		Male	Female	Total	Male	Female
A1-137, AN138-150, Y40-79	**All causes**	**3,618.8**	**2,825.8**	**3,232.8**	**7.7**	**8.5**
A1-44	Infective and parasitic diseases	256.8	233.1	245.2	7.8	8.3
A45-58	All malignant neoplasms	4.5	2.5	3.5	14.3	69.1
A59, 60	Neoplasms of lymphatic and haematopoietic tissues	1.0	1.4	1.2	11.3	1.3
A61	Benign neoplasms and neoplasms of unspecified nature	6.9	4.3	5.6	6.4	2.4
A62-66	Endocrine, nutritional and metabolic diseases	144.3	113.8	129.5	9.1	8.5
A67, 68	Diseases of blood and blood-forming organs	9.3	4.3	6.9	6.0	18.0
A69-71	Mental disorders	16.5	12.3	14.4	8.2	5.9
A72-74, A79 pt	Diseases of nervous system	26.7	27.5	27.1	12.1	13.1
A75-77, A79 pt	Diseases of eye	23.7	22.8	23.2	4.5	7.0
A78, A79 pt	Diseases of ear and mastoid process	36.7	24.2	30.6	5.5	5.6
A80-84	Rheumatic fever, hypertensive disease and heart disease	9.9	7.2	8.6	6.4	6.2
A85-88	Diseases of peripheral circulatory system	3.8	2.2	3.0	5.9	7.2
A89-96	Diseases of respiratory system	377.1	261.3	320.7	6.0	6.0
A97-104	Diseases of digestive system	170.7	66.9	120.2	5.4	5.9
A105-108, 111 pt	Diseases of urinary system	21.3	21.0	21.1	9.2	7.7
A109, 111 pt	Male genital disorders	29.5	—	15.1	2.0	—
A110, 111 pt	Diseases of breast and female genital system	0.3	5.1	2.6	0.0	3.4
A112-118 Y60, Y61	Conditions of pregnancy, childbirth and puerperium	—	—	—	—	—
A119, 120	Diseases of skin and subcutaneous tissue	46.3	34.0	40.3	7.6	6.5
A121-125	Diseases of musculoskeletal system and connective tissue	6.2	9.8	7.9	8.6	7.6
A126-130	Congenital anomalies	294.1	221.9	259.0	10.6	11.6
A131-135	Certain causes of perinatal morbidity	1,347.6	1,109.5	1,231.7	9.0	10.0
A136, 137	Symptoms and ill-defined conditions	587.9	473.4	532.2	5.9	6.3
AN138-142	Fractures, dislocations and sprains	18.2	14.8	16.5	8.5	5.9
AN143-150	Other injuries and reactions	92.9	78.4	85.9	5.5	4.4
Y43, Y40-52 rem Y62-79	Persons undergoing preventive measures and those without current complaint or sickness	86.7	74.1	80.6	5.8	4.5

Source: OPCS and DHSS, *Hospital In-patient Enquiry*

Table A10.1 Mortality of women in, or associated with, childbirth, England and Wales, 1891-1939

Year	Classification in use from 1911 onwards				Classification in use before 1911				Total mortality from, or associated with, pregnancy or childbirth◆
	Puerperal (including post-abortive) sepsis	Other puerperal causes including abortion◆	Total mortality from pregnancy and child-bearing◆	Associated causes*	Puerperal (including post-abortive) sepsis	Other puerperal causes including abortion◆	Total mortality from pregnancy and child-bearing◆	Associated causes†	
Rates per 1,000 live births									
1891-95	—	—	—	—	2.60	2.89	5.49	—	—
1896-1900	—	—	—	—	2.12	2.57	4.69	—	—
1901-05	—	—	—	—	1.95	2.32	4.27	1.29	5.56
1906-10	—	—	—	—	1.56	2.18	3.74	1.26	5.00
1911-15	1.42	2.61	4.03	0.99	1.50	2.31	3.81	1.21	5.02
1916-20	1.51	2.61	4.12	1.68	1.59	2.29	3.88	1.92	5.80
1921-25	1.40	2.50	3.90	1.14	1.48	2.21	3.69	1.35	5.04
1926-30	1.73	2.54	4.27	1.24	1.78	2.23	4.01	1.50	5.51
1931-35	1.76	2.54	4.30	1.29	1.83	2.29	4.12	1.48	5.60
1911	1.43	2.44	3.87	1.04	1.52	2.15	3.67	1.24	4.91
1912	1.39	2.59	3.98	0.97	1.47	2.31	3.78	1.17	4.95
1913	1.26	2.70	3.96	0.91	1.34	2.37	3.71	1.16	4.87
1914	1.55	2.62	4.17	0.95	1.63	2.32	3.95	1.17	5.12
1915	1.47	2.71	4.18	1.09	1.56	2.38	3.94	1.38	5.27
1916	1.38	2.74	4.12	0.94	1.47	2.40	3.87	1.19	5.06
1917	1.31	2.58	3.89	0.95	1.39	2.27	3.66	1.18	4.84
1918	1.28	2.51	3.79	3.81	1.35	2.20	3.55	4.05	7.60
1919	1.67	2.70	4.37	1.93	1.76	2.36	4.12	2.18	6.30
1920	1.81	2.52	4.33	1.13	1.87	2.25	4.12	1.34	5.46
1921	1.38	2.54	3.92	1.08	1.46	2.25	3.71	1.29	5.00
1922	1.39	2.42	3.81	1.35	1.46	2.12	3.58	1.58	5.16
1923	1.30	2.52	3.82	1.00	1.38	2.22	3.60	1.22	4.82
1924	1.39	2.51	3.90	1.16	1.48	2.22	3.70	1.36	5.06
1925	1.56	2.52	4.08	1.07	1.62	2.24	3.86	1.29	5.15
1926	1.60	2.52	4.12	1.02	1.64	2.23	3.87	1.27	5.14
1927	1.57	2.54	4.11	1.32	1.63	2.20	3.83	1.60	5.43
1928	1.79	2.63	4.42	1.20	1.85	2.30	4.15	1.47	5.62
1929	1.80	2.53	4.33	1.49	1.83	2.24	4.07	1.75	5.82
1930	1.92	2.48	4.40	1.19	1.96	2.19	4.16	1.43	5.59
1931	1.66	2.45	4.11	1.44	1.71	2.22	3.93	1.62	5.55
1932	1.61	2.60	4.21	1.16	1.68	2.33	4.01	1.36	5.37
1933	1.83	2.68	4.51	1.43	1.90	2.42	4.32	1.62	5.94
1934	2.03	2.57	4.60	1.25	2.10	2.30	4.39	1.45	5.85
1935	1.68	2.42	4.10	1.19	1.75	2.20	3.95	1.34	5.29
1936	1.39	2.41	3.80	1.10	1.47	2.18	3.65	1.25	4.90
1937	0.98	2.28	3.26	1.24	1.03	2.07	3.10	1.40	4.50
1938	0.89	2.19	3.09	1.01	0.93	2.04	2.97	1.13	4.10
1939	0.77	2.16	2.93	0.90	0.81	1.98	2.79	1.04	3.83

* 629 deaths in 1938 and 554 in 1939

† Adding in 1938 and 1939 respectively, 73 and 87 deaths from puerperal nephritis and albuminuria and 0 and 1 deaths from tetanus

◆ Excluding criminal abortion

Source: *Registrar General's Statistical Review* for 1938 and 1939

Table A10.2 Maternal deaths from principal causes and associated maternal deaths, England and Wales, 1931-81
(a) 1935-78

Year	Maternal deaths (complications of pregnancy, childbirth and puerperium, including abortion)								
	Puerperal phlebitis, thrombosis and embolism	Puerperal sepsis	Haemorrhage		Toxaemia	Prolonged labour	Trauma, shock: other complications of delivery	Other causes	Total maternal causes other than abortion
			Ante-partum	Post-partum					
	ICD code 671, 673	630, 635, 670	632, 651	652, 653	636, 639	654-657	658-661	Rem 630-639, 650-678	630-639, 650-678
Numbers									
1935	192	647	292		488	507			2,126
1936	183	561	302		510	455			2,011
1937	152	347	307		510	457			1,773
1938	178	277	312		472	503			1,742
1939	154	248	117	179	478	467			1,643
1940†	134	195	106	180	398	125	111	124	1,373
1941	134	141	101	210	381	155	109	122	1,353
1942	128	151	87	198	410	158	94	133	1,359
1943	136	132	86	187	375	165	106	112	1,299
1944	107	105	84	179	328	176	87	113	1,179
1945	86	82	68	158	321	148	72	92	1,027
1946	102	53	85	162	359	117	83	91	1,052
1947	110	33	56	156	312	110	63	77	917
1948	67	33	46	115	249	66	55	55	686
1949	56	32	38	90	199	69	60	65	609
1950†	62	26	44	38	185	42	54	66	517
1951	49	16	35	53	141	38	37	50	419
1952	52	10	19	39	122	32	43	56	373
1953	49	17	39	51	143	31	34	55	419
1954	51	13	32	44	104	32	41	53	370
1955	55	17	24	41	91	31	23	57	·339

* Excludes the following cases in which it was stated that the interval elapsing between the onset of the maternal condition and death exceeded 12 months: 1951-40, 1952-35, 1953-32, 1954-34, 1955-34, 1956-25, 1957-16, 1958-22, 1959-21, 1960-26, 1961-11, 1962-20, 1963-24, 1964-25, 1965-9, 1966-17, 1967-11, 1968-12, 1969-13, 1970-5, 1971-3, 1972-3, 1973-7, 1974-1, 1975-2, 1976-1, 1977-2, 1978-2.

† Revision of the ICD was made in these years

Abortion					Total mater-nal deaths*	Associated maternal deaths			Total attri-buted to, or associ-ated with, mater-nal causes	Year
Criminal		Other		All forms		Other than abortion	With abortion	Total		
With sepsis	With-out men-tion of sepsis	With sepsis	With-out men-tion of sepsis							
642.0, 642.2	Rem 642	640, 641, 643.0-645.2	640, 641 643.1-645.9	640-645	630-678					
Numbers										
64	30	262	108	464	2,590	638	74	712	3,302	1935
49	24	242	105	420	2,431	541	70	611	3,042	1936
56	28	176	109	369	2,142	585	104	689	2,831	1937
54	26	173	101	354	2,096	449	81	530	2,626	1938
80	28	167	79	354	1,997	429	49	478	2,475	1939
43	33	116	76	268	1,641	368	56	424	2,065	1940
66	24	145	90	325	1,678	358	47	405	2,083	1941
64	12	175	62	313	1,672	363	49	412	2,084	1942
76	15	166	64	321	1,620	437	57	494	2,114	1943
75	7	168	63	313	1,492	383	52	435	1,927	1944
65	9	109	50	233	1,260	342	19	361	1,621	1945
41	5	69	42	157	1,209	353	37	390	1,599	1946
37	3	54	49	143	1,060	264	44	308	1,368	1947
34	4	55	32	125	811	231	16	247	1,058	1948
20	9	58	31	118	727	157	19	176	903	1949
25	21	39	18	103	620	180	21	201	821	1950
33	26	34	14	107	526	151	9	160	686	1951
19	28	28	15	90	463	153	8	161	624	1952
17	24	22	13	76	495	121	7	128	623	1953
10	25	22	19	76	446	116	5	121	567	1954
17	15	19	15	66	405	108	7	115	520	1955

Year	Maternal deaths (complications of pregnancy, childbirth and puerperium, including abortion)								
	Puerperal phlebitis, thrombosis and embolism	Puerperal sepsis	Haemorrhage		Toxaemia	Prolonged labour	Trauma, shock: other complications of delivery	Other causes	Total maternal causes other than abortion
			Ante-partum	Post-partum					
	ICD code 671, 673	630, 635, 670	632, 651	652, 653	636, 639	654-657	658-661	Rem 630-639, 650-678	630-639, 650-678
	Numbers								
1956	32	13	33	24	93	34	15	58	302
1957	32	18	27	22	77	27	23	46	272
1958†	40	13	25	33	66	21	20	47	265
1959	30	17	21	23	57	18	26	51	243
1960	27	8	25	19	63	26	36	44	248
1961	24	6	20	23	55	15	32	45	220
1962	34	12	23	20	53	20	23	57	242
1963	20	8	17	21	46	9	18	55	194
1964	22	10	7	12	34	13	26	53	177
1965	17	5	13	11	48	12	23	40	169
1966	11	9	13	14	38	16	23	46	170
1967	10	3	7	5	44	12	13	44	138
1968†	28	7	11	8	33	16	5	42	150
1969	16	4	6	6	24	9	12	43	120
1970	10	9	7	5	24	8	15	36	114
1971	13	5	10	9	22	10	13	25	107
1972	13	3	7	4	21	4	8	26	86
1973	9	4	4	4	20	4	11	20	76
1974	8	2	2	4	16	6	7	25	70
1975	10	3	3	4	23	1	7	18	69
1976	11	4	1	5	16	3	15	16	71
1977	9	4	4	4	15	3	9	20	68
1978	11	1	3	1	23	2	9	13	63

* *Excludes the following cases in which it was stated that the interval elapsing between the onset of the maternal condition and death exceeded 12 months: 1951-40, 1952-35, 1953-32, 1954-34, 1955-34, 1956-25, 1957-16, 1958-22, 1959-21, 1960-26, 1961-11, 1962-20, 1963-24, 1964-25, 1965-9, 1966-17, 1967-11, 1968-12, 1969-13, 1970-5, 1971-3, 1972-3, 1973-7, 1974-1, 1975-2, 1976-1, 1977-2, 1978-2.*

† *Revision of the ICD was made in these years*

Abortion					Total maternal deaths*	Associated maternal deaths			Total attributed to, or associated with, maternal causes	Year
Criminal		Other		All forms		Other than abortion	With abortion	Total		
With sepsis	Without mention of sepsis	With sepsis	Without mention of sepsis							
642.0, 642.2	Rem 642	640, 641, 643.0-645.2	640, 641 643.1-645.9	640-645	630-678					

Numbers

20	16	20	16	72	374	119	6	125	499	1956
15	15	18	13	61	333	122	6	128	461	1957
8	12	27	16	63	328	94	4	98	426	1958
13	10	16	8	47	290	75	7	82	372	1959
12	18	21	11	62	310	70	5	75	385	1960
8	15	24	7	54	274	68	3	71	345	1961
11	18	17	11	57	299	75	2	77	376	1962
15	6	17	11	49	243	61	6	67	310	1963
13	11	16	10	50	227	54	1	55	282	1964
8	13	21	10	52	221	42	6	48	269	1965
12	18	17	6	53	223	53	3	56	279	1966
8	9	7	10	34	172	64	4	68	240	1967
10	12	16	12	50	200	41	3	44	244	1968
8	7	10	10	35	155	62	4	66	221	1969
4	7	17	4	32	146	55	1	56	202	1970
1	5	8	13	27	134	33	2	35	168	1971
3	4	10	9	26	112	27	1	28	140	1972
2	2	4	4	12	88	31	0	31	119	1973
1	1	3	6	11	81	19	2	21	102	1974
0	1	1	6	8	77	24	1	25	102	1975
1	0	2	4	7	78	22	1	23	101	1976
1	0	3	2	6	74	24	0	24	98	1977
0	0	2	3	5	68	21	1	22	90	1978

Table A10.2   Maternal deaths from principal causes and associated maternal deaths, England and Wales, 1931-78 – *continued*

(a) 1935-78

Year	Maternal deaths (complications of pregnancy, childbirth and puerperium, including abortion)								
	Puerperal phlebitis, thrombosis and embolism	Puerperal sepsis	Haemorrhage		Tox-aemia	Pro-longed labour	Trauma, shock: other complications of delivery	Other causes	Total maternal causes other than abortion
			Ante-partum	Post-partum					
ICD code	671, 673	630, 635, 670	632, 651	652, 653	636, 639	654-657	658-661	Rem 630-639, 650-678	630-639, 650-678
Rates per 100,000 total births									
1935	31	104	47		78	81			341
1936	29	89	48		81	72			319
1937	24	55	48		80	72			279
1938	28	43	48		73	78			270
1939	24	39	18	28	75	73			257
1940†	22	32	17	29	65	20	18	20	224
1941	22	24	17	35	64	26	18	20	226
1942	19	22	13	29	61	23	14	20	202
1943	19	19	12	27	53	23	15	16	184
1944	14	14	11	23	42	23	11	15	153
1945	12	12	10	23	46	21	10	13	147
1946	12	6	10	19	43	14	10	11	125
1947	12	4	6	17	35	12	7	9	102
1948	8	4	6	14	31	8	7	7	86
1949	7	4	5	12	27	9	8	9	81
1950†	9	4	6	5	26	6	8	9	72
1951	7	2	5	8	20	5	5	7	60
1952	8	1	3	6	18	5	6	8	54
1953	7	2	6	7	20	4	5	8	60
1954	7	2	5	6	15	5	6	8	54
1955	8	2	4	6	13	5	3	8	50

* *Excludes the following cases in which it was stated that the interval elapsing between the onset of the maternal condition and death exceeded 12 months: 1951-40, 1952-35, 1953-32, 1954-34, 1955-34, 1956-25, 1957-16, 1958-22, 1959-21, 1960-26, 1961-11, 1962-20, 1963-24, 1964-25, 1965-9, 1966-17, 1967-11, 1968-12, 1969-13, 1970-5, 1971-3, 1972-3, 1973-7, 1974-1, 1975-2, 1976-1, 1977-2, 1978-2.*

† *Revision of the ICD was made in these years*

Abortion					Total mater-nal deaths*	Associated maternal deaths			Total attri-buted to, or associ-ated with, mater-nal causes	Year
Criminal		Other		All forms		Other than abortion	With abortion	Total		
With sepsis	With-out men-tion of sepsis	With sepsis	With-out men-tion of sepsis							
642.0, 642.2	Rem 642	640, 641, 643.0-645.2	640, 641 643.1-645.9	640-645	630-678					
Rates per 100,000 total births										
10	5	42	17	74	415	102	12	114	529	1935
8	4	38	17	67	386	86	11	97	483	1936
9	4	28	17	58	337	92	16	108	446	1937
8	4	27	16	55	324	70	13	82	407	1938
13	4	26	12	55	313	67	8	75	387	1939
7	5	19	12	44	268	60	9	69	337	1940
11	4	24	15	54	280	60	8	68	347	1941
9	2	26	9	46	248	54	7	61	309	1942
11	2	24	9	45	230	62	8	70	300	1943
10	1	22	8	41	193	50	7	56	249	1944
9	1	16	9	33	180	49	3	52	232	1945
5	1	8	5	19	143	42	4	46	190	1946
4	0	6	5	16	117	29	5	34	152	1947
4	1	7	4	16	102	29	2	31	133	1948
3	1	8	4	16	97	21	3	24	121	1949
4	3	5	3	14	87	25	3	28	115	1950
5	4	5	2	15	76	22	1	23	99	1951
3	4	4	2	13	67	22	1	23	91	1952
2	3	3	2	11	71	17	1	18	89	1953
1	4	3	3	11	65	17	1	18	82	1954
2	2	3	2	10	59	16	1	17	76	1955

Table A10.2 **Maternal deaths from principal causes and associated maternal deaths, England and Wales, 1931-78** – *continued*

(a) **1935-78**

Year	Maternal deaths (complications of pregnancy, childbirth and puerperium, including abortion)								
	Puerperal phlebitis, thrombosis and embolism	Puerperal sepsis	Haemorrhage		Tox-aemia	Pro-longed labour	Trauma, shock: other complications of delivery	Other causes	Total maternal causes other than abortion
			Ante-partum	Post-partum					
	ICD code 671, 673	630, 635, 670	632, 651	652, 653	636, 639	654-657	658-661	Rem 630-639, 650-678	630-639, 650-678
Rates per 100,000 total births									
1956	4	2	5	3	13	5	2	8	42
1957	4	2	4	3	10	4	3	6	37
1958†	5	2	3	4	9	3	3	6	35
1959	4	2	3	3	7	2	3	7	32
1960	3	1	3	2	8	3	4	5	31
1961	3	1	2	3	7	2	4	5	27
1962	4	1	3	2	6	2	3	7	28
1963	2	1	2	2	5	1	2	6	22
1964	2	1	1	1	4	1	3	6	20
1965	2	1	1	1	5	1	3	5	19
1966	1	1	2	2	4	2	3	5	20
1967	1	0	1	1	5	1	2	5	16
1968†	3	1	1	1	4	2	1	5	18
1969	2	0	1	1	3	1	1	5	15
1970	1	1	1	1	3	1	2	5	14
1971	2	1	1	1	3	1	2	3	13
1972	2	0	1	1	3	1	1	4	12
1973	1	1	1	1	3	1	2	3	11
1974	1	0	0	1	2	1	1	4	11
1975	2	0	0	1	4	0	1	3	11
1976	2	1	0	1	3	1	3	3	12
1977	2	1	1	1	3	1	2	3	12
1978	2	0	0	0	4	0	1	2	10

* *Excludes the following cases in which it was stated that the interval elapsing between the onset of the maternal condition and death exceeded 12 months: 1951-40, 1952-35, 1953-32, 1954-34, 1955-34, 1956-25, 1957-16, 1958-22, 1959-21, 1960-26, 1961-11, 1962-20, 1963-24, 1964-25, 1965-9, 1966-17, 1967-11, 1968-12, 1969-13, 1970-5, 1971-3, 1972-3, 1973-7, 1974-1, 1975-2, 1976-1, 1977-2, 1978-2.*

† *Revision of the ICD was made in these years*

Rates per 100,000 total births

Abortion Criminal With sepsis	Without mention of sepsis	Other With sepsis	Without mention of sepsis	All forms	Total maternal deaths*	Associated maternal deaths Other than abortion	With abortion	Total	Total attributed to, or associated with, maternal causes	Year
42.0, 42.2	Rem 642	640, 641, 643.0-645.2	640, 641 643.1-645.9	640-645	630-678					
	2	3	2	10	52	17	1	17	70	1956
	2	2	2	8	45	16	1	17	62	1957
	2	4	2	8	43	12	1	13	56	1958
	1	2	1	6	38	10	1	11	49	1959
	2	3	1	8	39	9	1	9	48	1960
	2	3	1	7	33	8	0	9	42	1961
	1	2	1	7	35	9	0	9	44	1962
	2	2	1	6	28	7	1	8	36	1963
	1	2	1	6	25	6	0	6	32	1964
	1	2	1	6	25	5	1	5	31	1965
	2	2	1	6	26	6	0	7	32	1966
	1	1	1	4	20	8	0	8	28	1967
	1	2	1	6	24	5	0	5	29	1968
	1	1	1	4	19	8	0	8	27	1969
	1	2	0	4	18	7	0	7	25	1970
0	1	1	2	3	17	4	0	4	21	1971
0	1	1	1	4	15	4	0	4	19	1972
0	0	1	1	2	13	5	—	5	17	1973
0	0	0	1	2	13	3	0	3	16	1974
0	0	0	1	1	13	4	0	4	17	1975
0	—	0	1	1	13	4	0	4	17	1976
0	—	1	0	1	13	4	—	4	17	1977
0	—	0	0	1	11	3	0	4	15	1978

Table A10.2 – *continued*
(b) 1979-81

Year	Maternal deaths (complications of pregnancy, childbirth and puerperium, including abortion)								
	Compli-cations of preg-nancy, child-birth and the puer-perium*	Abortions					Direct obstetric causes		
		All	Ectopic preg-nancy	Spon-taneous	Legally induced	Illegally induced	All	Haemor-rhage of preg-nancy and child-birth	Toxaemia of preg-nancy
	ICD code 630-676	630-639	633	634	635	636	640-646, 651-676	640, 641, 660	642.4-64:
	Numbers								
1979†	74	9	3	1	2	0	58	8	13
1980	70	13	10	1	1	0	49	6	10
1981	57	10	6	1	1	0	36	4	12
	Rates per 100,000 total births								
1979†	12	1	0	0	0	—	9	1	2
1980	11	2	2	0	0	—	7	1	2
1981	9	1	1	0	0	—	6	1	2

* *Excludes the following cases in which it was stated that the interval elapsing between the onset of the maternal conditi*
and death exceeded 12 months: 1979 – 1

† *Revision of the ICD was made in this year*

Source: *OPCS mortality statistics*

fec-tions of nito-inary ...ct in ...eg-ncy	Indications for care in pregnancy, labour and delivery	Complications in labour and delivery	Complications of puerperium	Indirect obstetric causes		Associated maternal deaths			Total attributed to, or associated with maternal causes	Year
						Chorio-carcinoma	Other	Total		
46.6	651-659	660-669	670-676	647	648					
Numbers										
5	10	21	7	0	6	6	12	86	1979
3	11	18	1	7	3	5	8	78	1980
1	4	12	0	11	3	3	6	63	1981
Rates per 100,000 total births										
1	2	3	1	—	1	1	2	13	1979
0	2	3	0	1	0	1	1	12	1980
0	1	2	—	2	0	0	1	10	1981

Table A10.3   Maternal deaths by cause, Scotland, 1965-81

(a) 1965-78

Year	Puerperal phlebitis, thrombosis and embolism ICD Code 671, 673	Puerperal sepsis 630, 635 670	Haemorrhage		Toxaemia 636, 639	Prolonged labour 654-657
			Ante-partum 632, 651	Post-partum 652, 653		
	*Numbers**					
1965	5	0	1	3	10	4
1966	4	1	2	2	6	2
1967	1	1	2	2	3	2
1968	3	0	0	1	0	3
1969	2	3	0	0	0	0
1970	2	1	2	0	0	1
1971	3	1	1	1	0	3
1972	3	0	0	1	1	2
1973	0	1	0	0	1	1
1974	3	2	1	1	1	0
1975	0	1	1	1	1	0
1976	2	0	0	0	1	1
1977	1	1	0	0	0	2
1978	1	0	2	0	0	0

(b) 1979-81

Year	Complications of pregnancy, childbirth and the puerperium	Abortions				
		All	Ectopic pregnancy	Spontaneous	Legally induced	Illegally induced
	ICD Code 630-676	630-639	633	632	633	634
	*Numbers**					
1979	7	1	0	1	0	0
1980	10	1	0	0	1	0
1981	13	1	1	0	0	0

* *Rates can be calculated using data given in Table A3.5*
Source: *Annual Reports* of the Registrar General for Scotland

Trauma, shock: other complications of delivery	Other causes	Total causes other than abortion	Abortion, all forms	Total maternal deaths	Year
658-661	Rem. 630-639 650-678	630-639 650-678	640-645	630-678	
*Numbers**					
0	8	31	7	38	1965
0	3	20	4	24	1966
2	9	22	0	22	1967
3	3	13	1	14	1968
1	4	10	3	13	1969
1	10	17	0	17	1970
1	2	12	2	14	1971
0	3	10	3	13	1972
2	9	14	2	16	1973
0	5	13	2	16	1974
1	1	6	0	6	1975
1	5	10	0	10	1976
0	8	12	1	13	1977
0	3	3	1	4	1978

Direct obstetric causes							Indirect obstetric causes	Year
All	Haemorrhage of pregnancy and childbirth	Toxaemia of pregnancy	Infections of genito-urinary tract in pregnancy	Indications for care in pregnancy, labour and delivery	Complications in labour and delivery	Complications of puerperium		
640-646 651-676	640,641 660	642.4- 642.9, 643	646.6	651-659	660-669	670-676	647, 648	
*Numbers**								
6	1	2		0	2	1	0	1979
9	1	3		0	1	4	0	1980
10	1	0		1	6	2	2	1981

Table A10.4   Maternal mortality in administrative counties* of England and Wales, 1880-1914

Period 1880-84		Period 1890-94		Period 1900-04		Period 1910-14	
County* in ranked order	Rate†	County* in ranked order	Rate†	County* in ranked order	Rate†	County* in ranked order	Rate†
Rates of 5.00 and over							
Merionethshire	7.65	Merionethshire	9.62	Brecknockshire	8.06	Merionethshire	8.53
Cardiganshire	7.43	Cardiganshire	9.12	Cardiganshire	7.43	Cardiganshire	8.12
Montgomeryshire	6.91	Denbighshire	8.82	Denbighshire	7.22	Anglesey	7.47
Flintshire	6.80	Caernarvonshire	7.99	Carmarthenshire	6.82	Brecknockshire	6.69
Brecknockshire	6.71	Glamorganshire	7.60	Pembrokeshire	6.71	Carmarthenshire	6.35
Herefordshire	6.55	Brecknockshire	7.32	Montgomeryshire	6.56	Montgomeryshire	6.14
Caernarvonshire	6.37	Monmouthshire	6.97	Merionethshire	6.52	Denbighshire	6.04
Radnorshire	6.05	Lancashire	6.89	Glamorganshire	6.43	Pembrokeshire	6.00
Denbighshire	5.95	Montgomeryshire	6.76	Monmouthshire	6.01	Caernarvonshire	5.55
Glamorganshire	5.88	Cheshire	6.64	Westmorland	6.00	Westmorland	5.29
Northumberland	5.67	Derbyshire	6.62	Cumberland	5.75	Monmouthshire	5.24
Carmarthenshire	5.54	Anglesey	6.57	Flintshire	5.49	Flintshire	5.10
Salop	5.42	Radnorshire	6.52	Anglesey	5.44	Glamorganshire	5.06
Pembrokeshire	5.40	Yorks., W.R.	6.29	Cheshire	5.41		
Durham	5.38	Carmarthenshire	6.29	Yorks., W.R.	5.18		
Lancashire	5.31	Northumberland	6.28	Caernarvonshire	5.05		
Yorks., W.R.	5.31	Flintshire	6.18	Lancashire	5.04		
Cheshire	5.21	Gloucestershire	6.04				
Cumberland	5.19	Gloucestershire	6.04				
Derbyshire	5.13	Durham	5.86				
Yorks., N.R.	5.06	Cornwall	5.84				
Nottinghamshire	5.03	Nottinghamshire	5.76				
Monmouthshire	5.01	Herefordshire	5.75				
		Pembrokeshire	5.71				
		Staffordshire	5.63				
		Cumberland	5.51				
		Lincolnshire	5.23				
		Salop	5.19				
		Somerset	5.09				
		Yorks., N.R.	5.09				
		Yorks., E.R.	5.04				
		Westmorland	5.02				
Rates from 4.50 to 4.99							
Wiltshire	4.90	Worcestershire	4.99	Radnorshire	4.96	Herefordshire	4.87
Anglesey	4.80	Warwickshire	4.97	Derbyshire	4.91	Yorks., W.R.	4.72
Worcestershire	4.68	Norfolk	4.94	Durham	4.81	Lancashire	4.51
Norfolk	4.64	Rutlandshire	4.91	Yorks., N.R.	4.66		
Cambridgeshire	4.59	Northamptonshire	4.90	Cornwall	4.65		
Staffordshire	4.59	Dorsetshire	4.85	Staffordshire	4.65		
Surrey	4.57	Devonshire	4.84	Lincolnshire	4.61		
Leicestershire	4.54	Berkshire	4.82	Northumberland	4.59		

* *With their associated county borough, if any.*

† *Rate per 1,000 live births from all puerperal causes.*

Table A10.4 Maternal mortality in administrative counties* of England and Wales, 1880-1914 - *continued*

Period 1880-84		Period 1890-94		Period 1900-04		Period 1910-14	
County* in ranked order	Rate†	County* in ranked order	Rate†	County* in ranked order	Rate†	County* in ranked order	Rate†

Rates of 5.00 and over

Period 1880-84		Period 1890-94		Period 1900-04		Period 1910-14	
Oxfordshire	4.51	Leicestershire	4.71	Nottinghamshire	4.55		
		Wiltshire	4.70	Wiltshire	4.50		
		Surrey	4.67				
		Essex	4.56				
		Middlesex	4.54				
		Cambridgeshire	4.51				

Rates from 4.00 to 4.49

Period 1880-84		Period 1890-94		Period 1900-04		Period 1910-14	
Dorsetshire	4.45	Sussex	4.45	Devonshire	4.49	Cumberland	4.47
Northamptonshire	4.45	London	4.44	Rutlandshire	4.46	Cheshire	4.45
Gloucestershire	4.44	Kent	4.37	Yorks., E.R.	4.34	Cornwall	4.45
Warwickshire	4.37	Hertfordshire	4.36	Warwickshire	4.22	Durham	4.29
Sussex	4.32	Hampshire	4.35	Gloucestershire	4.13	Devonshire	4.24
Buckinghamshire	4.30	Bedfordshire	4.34	Sussex	4.08	Radnorshire	4.19
Lincolnshire	4.30	Oxfordshire	4.33	Dorsetshire	4.07	Northumberland	4.14
Huntingdonshire	4.27	Suffolk	4.31	Northamptonshire	4.06		
Middlesex	4.26	Buckinghamshire	4.30	Worcestershire	4.06		
Berkshire	4.21						
Devonshire	4.21						
Cornwall	4.16						
Yorks., E.R.	4.13						
Westmorland	4.12						
London	4.09						
Somerset	4.09						
Hampshire	4.05						

Rates from 3.50 to 3.99

Period 1880-84		Period 1890-94		Period 1900-04		Period 1910-14	
Kent	3.95			Oxfordshire	3.98	Gloucestershire	3.99
Suffolk	3.80			Somerset	3.95	Yorks., N.R.	3.94
Essex	3.71			Herefordshire	3.88	Staffordshire	3.90
Hertfordshire	3.51			Berkshire	3.78	Derbyshire	3.86
				Norfolk	3.76	Leicestershire	3.77
				Leicestershire	3.70	Berkshire	3.75
				Suffolk	3.62	Cambridgeshire	3.68
				Cambridgeshire	3.59	Warwickshire	3.63
				Kent	3.57	Northamptonshire	3.61
						Suffolk	3.57
						Dorsetshire	3.55
						Huntingdonshire	3.51
						Nottinghamshire	3.50

* *With their associated county borough, if any.*
† *Rate per 1,000 live births from all puerperal causes.*

Table A10.4 Maternal mortality in administrative counties* of England and Wales, 1880-1914 - *continued*

Period 1880-84		Period 1890-94		Period 1900-04		Period 1910-14	
County* in ranked order	Rate†	County* in ranked order	Rate†	County* in ranked order	Rate†	County* in ranked order	Rate†
Rates of 3.49 and under							
Bedfordshire	3.35	Huntingdonshire	3.39	Bedfordshire	3.43	Surrey	3.48
Rutlandshire	3.28			Salop	3.43	Lincolnshire	3.45
				Buckinghamshire	3.41	Salop	3.44
				Surrey	3.41	Bedfordshire	3.33
				Hertfordshire	3.36	Sussex	3.30
				Essex	3.22	Yorks., E.R.	3.30
				Hampshire	3.22	Somerset	3.28
				London	3.20	Worcestershire	3.27
				Middlesex	3.15	Wiltshire	3.25
				Huntingdonshire	2.62	Norfolk	3.18
						Hertfordshire	3.11
						Kent	3.07
						Essex	3.04
						London	2.99
						Isle of Wight	2.97
						Middlesex	2.95
						Hampshire	2.81
						Buckinghamshire	2.67
						Oxfordshire	2.58
						Rutlandshire	2.49
						Isle of Ely	2.04

* *With their associated county borough, if any.*

† *Rate per 1,000 live births from all puerperal causes.*

Source: Ministry of Health, *Report on an investigation into maternal mortality,* 1937.

Table A10.5 **Maternal mortality in administrative counties* of England and Wales, 1924-33**

ADMINISTRATIVE COUNTIES WITH THEIR ASSOCIATED COUNTY BOROUGHS, if any, ranked in order of their puerperal mortality rates per 1,000 live births during the decennium 1924-33, in comparison with the corresponding rate in England and Wales during the same period, having regard to the statistical significance of the local figures.

County* (in ranked order of rate)	Rate†	Standard error	Difference from national rate† (that is 4.21)	
			Actual	Multiples of standard error

Group I *Areas in which the mortality rate was higher than that of England and Wales by an amount equivalent to at least twice the standard error of the local rate. (Note: In this group the difference of the local rates from that of England and Wales may be regarded as definitely significant.)*

1. Anglesey	6.79	0.92	+2.58	2.80
2. Denbigh	6.56	0.50	+2.35	4.70
3. Cardigan	6.39	0.92	+2.18	2.37
4. Carmarthen	6.34	0.45	+2.13	4.73
5. Pembroke	5.70	0.62	+1.49	2.40
6. Flint	5.63	0.54	+1.42	2.63
7. Glamorgan	5.61	0.15	+1.40	9.33
8. West Riding	5.26	0.10	+1.05	10.50
9. Cumberland	5.18	0.33	+0.97	2.94
10. Monmouth	4.95	0.24	+0.74	3.08
11. Lancashire	4.81	0.08	+0.60	7.50
12. Durham	4.72	0.12	+0.51	4.25

Group II *Areas in which the mortality rate was higher than that of England and Wales by an amount equivalent to at least 1.35 times the standard error (that is, approximately twice the 'probable error') but less than twice the standard error. (Note: In this group the difference of the local rates from that of England and Wales may be regarded as very probably significant.)*

13. Merioneth	5.84	0.92	+1.63	1.77
14. Westmorland	5.36	0.74	+1.15	1.55
15. Caernarvon	5.05	0.53	+0.84	1.58
16. North Riding	4.52	0.23	+0.31	1.35
17. Devon	4.50	0.21	+0.29	1.38

* *With their associated county borough, if any.*

† *Rate per 1,000 live births from all puerperal causes.*

Table A10.5   Maternal mortality in administrative counties* of England and Wales, 1924-33 - *continued*

County* (in ranked order of rate)	Rate†	Standard error	Difference from national rate† (that is 4.21)	
			Actual	Multiples of standard error

Group III *Areas in which the mortality rate differed from that of England and Wales by an amount equivalent to less than 1.35 times the standard error. (Note: In this group the local rates do not differ significantly from that of England and Wales).*

County* (in ranked order of rate)	Rate†	Standard error	Actual	Multiples of standard error
18. Radnor	5.27	0.21	+1.06	0.88
19. Isle of Wight	5.09	0.67	+0.88	1.31
20. Montgomery	4.76	0.75	+0.55	0.73
21. Cornwall	4.52	0.31	+0.31	1.00
22. Hunts.	4.49	0.78	+0.28	0.36
23. Brecon	4.48	0.67	+0.27	0.40
24. Cambridge	4.36	0.48	+0.15	0.31
25. Hereford	4.28	0.48	+0.07	0.15
26. Northumberland	4.27	0.17	+0.06	0.35
27. Soke of Peterboro.	4.25	0.74	+0.04	0.05
28. East Riding	4.24	0.20	+0.03	0.15
29. Shropshire	4.22	0.32	+0.01	0.03
30. Cheshire	4.20	0.16	−0.01	0.06
31. Worcester	4.19	0.24	−0.02	0.08
32. Lincs, Lindsey	4.17	0.24	−0.04	0.17
33. Somerset	4.15	0.25	−0.06	0.24
34. Derby	4.08	0.17	−0.13	0.76
35. Rutland	4.05	1.22	−0.16	0.13
36. Gloucester	4.00	0.18	−0.21	1.17
37. Leicester	4.00	0.21	−0.21	1.00
38. Dorset	3.96	0.33	−0.25	0.76
39. Northants.	3.95	0.30	−0.26	0.87
40. Bedford	3.86	0.35	−0.35	1.00
41. Berks.	3.86	0.29	−0.35	1.21
42. Isle of Ely	3.85	0.52	−0.36	0.69
43. West Sussex	3.84	0.36	−0.37	1.03

Group IV *Areas in which the mortality rate was lower than that of England and Wales by an amount equivalent to at least 1.35 times the standard error (that is, approximately twice the 'probable error') but less than twice the standard error. (Note: In this group the difference of the local rates from that of England and Wales may be regarded as very probably significant.)*

County* (in ranked order of rate)	Rate†	Standard error	Actual	Multiples of standard error
44. Notts.	3.87	0.18	−0.34	1.89
45. East Suffolk	3.77	0.28	−0.44	1.57
46. Bucks.	3.62	0.30	−0.59	1.97
47. West Suffolk	3.39	0.46	−0.82	1.78

* *With their associated county borough, if any.*

† *Rate per 1,000 live births from all puerperal causes.*

County* (in ranked order of rate)	Rate†	Standard error	Difference from national rate† (that is 4.21)	
			Actual	Multiples of standard error

Group V *Areas in which the mortality rate was lower than that of England and Wales by an amount equivalent to at least twice the standard error of the local rate. (Note: In this group the difference of the local rates from that of England and Wales may be regarded as definitely significant.)*

County* (in ranked order of rate)	Rate†	Standard error	Actual	Multiples of standard error
48. Warwick	3.87	0.12	−0.34	2.83
49. Staffs.	3.74	0.12	−0.47	3.75
50. Surrey	3.62	0.15	−0.59	3.93
51. Herts.	3.61	0.25	−0.60	2.40
52. Southants.	3.60	0.15	−0.61	4.07
53. Wilts.	3.52	0.27	−0.69	2.55
54. Middlesex	3.51	0.12	−0.70	5.83
55. Kent	3.47	0.14	−0.74	5.29
56. East Sussex	3.44	0.22	−0.77	3.50
57. Oxford	3.41	0.33	−0.80	2.42
58. Essex	3.40	0.11	−0.81	7.30
59. Lincs, Kesteven	3.34	0.42	−0.87	2.07
60. London	3.34	0.07	−0.87	12.43
61. Norfolk	3.27	0.20	−0.94	4.70
62. Lincs. Holland	3.02	0.41	−1.19	2.90

* *With their associated county borough, if any.*

† *Rate per 1,000 live births from all puerperal causes.*

Source: Ministry of Health, *Report on an investigation into maternal mortality,* 1937

Table A10.6 Main causes of true maternal deaths reported to confidential enquiries, England and Wales, 1952-78

Cause	1952-54	1955-57	1958-60	1961-63	1964-66	1967-69	1970-72	1973-75	1976-78	Excluded under international definition 1976-78
	Numbers									
Abortion	153	141	135	139	133	117	81	29	19†	1
Pulmonary embolism	138	157	132	129	91	75	61	35	45	2
Haemorrhage	220*	138	130	92	68	41	27	21	26	1
Hypertensive diseases of pregnancy	246	171	118	104	67	53	47	39	29	0
All other causes	369	254	227	228	220	169	139	111	108	5
Total	**1,094**	**861**	**742**	**692**	**579**	**455**	**355**	**235**	**227**	**9**
	Rates per million maternities									
Abortion	74.5	66.7	58.8	55.1	51.1	47.6	35.2	15.1	10.9	
Pulmonary embolism	67.2	74.3	57.5	51.2	35.0	30.5	26.5	18.2	25.7	
Haemorrhage	107.2*	65.3	56.7	36.5	26.2	16.7	11.7	10.9	14.9	
Hypertensive diseases of pregnancy	119.8	80.9	51.4	41.3	25.8	21.6	20.5	20.3	16.6	
All other causes	179.7	120.2	98.9	90.5	84.6	68.8	60.5	57.8	61.7	
Total	**532.9**	**407.4**	**323.4**	**274.6**	**222.7**	**185.2**	**154.5**	**122.3**	**129.8**	
Deaths known to Registrar General	1,404	1,112	928	816	671	527	387	254	228	
Percentage reported to enquiry	77.9	77.4	80.0	84.8	86.3	86.3	91.7	92.5	99.6	

* Corrected figures

† Including 5 deaths from anaesthesia associated with operations for abortion for comparison with previous triennia

Source: Confidential enquiries into maternal deaths in England and Wales

Table A10.7   Main causes of true maternal deaths reported to confidential enquiries, Scotland, 1965-75

Cause	1965-71		1972-75	
	Number	Rate*	Number	Rate*
Abortion	14	2.1	12	4.1
Vesicular mole	1	0.2	1	0.3
Ectopic pregnancy	3	0.4	6	2.0
Haemhorrage	9	1.4	7	2.4
Toxaemia of pregnancy	17	2.6	3	1.0
Dyslocia, birth trauma	19	2.9	5	1.7
Sepsis	18	2.7	5	1.7
Thrombosis and embolism	32	4.8	8	2.7
Cardiac disease	18	2.7	5	1.7
Other causes	57	8.6	40	13.6
Total deaths in enquiry	**188**	**28.4**	**92**	**31.2**
Total deaths known to Registrar General	232		93	
Percentage reported to enquiry	81		97	

* Rate per 100,000 total births

Source: Confidential enquiries into maternal deaths in Scotland

Table A10.8 Main causes of true maternal deaths reported to confidential enquiries, Northern Ireland, 1956-77

Cause	1956-59		1960-63		1964-67		1968-77	
	Number	Per cent	Number	Per cent	Number	Per cent	Number	Per cent
Abortion	1	1	2	3	5	14	7	13
Ectopic pregnancy	1	1	1	2	1	3	2	4
Haemorrhage	23	20	9	15	2	5	9	17
Toxaemia	25	22	15	25	9	24	6	11
Pulmonary embolism	12	10	6	10	11	30	3	5
Sepsis	15	13	3	5	2	5	2	4
Associated with anaesthesia	3	5	3	5	2	3	5	9
Associated with, but not necessarily due to caesarean section	15	13	10	16	1	3	14	26
Rupture of the uterus	3	3	3	5	1	3	2	4
Hyperemesis gravidarum	0	—	0	—	0	—	1	2
Cardiac disease†	13	..	13	..	11	..	6	..
Total deaths reported to the enquiry*	**116**	**100**	**61**	**100**	**37**	**100**	**54**	**100**

† No percentages are given as this category was not classified as a true maternal death in the enquiries for 1956-67

* Numbers and percentages may exceed the total as some deaths were included in more than one category.

Source: Confidential enquiries into maternal deaths in Northern Ireland

Table A10.9 Reported new cases of sexually transmitted diseases, constituent countries of United Kingdom, 1975-81

Disease	1975 Male	1975 Female	1976 Male	1976 Female	1977 Male	1977 Female	1978 Male	1978 Female	1979 Male	1979 Female	1980 Male	1980 Female	1981 Male	1981 Female
England and Wales														
Syphilis	2,876	859	3,110	927	3,380	1,075	3,538	975	3,196	911	3,213	954	3,046	882
Gonorrhea	38,452	22,134	38,115	22,011	37,793	22,289	36,484	21,511	35,761	20,469	34,853	20,744	34,179	19,122
Non-specific genital infections	71,401	16,704	75,214	19,770	77,998	19,882	80,439	20,077	82,797	21,924	89,193	27,665	92,436	30,341
Trichomoniasis	1,514	18,728	1,714	18,602	1,722	18,693	1,680	18,387	1,601	18,229	1,920	19,018	1,666	18,878
Candidiasis	5,881	29,857	6,891	30,433	7,757	31,171	8,492	31,859	8,317	32,247	9,518	36,122	9,898	38,491
Pubic lice	3,787	1,528	4,053	1,633	4,363	1,854	4,802	2,130	5,310	2,328	5,601	2,555	6,117	2,794
Herpes simplex	4,244	2,103	4,504	2,526	5,127	2,772	5,383	3,206	5,609	3,439	6,308	3,953	6,891	4,648
Warts	13,531	7,221	14,769	7,726	15,241	8,145	15,991	8,687	16,138	8,966	18,430	10,509	19,336	11,126
Other sexually transmitted conditions	3,605	1,199	3,466	1,208	3,322	1,160	3,275	1,161	3,196	1,139	3,254	1,290	3,210	1,285
Other conditions requiring treatment	26,862	12,999	26,138	13,829	28,411	15,213	30,073	17,649	30,554	20,382	35,963	25,568	38,450	30,848
Other conditions not requiring treatment	54,093	32,903	56,931	34,458	61,252	36,763	63,984	37,711	63,501	38,693	68,663	41,075	71,637	42,725
Total new cases	**226,246**	**146,235**	**235,005**	**153,123**	**246,366**	**159,017**	**254,141**	**163,353**	**255,980**	**168,727**	**276,916**	**189,453**	**286,866**	**201,140**
Scotland														
Syphilis	120	44	150	47	170	62	171	57	155	77	150	56	146	69
Gonorrhea	3,044	1,797	2,964	1,900	3,492	2,036	3,241	1,894	3,114	1,824	3,077	1,788	2,914	1,678
Non-specific genital infections	4,705	501	4,922	505	5,598	590	5,367	793	5,564	1,120	5,517	1,199	5,957	1,477
Trichomoniasis	50	1,405	44	1,352	72	1,527	52	1,373	39	1,425	21	1,160	60	1,168
Candidiasis	342	1,213	281	1,356	410	1,373	424	1,356	437	1,356	416	1,311	506	1,453
Pubic lice	417	64	374	66	404	92	430	92	469	98	560	97	578	110
Herpes simplex	298	114	309	102	374	119	312	123	364	123	337	146	348	145
Warts	1,478	573	1,541	619	1,613	729	1,569	638	1,443	679	1,579	811	1,698	836
Other sexually transmitted conditions	192	47	217	53	255	53	248	63	184	68	198	66	185	45
Other conditions requiring treatment	3,540	844	3,450	1,139	3,275	1,323	2,992	1,114	2,824	1,321	2,918	1,252	3,043	1,258
Other conditions not requiring treatment	3,327	1,672	3,747	1,547	4,015	1,602	4,155	1,523	3,969	1,611	4,266	1,788	4,308	1,865
Total new cases	**17,513**	**8,274**	**17,999**	**8,701**	**19,678**	**9,511**	**18,961**	**9,109**	**18,652**	**9,388**	**19,039**	**9,826**	**19,743**	**9,739**

293

Table A10.9 Reported new cases of sexually transmitted diseases, constituent countries of United Kingdom, 1975-81 - *continued*

Disease	1975 Male	1975 Female	1976 Male	1976 Female	1977 Male	1977 Female	1978 Male	1978 Female	1979 Male	1979 Female	1980 Male	1980 Female	1981 Male	1981 Female
Northern Ireland														
Syphilis	31	34	33	24	49	49	56	49	35	35	37	33	36	32
Gonorrhea	318	135	202	89	257	96	315	124	312	136	280	108	263	145
Non-specific genital infections	878	294	905	335	827	315	914	365	1,123	520	1,303	599	1,410	770
Trichomoniasis	87	128	79	112	44	87	59	129	80	113	54	104	52	98
Candidiasis	99	348	102	351	121	312	107	286	86	269	184	367	338	373
Pubic lice	32	10	33	9	42	14	37	8	53	15	65	37	96	31
Herpes simplex	2	1	3	3	5	2	11	1	15	3	24	13	28	6
Warts	240	83	266	114	235	100	281	106	300	128	301	150	303	181
Other sexually transmitted conditions	32	15	30	5	42	4	41	15	45	19	48	34	52	16
Other conditions requiring treatment	185	85	218	74	217	22	282	30	286	41	222	68	171	47
Other conditions not requiring treatment	638	322	588	220	619	288	845	378	825	451	879	399	878	505
Total new cases	**2,542**	**1,455**	**2,459**	**1,336**	**2,458**	**1,289**	**2,948**	**1,491**	**3,160**	**1,730**	**3,397**	**1,912**	**3,627**	**2,204**

Source: Returns from sexually transmitted disease clinics

Table A10.10 Cancers of the reproductive organs: standardised registration ratios*, by sex and site, England and Wales, 1968-77

ICD Code (8th Revision)	Site	Year of registration									
		1963	1969	1970	1971	1972	1973	1974	1975	1976	1977
Females											
180	Cervix uteri, excluding in-situ	100	95	96	95	92	94	94	94	93	94
181	Chorionepithelioma	100	132	158	63	93	123	171	134	198	173
182	Other malignant neoplasm of uterus	100	98	98	99	100	108	115	111	116	115
183	Ovary, fallopian tube and broad ligament	100	104	106	105	104	101	111	109	111	116
184	Other and unspecified genital organs	100	100	98	100	105	103	111	111	111	108
234.0	Carcinoma in-situ of cervix uteri	100	95	80	80	83	91	105	112	129	141
Males											
185	Prostate	100	101	100	107	110	117	128	126	130	130
186	Testis	100	104	116	113	114	119	133	129	129	130

* For each cancer site the standardised registration ratio is defined as

$$\frac{\textit{Number of cancers at that site registered in year} \times 100}{\textit{Sum over all age-groups of} \left(\begin{array}{c} \textit{Population in age-group} \times \textit{registration} \\ \textit{rate of cancer at that site in age-group} \\ \textit{in 1968} \end{array} \right)}$$

For a fuller definition see *OPCS Cancer statistics, registrations 1977*, page xii

Source: OPCS, *Cancer statistics, registrations, 1977*

Table A10.11 Deaths attributed to cancers of the reproductive organs, England and Wales, 1980

ICD Code (8th Revision)	Site of malignant neoplasm	Age							All ages
		0-14	15-24	25-34	35-44	45-54	55-64	65 and over	
Females		*Numbers*							
179	Uterus, part unspecified	0	0	2	2	33	69	227	333
180	Cervix uteri	0	10	104	161	305	545	943	2,068
181	Placenta	0	1	1	2	0	0	0	4
182	Body of uterus	0	0	2	16	74	219	860	1,171
183	Ovary and other uterine adnexa	5	15	31	129	531	1,024	1,976	3,711
183.0	Ovary	5	15	31	127	524	1,015	1,964	3,681
183.2	Fallopian tube	0	0	0	2	5	9	10	26
184	Other and unspecified female genital organs	0	2	1	6	22	69	420	520
184.0	Vagina	0	2	0	1	12	19	95	129
184.4	Vulva, unspecified	0	0	1	5	10	46	317	379
		Rates per million in each age-group							
179-184	Female genital organs	—	—	41	109	347	672	981	309
179	Uterus, part unspecified	—	—	1	1	12	24	50	13
180	Cervix uteri	—	—	30	56	110	190	209	82
182	Body of uterus	—	—	1	6	27	76	191	46
183	Ovary and other uterine adnexa	—	—	9	45	191	357	438	147
184	Other and unspecified female genital organs	—	—	—	2	8	24	93	21
	Population	*Thousands* 5,005.0	3,730.4	3,468.3	2,896.2	2,783.9	2,864.7	4,511.0	25,259.5

Table A10.11 Deaths attributed to cancers of the reproductive organs, England and Wales, 1980 - *continued*

ICD Code (8th Revision)	Site of malignant neoplasm	Age							All ages
		0-14	15-24	25-34	35-44	45-54	55-64	65 and over	
Males		*Numbers*							
185	Prostate	0	0	0	3	60	484	4,491	5,038
186	Testis	3	35	76	43	15	15	32	219
		Rates per million in each age-group							
185-186	Male genital organs	—	—	22	16	27	190	1,553	219
185	Prostate	—	—	—	1	22	184	1,542	210
186	Testis	—	—	22	15	5	6	11	9
		Thousands							
	Population	5,284.6	3,893.9	3,530.5	2,964.8	2,770.9	2,627.8	2,912.3	23,984.8

Source: OPCS, *Mortality statistics, Series DH2*

Table A10.12 Survival at one, three and five years after registration of cancer of the reproductive organs, England and Wales, 1975 registrations

ICD Code (8th Revision)	Site and age	Number of 1975 registrations	Survival rates					
			One year		Three years		Five years	
			Crude	Relative	Crude	Relative	Crude	Relative
Females								
180	Cervix uteri, excluding in-situ							
	All ages	3,879	74.4	75.8	54.0	57.3	46.7	51.7
	25-34	311	89.4	89.4	76.7	76.8	75.0	75.3
	35-44	456	86.0	86.1	71.5	71.9	66.9	67.6
	45-54	906	78.1	78.5	58.8	59.7	52.0	53.5
	55-64	1,051	77.3	78.1	56.3	58.3	46.9	50.0
	65-74	719	67.2	69.0	40.9	44.9	31.0	36.8
	75-84	341	50.2	54.0	24.6	31.4	17.6	27.5
181	Chorionepithelioma							
	All ages	22	81.8	81.9	77.3	77.6	77.3	77.8
182	Other malignant neoplasm of uterus							
	All ages	3,632	77.7	79.8	63.9	69.7	57.3	66.8
183	Ovary, fallopian tube and broad ligament							
	All ages	3,895	44.6	45.8	24.9	26.9	20.5	23.5
	25-34	94	72.3	72.4	51.1	51.2	47.9	48.1
	35-44	317	67.8	68.0	43.5	43.8	39.4	39.9
	45-54	821	58.3	58.6	33.9	34.4	28.4	29.2
	55-64	997	44.0	44.4	22.9	23.7	18.5	19.8
	65-74	1,045	36.5	37.5	18.5	20.3	14.6	17.3
	75-84	491	24.4	26.3	12.6	16.1	8.6	13.4
184	Other and unspecified genital organs							
	All ages	1,029	62.4	65.9	44.6	52.8	36.9	49.3
234	Carcinoma in-situ of cervix uteri							
	All ages	3,072	99.5	99.7	98.5	99.3	97.8	99.2
	15-24	234	100.0	100.0	99.6	99.7	99.6	99.8
	25-34	1,357	100.0	100.0	99.5	99.7	99.5	99.8
	35-44	838	99.9	100.0	99.2	99.7	98.4	99.4
	45-54	444	98.6	99.1	97.3	98.7	96.2	98.6
	55-64	130	98.5	99.4	93.1	95.9	89.3	94.4

Table A10.12 Survival at one, three and five years after registration of cancer of the reproductive organs, England and Wales, 1975 registrations - *continued*

ICD Code (8th Revision)	Site and age	Number of 1975 registrations	Survival rates					
			One year		Three years		Five years	
			Crude	Relative	Crude	Relative	Crude	Relative
Males								
185	Prostate							
	All ages	6,760	62.2	67.9	34.2	45.0	21.8	35.1
	45-54	119	79.8	80.6	41.2	42.5	31.9	33.9
	55-64	901	74.4	76.2	46.3	50.3	31.9	37.1
	65-74	2,800	68.7	72.8	41.1	49.8	27.7	39.2
	75-84	2,362	54.8	61.9	25.7	37.9	14.2	28.5
	85 and over	563	37.5	47.4	14.2	30.1	6.2	23.4
186	Testis							
	All ages	738	80.1	80.9	67.5	69.6	63.9	67.3

Source: OPCS, *Cancer statistics, survival 1971-1975 Series MB1 No. 9* (Tables 1 and 2)

Table A10.13 Cervical cytology: estimated numbers of smears by age, England and Wales, 1975-81

Year	Age				All ages
	Under 25	25-29	30-34	35 and over	
	Thousands				
1973	487	455	328	1,068	2,338
1974	560	490	354	1,072	2,476
1975	592	482	380	1,044	2,498
1976	566	476	429	1,097	2,568
1977	616	458	385	1,086	2,545
1978	600	441	383	1,163	2,587
1979	632	467	406	1,244	2,749
1980	701	469	404	1,354	2,928
1981	717	495	471	1,316	2,999
	Positive cases per 1,000 smears examined				
1973	1.8	3.5	4.5	5.7	4.3
1974	2.5	4.2	5.6	5.9	4.7
1975	2.1	4.5	5.5	6.2	4.8
1976	2.4	5.1	6.1	6.3	5.2
1977	2.5	6.0	7.8	7.1	5.9
1978	2.8	7.3	9.3	6.7	6.3
1979	2.6	7.2	9.7	6.7	6.3
1980	3.0	8.6	11.4	6.8	6.8
1981	2.9	9.0	10.8	7.4	7.1

Source: DHSS, SBH 140 return (positive cases)
NHSCR, cervical cytology recall scheme (negative cases)

Table A11.1 Changes in prices, United Kingdom, 1973-80

Year	Retail price index* (annual averages)		Hospital prices index†	Health Service prices index†	Maternity costs index‡
	(1972 = 100)	(1974 = 100)	(1974 = 100)	(1978 = 100)	(1972 = 100)
1973	109.1				102.3
1974	126.6	108.5			148.1
1975	157.2	134.8	126.63		174.4
1976	183.2	157.1	160.01		188.5
1977	212.3	182.0	188.20		225.6
1978	229.9	197.1	207.41		251.6
1979	256.2	223.5	225.41	102.24	320.5
1980	..	263.7	..	127.56	366.0

* *The retail price index is constructed from data about prices and 'typical' household expenditure patterns derived from the Family Expenditure Survey.*

† *Calculated from data supplied by regional and area health authority treasurers, by DHSS and based on prices and purchasing patterns for goods and services purchased by the health authorities. Index of hospital prices relate to January each year; index of Health Service prices relate to November.*

‡ *Index of prices of goods purchased by mothers for a new baby, based on prices in catalogue of Mothercare Ltd.*

Table A11.2 Identifiable current expenditure on maternity and child health services*, England, 1975/76 to 1977/78

	1975/76	1976/77	1977/78
Maternity services			
	£ millions		
Hospital and community health services			
Obstetric in-patients	199.4	198.3	198.0
Obstetric out-patients	25.6	27.2	29.1
Health visiting	6.5	6.5	6.9
Midwives	31.2	30.2	30.6
Clinics, administration, ambulances, etc	39.1	40.2	39.6
Total	301.8	302.4	304.2
Family practitioner services			
General medical services	17.5	18.3	18.9
Total identifiable current expenditure on maternity services	**319.3**	**320.7**	**323.1**
Percentage of total current expenditure on hospital, community health and family practitioner services	*percent* 5.9	5.8	5.7
Expenditure per birth	*£* 555.40	574.80	595.90
Services for children aged 0-4 years			
Hospital and community health services	*£ millions*		
Acute in-patient	163.1	152.2	155.4
Acute out-patient	40.3	33.6	35.3
Non-psychiatric day patients	0.3	0.3	0.3
Mental handicap in-patients/out-patients	1.1	1.1	0.9
Health visiting	32.0	31.9	3.38
District nursing	21.6	23.3	23.6
Prevention	10.9	6.4	6.1
Clinics, administration, ambulances, etc.	37.5	37.5	34.3
Total	306.8	286.3	289.7

* *The table sets out estimates of identifiable current expenditure in England on maternity services and on services for children aged 0-4 years. All figures are at 'Survey 1979' prices (the price basis of the November 1979 Expenditure White Paper, Cmnd 7746, broadly the pay and price levels of November 1978). A similar breakdown is not available for Wales.*

Table A11.2   Identifiable current expenditure on maternity and child health services*, England, 1975/76 to 1977/78 - *continued*

	1975/76	1976/77	1977/78
Services for children aged 0-4 years - continued			
Family practitioner services			
General medical services	34.9	36.7	37.7
General dental services	8.7	8.8	8.2
General ophthalmic services	0.2	0.2	0.1
Pharmaceutical services	31.5	34.4	35.7
Total	75.3	80.1	81.7
Total identifiable current expenditure on children 0-4	**382**	**366.4**	**371.4**
Percentage of total current expenditure on hospital, community health and family practitioner services	*percent* 7.1	6.7	6.6
Expenditure per child aged 0-4	£ 117.80	119.70	128.20

* *The table sets out estimates of identifiable current expenditure in England on maternity services and on services for children aged 0-4 years. All figures are at 'Survey 1979' prices (the price basis of the November 1979 Expenditure White Paper, Cmnd 7746, broadly the pay and price levels of November 1978). A similar breakdown is not available for Wales.*

Source: *Second Report from the Social Services Committee. Perinatal and Neonatal Mortality. Vol IV. Session 1979-80.*

Table A11.3 **Estimated expenditure on selected programmes in hospital and community health services, England, 1975/76 to 1980/81**

Programme	1975/76	1976/77	1977/78	1978/79	1979/80	1980/81*
	£ millions					
Obstetric in-patients						
At 1979 prices	243.3	242.0	241.6	237.3	240.4	..
At 1980 prices	305.7	303.9	303.5	297.9	302.1	306.4
Obstetric out-patients						
At 1979 prices	31.3	33.3	35.5	34.9	33.2	..
At 1980 prices	39.3	41.8	44.5	43.9	41.8	43.8
Health visiting						
At 1979 prices	66.2	66.0	69.9	70.9	71.2	..
At 1980 prices	83.2	82.9	87.8	89.0	89.4	90.9
Community midwifery						
At 1979 prices	38.2	37.0	37.4	34.9	35.4	..
At 1980 prices	48.0	46.4	46.9	43.8	44.5	48.7
Family planning						
At 1979 prices	17.5	17.4	17.1	17.6	17.3	..
At 1980 prices	22.0	21.9	21.5	22.1	21.8	21.8
Day nurseries						
All 1980 prices	47.3	51.7	52.2	53.9	53.5	58.8
Other day care for children						
At 1980 prices	5.4	5.9	6.0	7.0	7.6	8.0

*   *Provisional*

Apportionment of hospital expenditure is calculated by applying unit costs in single specialty hospitals to all cases in the maternity specialty, whether or not treated in a single specialty hospital.

Hospital activity data for calendar year is assumed to be the same as for the relevant financial year.

Source: Reports from the Social Services Committee. *Third Report 1980-1. Vol II* p 101. *Second Report 1981-2 Vol II* p 19.

Table A11.4 Pay scales in the National Health Service:
(a) Examples of pay scales* of selected NHS staff at April 1982

Category of staff	Usual full-time hours	Range of gross annual salary (£)	Extra payments (£)
Ancillary	40		
Unskilled		3,070-3,658	
Skilled or supervisor		3,696-4,148	Bonuses for shift or weekend work*
Nursing	37.5		
Auxiliary		3,143-4,017	
Student nurse		3,290-3,593	
Nursery nurse (NNEB)		3,583-4,375	
Enrolled nurse		4,008-4,835	
Staff nurse		4,450-5,426	
Sister/SCM		5,028-7,215	
Nursing Officer I		6,523-7,791	
Nursing Officer II, Health Visitor		6,248-7,551	
Senior Nursing Officer I		6,954-8,148	
Senior Nursing Officer II		7,280-8,462	
Administrative and clerical	37		
Administrator (large district)		20,066-23,034	
Administrator (small hospital)		8,490-10,323	
Administrative assistant (lowest scale)		5,119-6,684	
Clerical assistant (lowest scale)		2,308-3,861	
Professional, technical, paramedical	39		
Physiotherapist		6,371-9,977	Extra payments for weekend
Lab. technician: student		2,566-	or nights and 'on call'
principal		-11,092	
Scientific Officer: probationary		5,129-	
principal		-19,239	
Hospital medical staff	40		
House Officer		6,180-6,980	185.40-209.40 per UMT
Senior House Officer		7,700-8,730	231.00-261.90 per UMT
Registrar		8,730-10,570	261.90-317.10 per UMT
Senior Registrar		10,050-12,670	301.50-380.10 per UMT
Consultant		17,370-22,270	Additional awards may be made to individuals for special merit as follows:

Class	Amounts £ pa
A+	19,645
A	15,130
B	9,060
C	4,040

All rates exclude 1982 pay awards. There are considerable variations between categories of staff in conditions of employment such as holiday allowances or superannuation.

* *A parliamentary reply on the 28 July 1982 gave information about overtime payments to ancillary staff from 1979-1981. In 1982 average overtime payments were £17.21 per week for men and £4.48 per week for women.*

† *UMT, unit of medical time is equivalent to 4 hours per week beyond full time hours. Class A UMT refers to time on call in hospital. Rates given are annual amounts.*

Table 11.4 Pay scales in the National Health Service - *continued*
(b) NHS consultants: numbers of distinction award holders in England and Wales at 31 December 1981

Specialty	Number of eligible practitioners		Award holders					Non-award holders
			Total	A+	A	B	C	
All specialties	13,903	Number	4,962	125	462	1,324	3,051	8,941
		Per cent*	35.7	0.9	3.3	9.5	22.0	64.3
Obstetrics and gynaecology	699	Number	269	9	25	69	166	439
		Per cent*	38.5	1.3	3.6	9.9	23.8	61.5
Paediatrics	532	Number	190	6	15	54	115	342
		Per cent*	35.7	1.1	2.8	10.2	21.6	64.3
Paediatric surgery	39	Number	22	1	3	5	13	17
		Per cent*	56.4	2.6	7.7	12.8	33.3	43.6

* *Percentage of eligible practitioners in specialty*

Source: Whitley Council handbooks of pay scales and allowances.
Health Trends, 1982; 14(3): 75

Table A12.1 Infant mortality rates: selected countries, years from 1955 for (a) all causes, (b) congenital malformations† and (c) other causes

Country		1955	1965	1970	1971	1972	1973	1974	1975	1976	1977	1978	1979
Canada	a	31.2	23.6	18.8	17.6	17.1	15.6	15.0	13.7	13.5	12.4	12.0	‥
	b	4.9	4.4	3.8	3.7	3.8	3.5	3.5	3.0	‥	‥	‥	‥
	c	26.3	19.2	15.0	13.9	13.3	12.0	11.5	10.7	‥	‥	‥	‥
USA	a	26.4	24.7	20.0	19.1	18.5	17.7	16.7	16.1	15.2	14.0*	13.6*	13.0*
	b	3.8	3.6	3.0	3.0	2.9	2.9	2.7	2.7	2.6	‥	‥	‥
	c	22.6	21.1	17.0	16.1	15.6	14.9	14.0	13.3	12.6	‥	‥	‥
Japan	a	39.8	18.5	13.2	12.5	11.7	11.3	10.8	10.1	9.3	8.9	8.4	8.0*
	b	2.1	2.0	2.0	2.2	2.1	2.2	2.2	2.1	2.1	2.2	2.2	‥
	c	37.7	16.5	11.2	10.3	9.5	9.2	8.6	7.9	7.2	6.7	‥	‥
Belgium	a	40.7	23.7	21.1	20.4	18.8	17.7	17.4	16.1	15.3	11.8	11.7*	‥
	b	5.2	4.7	4.4	4.5	4.1	4.0	4.2	3.6	4.0	‥	‥	‥
	c	35.5	19.0	16.7	15.9	14.7	13.7	13.2	12.7	11.2	‥	‥	‥
Czechoslovakia	a	34.1	25.5	22.1	21.7	21.6	21.3	20.5	20.8	21.0	19.7	18.7*	‥
	b	4.1	4.8	4.4	4.2	3.9	3.8	3.7	3.8	‥	‥	‥	‥
	c	30.0	20.6	17.8	17.5	17.7	17.5	16.8	17.0	‥	‥	‥	‥
Denmark	a	25.2	18.7	14.2	13.5	12.2	11.5	10.7	10.4	10.2	8.7	8.8	9.1*
	b	4.0	3.9	3.9	3.7	3.2	3.3	2.9	2.7	3.2	2.7	‥	‥
	c	21.2	14.8	10.3	9.8	9.3	8.2	7.8	7.7	6.9	6.0	‥	‥
Finland	a	29.7	17.6	13.2	12.7	12.1	10.6	11.0	9.6	9.9	9.1	7.6	‥
	b	3.9	3.5	3.2	3.3	2.7	2.8	3.2	2.8	‥	‥	‥	‥
	c	25.8	14.1	10.1	9.4	9.4	7.8	7.8	7.8	‥	‥	‥	‥
France	a	34.3	18.1	15.1	14.2	13.3	12.6	12.2	13.8	12.5	11.4	10.6*‡	9.8*‡
	b	3.6	3.4	3.1	3.0	2.7	2.7	2.7	2.6	2.5	‥	‥	‥
	c	30.7	14.7	12.1	11.2	10.7	9.9	9.5	11.2	8.8	‥	‥	‥
German Democratic Republic	a			18.5	18.0	17.6	15.6	15.9	15.9	14.0	13.1	13.1	13.0*
	b			3.3	3.1	3.3	3.1	3.0	3.6	2.9	‥	‥	‥
	c			15.2	14.9	14.3	12.5	12.9	12.3	11.1	‥	‥	‥
German Federal Republic	a	41.5	23.9	23.6	23.3	22.7	22.9	22.0	19.8	17.4	15.5	14.7	‥
	b	5.1	4.1	4.0	4.2	4.1	4.3	4.2	4.0	3.7	3.6	3.4	‥
	c	36.4	19.8	19.7	19.1	18.6	18.7	17.8	15.8	13.7	11.9	11.3	‥

* Provisional
† Congenital malformations: deaths classified to causes coded 740-759 (ICD8)
‡ Excluding liveborn infants dying before registration

Table A12.1 Infant mortality rates: selected countries, years from 1955 for (a) all causes, (b) congenital malformations† and (c) other causes – *continued*

Country		1955	1965	1970	1971	1972	1973	1974	1975	1976	1977	1978	1979
Greece	a		34.3	29.6	26.9	27.3	24.1	23.9	24.0	22.5	20.4	19.3	18.7*
	b		3.4	3.8	4.4	4.3	4.2	4.7	4.7	4.6	4.2	4.4	..
	c		30.9	25.8	22.5	23.0	19.9	19.2	19.3	17.9	16.2	14.9	..
Hungary	a	60.0	38.8	35.9	35.1	33.2	33.8	34.3	32.9	29.8	26.2	24.4	23.7*
	b	6.3	6.9	6.1	5.7	5.5	5.1	5.3	5.7	5.3	5.4	5.2	..
	c	53.6	32.0	29.8	29.5	27.7	28.8	29.0	27.2	24.5	20.9	19.2	..
Italy	a	50.9	36.0	29.6	28.5	26.9	26.2	22.3	21.2	19.5	18.1	16.9	15.3*
	b	4.0	3.6	3.4	3.5	3.5	3.6	3.3	..	..			..
	c	46.9	32.4	26.2	25.0	23.4	22.6	19.0	..	..			..
Netherland	a	20.1	14.4	12.8	12.1	11.7	11.5	11.3	10.6	10.7	9.5	9.6	8.5*
	b	5.1	3.6	3.6	3.5	2.9	3.1	2.8	2.8	3.2	2.9	2.9	..
	c	15.0	10.8	9.1	8.7	8.8	8.4	8.5	7.9	7.5	6.6	6.7	..
Norway	a	20.6	16.8	12.8	12.8	11.7	11.9	10.4	11.1	10.5	9.2	8.6	..
	b	3.4	3.3	2.5	3.1	2.4	2.6	2.9	3.2	3.1	2.8	2.5	..
	c	17.2	13.5	10.2	9.7	9.4	9.3	7.5	7.9	7.4	6.4	6.1	..
Poland	a		41.7	33.2	29.5	28.5	25.8	23.5	24.9	23.8	24.6	22.5	..
	b		4.6	5.0	5.1	5.0	4.8	4.5	4.8	4.8	5.2	5.0	..
	c		37.1	28.2	24.4	23.5	21.0	19.0	20.1	19.0	19.4	17.5	..
Spain	a		29.5	20.8	18.9	16.3	15.2	13.8	18.9	17.1	15.6*	15.1*	..
	b		2.1	1.9	2.1	2.4	2.6	2.7	4.1	3.7	..	..	..
	c		27.4	18.9	16.7	13.9	12.6	11.1	14.8	13.4	..	..	..
Sweden	a	17.4	13.4	11.0	11.1	10.8	9.9	9.5	8.6	8.3	8.0	7.8	7.3*
	b	3.3	3.1	3.0	3.1	3.3	3.1	2.9	2.7	3.0	2.8	2.8	..
	c	14.2	10.3	8.0	8.0	7.5	6.8	6.7	5.9	5.3	5.2	5.0	..
England and Wales	a	24.9	19.0	18.2	17.5	17.2	16.9	16.4	15.7	14.3	13.8	13.2	12.8
	b	4.6	3.9	3.7	3.8	3.8	3.8	3.9	3.8	3.5	3.4	3.3	3.3
	c	20.3	15.1	14.5	13.8	13.4	13.1	12.4	11.9	10.8	10.2	9.9	9.5

* *Provisional*

† *Congenital malformations: deaths classified to causes coded 740-759 (ICD8)*

‡ *Excluding liveborn infants dying before registration*

Table A12.1 Infant mortality rates: selected countries, years from 1955 for (a) all causes, (b) congenital malformations† and (c) other causes – *continued*

Country		1955	1965	1970	1971	1972	1973	1974	1975	1976	1977	1978	1979
Northern	a	32.4	25.1	22.9	22.7	20.5	20.9	20.9	20.4	18.3	17.2	16.1*	..
Ireland∅	b	6.6	5.7	5.5	5.8	4.9	4.6	4.8	5.3	4.1	5.2	..	..
	c	25.8	19.4	17.4	17.0	15.7	16.3	16.1	15.2	14.2	12.0	..	..
Scotland	a	30.4	23.1	19.6	19.9	18.8	19.0	18.9	17.2	14.8	16.1	12.9*	12.8*
	b	5.2	5.2	4.5	5.3	4.3	4.8	5.0	4.2	3.7	4.6	..	..
	c	25.2	17.9	15.1	14.6	14.6	14.1	13.9	13.0	11.1	11.5	..	..
Yugoslavia	a		71.8	55.5	49.6	44.4	44.0	41.3	39.8	36.8	35.6	33.8*	32.2*
	b		1.8	2.6	2.4	2.4	2.4	2.5	2.2	2.6	2.5	..	..
	c		70.0	52.9	47.2	42.0	41.7	38.8	37.5	34.2	..	..	..
USSR	a		27.2	24.7	22.9	24.7	26.4	27.9	..	..	..	..	..
	b		..	..	..	..	..	..	..	..	..	..	..
	c		..	..	..	..	..	..	..	..	..	..	..
Australia	a	22.0	18.5	17.9	17.3	16.7	16.5	16.1	14.3	13.8	12.5	..	..
	b	3.9	3.4	3.5	3.4	3.4	3.4	3.6	3.2	3.6	3.4	..	..
	c	18.1	15.0	14.4	13.3	13.3	13.1	12.6	11.1	10.3	9.0	..	..
New	a	24.5	19.5	16.7	16.6	15.6	16.2	15.6	16.0	14.0	14.2	13.8	..
Zealand	b	3.8	3.7	3.6	3.2	3.1	3.5	3.8	3.8	..	..	..	..
	c	20.7	15.8	13.2	13.4	12.5	12.7	11.8	12.2	..	..	..	..

* Provisional
† Congenital malformations: deaths classified to causes coded 740-759 (ICD8)
‡ Excluding liveborn infants dying before registration
∅ Deaths occurring by date of registration

Sources: World Health Organisation
OPCS *Mortality statistics, Series DH3*

Table A12.2 Trends in low birthweight in selected countries

Year	Percentage of live births weighing 2,500 g or less				
	England and Wales	Hungary	USA	Finland	Sweden
1950	..	4.6	8.1	5.3	4.0
1951	..	..	8.2	5.0	4.4
1952	..	..	8.2	5.2	4.6
1953	6.6	..	8.2	5.1	4.7
1954	6.9	..	8.1	5.3	4.9
1955	6.9	5.1	8.3	5.3	5.0
1956	6.8	..	8.2	5.4	5.0
1957	7.0	..	8.3	5.8	5.2
1958	6.8	..	8.4	5.8	4.9
1959	6.7	..	8.4	5.8	4.9
1960	6.7	6.9	8.4	5.3	5.1
1961	6.7	..	8.3	5.5	5.0
1962	6.7	..	8.7	5.8	5.0
1963	6.6	..	8.9	5.8	5.1
1964	6.4	..	9.0	5.3	5.1
1965	6.4	9.6	9.1	5.8	4.9*
1966	6.5	..	8.7	5.3	4.9*
1967	6.5	..	9.0	5.3	4.9*
1968	6.7	..	8.9	5.3	5.0*
1969	6.7	..	8.8	5.1	4.7*
1970	6.8	10.4	8.6	5.1	4.7*
1971	6.4	..	8.3	5.0	4.5*
1972	6.6	..	8.3	5.1	..
1973	6.5	11.6	8.1	4.9	4.6†
1974	6.5	11.7	8.0	5.0	4.7†
1975	6.4	11.2	7.9	5.0	4.7†
1976	6.4	11.0	7.8	4.8	4.6†
1977	6.5	10.6	7.6	4.2	..
1978	6.5	10.5	..	4.2	..
1979	6.7	10.5	..	..	..

* *Incomplete coverage*
† *New source of data*
Source: E Hemminki, personal communication (Finland, Sweden)
         United States National Center for Health Statistics
         DHSS, LHS 27/1 returns
         L Lampe, personal communication (Hungary)

Table A12.3 Birthweight and infant mortality, selected countries with available data

Country	Infant mortality rate (per 1,000 live births)	Percentage of live births weighing 2,500 g or less	Year
Canada	12.4	6.4	1977
USA	14.0	7.4	1977
Japan	10.8	5.1	1974
Denmark	11.5	6.4	1973
Finland	9.1	3.9	1977
Norway	11.7	4.2	1972
Sweden	9.9	3.6	1973
England and Wales	15.7	6.4	1975
Scotland	17.2	6.9	1975
FRG	22.9	6.7	1973
Czech	21.3	6.1	1973
GDR	15.9	6.3	1974
Hungary	34.3	11.7	1974
Poland	23.5	8.0	1974
New Zealand	14.0	4.9	1976
USSR	27.9*	8.0	1975

* *Data for 1974*
Source: World Health Organisation

EAST GLAMORGAN GENERAL HOSPITAL
CHURCH VILLAGE, near PONTYPRIDD

Printed in UK for HMSO
(1029) Dd736363 C10 4/84 G381